CLINICAL TRANSESOPHAGEAL ECHOCARDIOGRAPHY

Clinical Transesophageal Echocardiography

HOWARD C. DITTRICH, M.D.
Associate Professor of Medicine (Cardiology)
Director, Cardiology Noninvasive Laboratory
University of California at San Diego
San Diego, California

Foreword by:

RICHARD L. POPP, M.D.
Professor of Medicine (Cardiology)
Stanford University School of Medicine
Stanford, California

Mosby Year Book

St. Louis Baltimore Boston Chicago London Philadelphia Sydney Toronto

Mosby Year Book
Dedicated to Publishing Excellence

Sponsoring Editor: Stephanie Manning
Assistant Editor: Jane Petrash
Assistant Director, Manuscript Services: Frances M. Perveiler
Production Supervisor: Carol A. Reynolds
Proofroom Manager: Barbara Kelly

Mosby–Year Book, Inc.
11830 Westline Industrial Drive
St. Louis, MO 63146

1 2 3 4 5 6 7 8 9 0 CL CL KP 96 95 94 93 92

Library of Congress Cataloging-in-Publication Data
Clinical transesophageal echocardiography / [edited by] Howard C. Dittrich.
p. cm.
Includes bibliographical references and index.
ISBN 0-8016-1211-X
1. Transesophageal echocardiography. I. Dittrich, Howard C.
[DNLM: 1. Echocardiography—methods. 2. Heart Diseases–
-diagnosis. WG 141.5.E2 C6413]
RC683.5.T83C 1992 91-46280
616.1'207'543—dc20 CIP
DNLM/DLC
for Library of Congress

To my wife Sharon and my children, Jessica and Mark, who lovingly gave their support and time so that I could complete this work.

CONTRIBUTORS LIST

Ramesh C. Bansal, M.D.
Professor of Medicine (Cardiology)
Director, Echocardiography Laboratory
Loma Linda University School of Medicine
Loma Linda, California

Klaus Bargheer, M.D.
Division of Cardiology
Department of Internal Medicine
Hannover Medical School
Hannover, Germany

Daniel G. Blanchard, M.D.
Assistant Professor of Medicine
Associate Director
Cardiology Noninvasive Laboratory
University of California at San Diego
San Diego, California

Michael K. Cahalan, M.D.
Associate Professor of Anesthesia
Director, Anesthesia for Cardiac Surgery
University of California at San Francisco
San Francisco, California

Alan Camp, M.D.
Division of Cardiology
Department of Medicine
St. Louis University School of Medicine
St. Louis, Missouri

Gerald I. Cohen, M.D.
Assistant Staff Physician
Department of Cardiology
The Cleveland Clinic Foundation
Cleveland, Ohio

Werner G. Daniel, M.D.
Professor of Medicine and Cardiology
Director, Noninvasive Laboratory
Hannover Medical School
Hannover, Germany

Howard C. Dittrich, M.D.
Associate Professor of Medicine (Cardiology)
Director, Cardiology Noninvasive Laboratory
University of California at San Diego
San Diego, California

Elyse Foster, M.D.
Assistant Clinical Professor of Medicine (Cardiology)
Associate Director
Adult Echocardiology Laboratory
University of California at San Francisco
San Francisco, California

Allan L. Klein, M.D.
Staff Physician
Department of Cardiology
The Cleveland Clinic Foundation
Cleveland, Ohio

Arthur J. Labovitz, M.D.
Professor of Medicine (Cardiology)
Director, Echocardiography and Noninvasive Hemodynamics
St. Louis University School of Medicine
St. Louis, Missouri

Hugh A. McCann, M.B., M.R.C.P.I.
Assistant Professor of Medicine (Cardiology)
University of California at San Diego
San Diego, California

Mark M. Mitchell, M.D.
Professor of Anesthesiology
University of California at San Diego
San Diego, California

Andreas Mügge, M.D.
Associate, Division of Cardiology
Department of Internal Medicine
Hannover Medical School
Hannover, Germany

David J. Sahn, M.D.
Professor of Pediatrics and Radiology
University of California at San Diego
San Diego, California

Ernesto E. Salcedo, M.D.
Staff Physician
Department of Cardiology
The Cleveland Clinic Foundation
Cleveland, Ohio

Nelson B. Schiller, M.D.
Professor of Medicine
Co-Director, Adult Echocardiography Laboratory
University of California at San Francisco
San Francisco, California

William J. Stewart, M.D.
Staff Physician
Department of Cardiology
The Cleveland Clinic Foundation
Cleveland, Ohio

Christoph Stottmeister, M.D.
Division of Cardiology
Department of Internal Medicine
Hannover Medical School
Hannover, Germany

Oliver F.W. Stümper, M.D.
Western General Hospital
Edinburgh, Scotland

George R. Sutherland, F.E.C.S., F.R.C.P. (Edin)
British Heart Foundation Senior Research Fellow
Consultant Cardiologist
Department of Cardiology
Western General Hospital
Edinburgh, Scotland

FOREWORD

Anyone in the field of echocardiography now realizes the time of transesophageal echocardiography has arrived. This technique developed slowly, as is the rule for virtually all new methods. Yet compared to many others, transesophageal echocardiography has proven its clinical worth very early. I remember well a paper on M-mode echocardiography from the esophagus presented at the first meeting totally dedicated to echocardiography that I attended in 1967. The image quality and detail available recently with relatively high frequency transducers mounted on endoscopes have provided information not previously available. The growing literature on this subject has aroused the interest of virtually all members of the cardiology community. Additionally, many cardiovascular surgeons, intensive care specialists, anesthesiologists, and internists have become enthused with the technique because of its potential for improved patient care. This set of circumstances makes this an especially auspicious time to develop a textbook providing the consensus of experts in the field.

It is in the nature of the early textbooks in a new field that the expansion of information continues so the textbook provides the basis of accepted information upon which more is developed. An especially important feature of this textbook, however, is the fact that it is the work of many authors. The contributors to this text are some of the most prominent investigators and most experienced practitioners of this method. Their personal comments and experiences are related in the context of the published formal papers. A chapter in a textbook such as this one provides an excellent opportunity for the authors to expand on what they already have written in the constrained format of journal articles. The student of transesophageal echocardiography reading this book will notice that not all authors agree on all points. Many cite the same articles from the literature and emphasize different aspects of the published material. While this obviously produces some redundancy in the text, it is a very beneficial redundancy because many different facets of the work are highlighted. The lack of perfect agreement among experts accurately reflects the field. The broad picture of the worth of transesophageal echocardiography in areas such as assessment of prosthetic valves, work up of the patient with suspected infective endocarditis, and the patient with suspected cardiac source of emboli gradually is emerging.

Some of the most basic areas of the field will be helped by the stabilizing influence of the American Society of Echocardiography, which is developing guidelines for physician training and for image orientation, for example. However, the reader will appreciate that even a description of the basic techniques for performance of this study are not absolutely uniform among the authors of this book. There still remains some lack of agreement regarding the optimal technique, the safety of the procedure, training for those in formal fellowship and those wishing to learn the technique who are primarily in clinical practice, and the standardization of the presentation of images. It is obvious to most of us working in the field that there still is an inadequate definition of which patient should undergo this procedure when an embolism from a cardiac source is part of the differential diagnosis. In this example one can recognize why there is so much excitement about transesophageal echocardiography now. It is well established that patients with clinically evident stroke or transient cerebral ischemic episodes more commonly have interatrial septal aneurysms, spontaneous swirling contrast in the left atrium, and strand-like projections extending on the atrial side of the mitral valve by transesophageal echocardiography. But we do not yet truly know what the mechanism is for embolism resulting from intraatrial septal aneurysm. There is general agreement developing about the mechanism of spontaneous contrast in the left atrial images, but their etiologic role in these syndromes is not clear. The strand-like structures on the mitral valve have only rarely been documented by pathology since one does not do cardiac surgery in this setting as a rule. This book very well documents the information that is known on this subject and others. The exciting part of the field is the promise that this sort of tantalizing information will lead to a more full understanding of the etiology of these clinical syndromes which might lead to better treatment of them.

One of the most frustrating problems in general echocardiography is the quantitation of valvular regurgitation. Transesophageal echocardiography shares that problem to some extent but improves upon it as well. The proximity of the transducer to the mitral valve with transesophageal echocardiography seems to standardize the studies in a way because the variability of attenuation of the sound by adipose tissue or nearby lung does not contaminate this study as it does transthoracic echocardiography. Yet a true understanding of the complex variables involved in quantitation of a color flow velocity map throughout systole makes those interpreting transesophageal studies for quantitating mitral regurgitation appropriately humble. Accessibility of the pulmonary veins and increased understanding of the flow velocity patterns in them with different cardiac abnormalities can potentially help in this regard. The full understanding of all these patterns is yet to come.

These are examples of problems that one must appreciate and adjust to when carrying out transesophageal echocardiography clinically. The chapter in this book on pitfalls of the technique is especially valuable. One seldom sees a journal article expounding on the mistakes one can make, yet there are well recognized problems that can potentially lead to major misdiagnoses that can be avoided if the echocardiographer is aware of them. This is a very helpful chapter. My personal opinion is that while all of the individual chapters are excellent, some of them are especially helpful just because they are not so fully developed elsewhere. The introduction and detailed discussion of the technique is one such chapter. Obviously the authors have had some striking clinical experiences that lead them to say some recommendations they make are "absolutely essential" and yet other laboratories seem to not put these same features in those categories. The use of a suction device in every patient is one such example. Another is the use of an oximiter. I think it is best to recognize that these recommendations are coming from experts who may have had some "close calls" and we all should benefit from their experience by taking their advice to the extent to which it is practical in our own laboratories. This may become more coherent in the future as shown by the history of the controversy of antibiotic use in the setting of transesophageal echocardiography. At the beginning of the use of this technique, there were strong views voiced, both pro and con, over the use of antibiotics in all patients or in some subcategories. As well designed studies were completed, and one multicenter study involving over 10,000 patients was reported, we developed a good deal of comfort about the lack of bacteremia associated with this method. The recommendation that the American Heart Association Guidelines for endocarditis prophylaxis be applied is made in this text and receives a very broad consensus now.

The role of transesophageal echocardiography in the operating room is another expanding and somewhat controversial topic. This is discussed beautifully in this text. I draw the readers' attention to the discussions of intraoperative direct epicardial imaging versus intraoperative transesophageal imaging in this book. Some of the anesthesiologists most experienced with transesophageal echocardiography tell us of their experience here. The relationship between physicians in anesthesia and those in cardiology, as well as cardiovascular surgery and general surgery, are not well defined with respect to who is responsible for what currently. I believe this will be sorted out more on a local level than on a national level because of the practicalities of every day life. Similarly, the excellent compilation of experience of some physicians in the intensive care setting shows the broad application of the technique and implies that local arrangements for designated responsibility regarding transesophageal echocardiography will have to be worked out there as well.

The role of transesophageal echocardiography in congenital heart disease is one of the least well-defined areas in my view. This is not because the technique lacks value here. On the contrary, the detailed anatomic and flow information available by transesophageal ultrasound is a major step forward for the diagnosis of these conditions in larger patients and adults. But the technology for high resolution images using transducers of the size that would be appropriate for neonates and infants is not yet available. Surely the manufacturers must continue to help us. Higher frequency transducers with well formed beams have been the key to providing the spectacular images we now enjoy. The relatively recent addition of biplane imaging was a major step forward as well. The ability to simultaneously display the biplane images side-by-side has some definite advantages for mental understanding of the size and location of abnormal structures within the heart. The most recent addition of "omniplane" transducers, which allow control of the imaging plane with a great degree of freedom in three dimensional space should further enhance our use of the technique and the benefit for patients. Further technological breakthroughs will be necessary, both for improved pediatric imaging and for reconstruction of the images to help understanding of complex anatomy. This leads me to a final comment.

The images obtained with transesophageal echocardiography usually are so crisp, so clear, so detailed, and so available that they may seem easy to interpret. I believe that is not true. We traditionally look at these images on a scale that tends to distort our understanding of the structures. Everything seems much bigger than life and the detail may go beyond our general understanding of the anatomy. Color flow imaging and transesophageal echocardiography often seems to provide information overload. I believe there should be well defined training for and experience with the technique before physicians try to interpret the images on their own. This book makes recommendations in that regard and the Guidelines offered by the American Society of Echocardiography will probably become the standard. However, this technique is not for people who are unfamiliar with echocardiography, in my opinion. After all, the images are not direct anatomy or direct flow images, but are electronic representations of these phenomena that are developed using sound. This fact, along with the inherent difficulty in understanding arbitrary two-dimensional slices of three-dimensional structures present a formidable challenge. However, the technique is so powerful that those devoting themselves to getting proper training and experience will be rewarded by obtaining information which often simply is not available otherwise. As this book illustrates, transesophageal echocardiography already has become the method of choice for some indications. It continues to grow in terms of patient benefit as more and more people work with it and develop new information. Dr. Dittrich and his co-authors are due a debt of gratitude for taking the time and energy to create this book. It serves as an excellent basis upon which we can build.

Richard L. Popp, M.D.
Professor of Medicine
Stanford University
Stanford, California

PREFACE

This is a book for individuals interested in clinical applications of the relatively new technology of transesophageal echocardiography (TEE). The contributors include cardiologists and anesthesiologists from the United States and Europe who have made important contributions to the literature describing TEE and who have a substantial combined experience with clinical applications of the technology. The information provided in this text is intended not only for individuals in training in cardiology and anesthesiology, but also for cardiovascular technologists, as well as practicing cardiologists, anesthesiologists, and cardiovascular surgeons. Given the heterogeneous educational experiences of these specialties, it can sometimes be difficult to provide the appropriate amount and type of background information. I have chosen not to present the physics of ultrasound and its instrumentation. Instead, I refer the interested reader to textbooks on standard echocardiography for such information since the same principles, in general, apply to TEE.

Those lacking experience with standard surface echocardiography should not fear this new technology or assume that their background precludes their use of this technique. Although there are certainly benefits for readers who have a thorough background in cardiac ultrasound, the new orientation of imaging planes and the superiority of image resolution with TEE require that those familiar with standard surface echocardiography develop a new frame of reference in distinguishing what is normal from what is pathologic. In this respect, a lack of background in reading surface echocardiography may provide a certain advantage.

The book is presented in four parts. The first, on technical aspects, opens with a chapter on basic technique and indications. Following a brief account of the short history of this technology, it provides detailed discussions of the proper setup for studies in the awake patient, the technique for inserting the endoscopic probe, and indications for TEE. Chapter 2 reviews normal anatomy in both transverse and longitudinal planes with detailed instruction on transducer positioning for all standard views as well as manipulation of the probe between views. The section concludes with a chapter devoted to pitfalls in TEE, particularly images that are sometimes misread by individuals new to the technology.

The second section deals with the most common indications for which TEE is performed in the awake patient. It focuses in detail on pathologic conditions and the associated findings on TEE with careful reviews of the literature pertinent to these conditions. Included in this section are chapters on native and prosthetic valve disease, sources of cardiac emboli, cardiac and paracardiac masses, evaluation of the aorta, and the TEE assessment of congenital heart disease. In all cases, numerous figures demonstrating the pathology are included.

Part III addresses clinical applications of TEE during surgery and in critically ill patients. This section should have the greatest appeal to anesthesiologists, surgeons, and intensivists. The information presented in this section makes clear that TEE can and should bring useful clinical information to all participants in the multidisciplinary arena of the surgical theater and intensive care unit.

The final section presents a chapter on future

advances in this rapidly evolving technology. The astounding pace of new developments requires that the interested individual be aware of changes that are likely to take place as a consequence of technological advances.

Above all, this textbook is intended to provide cardiovascular health care professionals with a thorough perspective on TEE as it is applied clinically. Individuals interested in performing and interpreting TEE will find in these pages all the information they need. Those simply interested in how TEE may impact on a particular clinical question will likely discover the answer here.

HOWARD C. DITTRICH, M.D.

ACKNOWLEDGMENTS

I would like to express my appreciation to John H. K. Vogel, M.D., for encouraging me in this effort and to Linda Carlson for her help with our initial efforts in TEE and her continued support. I also wish to thank G. Douglas Moir, M.D., who provided support one day at a time for my efforts on this textbook.

The secretarial and organizational skills of Dorothea Sisto were invaluable. Her calm, reassuring approach made this difficult process much easier.

I would like to thank manufacturers of ultrasound equipment, Hewlett Packard and Acuson, for the support they have provided.

Finally, I wish to express my appreciation to Linda Donaghey, R.D.C.S., Teri Kuvelas, R.D.C.S., and Karen Wheeler, R.D.C.S., for the many hours of work and their superior skills as technologists. Their support for this effort was vital to its success.

Howard C. Dittrich, M.D.

CONTENTS

PART I

Technical Aspects

Chapter 1

Basic Technique and Indications in the Awake Patient

Howard C. Dittrich, M.D.

Transesophageal echocardiography (TEE) incorporating M-mode echo was first introduced by Frazin and associates in the mid-1970s[1] but failed to gain widespread use because of the limitations inherent in M-mode imaging. Early applications of TEE included assessment of wall motion, which was limited;[2] evaluation of the mitral valve;[3] and assessment of left ventricular performance during supine exercise.[4] With the advent of phased-array two-dimensional imaging, more consideration was given to TEE and the possibilities of defining posteriorly situated structures.[5–7] Unfortunately, transducer size limited this application until the early 1980s when prototypic probes were developed in Europe and Japan. With the addition of color Doppler flow imaging, TEE became increasingly used in the intraoperative setting for monitoring ischemia, assessing intracardiac air in upright patients undergoing neurosurgical procedures, and determining left ventricular volume status and mitral valvular repair.[8] Soon, investigators in Europe began to appreciate the utility of this technique in ambulatory patients.

The current widespread use of this diagnostic modality can be measured by the intense interest in clinical studies involving TEE that have recently been presented at scientific meetings and have appeared in peer-reviewed journals. With the increased use of this test, which incorporates cardiac ultrasound and upper gastrointestinal endoscopy, concern has risen about proper application of the technique by individuals adequately trained in all aspects of TEE.

TRAINING IN PERFORMANCE AND INTERPRETATION OF TEE

The transition from interpreting surface or transthoracic cardiac ultrasound images to TEE is relatively straightforward but requires pattern recognition, which can only be accomplished by reviewing a large number of studies. Only then can one begin to appreciate the imaging plane from either monoplane or biplane transesophageal probes. (See Chapter 2 for standard monoplane and biplane images.) For those individuals not trained in cardiac ultrasound who are interested in learning this technology, the task can be much more difficult. Few sites exist either in the United States or elsewhere that provide adequate training. This training should ideally take place over a period of months in a setting of rigorous daily interpretation under the guidance of an experienced echocardiographer. To date, no specific guidelines exist that define adequate training for interpretation of TEE images for any of these groups. It is anticipated that organizations such as the American Society of Echocardiography, the American Heart Association, and the American College of Cardiology will come forth with specific recommendations concerning training of individuals in the interpretation of TEE images. Certainly, a significant component of training will involve obtaining images in unconscious patients undergoing surgical procedures, especially those with underlying cardiac disease who are undergoing noncardiac surgery in which TEE monitoring for ischemia is being performed. This setting allows the trainee sufficient time for performing a detailed examination and becoming familiar with transducer manipulation.

The individual performing the endoscopic procedure has been and presumably will continue to be a physician. Adequate training mandates that this person receive instruction from an individual fully qualified in upper gastrointestinal endoscopy. The number of endoscopic procedures required to become proficient will vary. A minimum of 30 to 40 endoscopic insertions has been recommended.[9, 10] Certainly, some minimum number is required, but proficiency in this technique should be determined by the instructor. Certification for performing the procedure is an institutional decision that may be based on guidelines provided by organizations such as the American Society of Echocardiography, but to date these have not been developed.

ESSENTIALS FOR TRANSESOPHAGEAL ECHOCARDIOGRAPHY IN THE AWAKE PATIENT

Universal precautions for individuals working in the laboratory should be followed, including hepatitis B vaccinations and the routine use of gloves and gowns to protect personnel. A bite block should always be used (unless the patient is edentulous) to prevent the physician or probe from being inadvertently bitten by the patient.

Personnel in the Laboratory

In addition to the physician performing the procedure, it is important that at least one other assistant be available. In general, two technologists assist in the performance of the procedure, with one adjusting the ultrasound equipment while the physician manipulates the esophageal probe. The other technologist assists in monitoring the patient and providing suctioning, as well as in making the contrast agent available for injection.

At the beginning of studies in our outpatient laboratory, an anesthesiologist was available for all cases until such time that we became comfortable with the use of intravenous (IV) sedation and monitoring of the patient. In some situations, a nurse or physician trainee can assist with the procedure.

Some studies are being performed in pre-existing endoscopy suites. These suites are fully equipped with all necessary monitoring equipment and are staffed by nurses or technologists well trained in endoscopy. The advantage for the cardiologist performing outpatient TEE in an endoscopy suite is of course the experience brought to the procedure by these individuals. An important disadvantage, however, is the additional cost that must be borne by the patient for the use of an endoscopy suite and ancillary personnel. In addition, the endoscopy suites may not be located strategically with regard to the echocardiographic suite.

Patient Preparation

As with all procedures involving potential risks, informed consent should be obtained. This medicolegal issue continues to take on increasing importance and therefore requires careful attention with patients undergoing TEE. Basics of informed consent include a discussion of risks, benefits, and alternatives to the procedure. At our institution, a form is used that is generic for surgical and other procedures. In addition, a form has been developed for describing the entire procedure and also documenting the fact that the essential components of informed consent were obtained prior to the procedure.

The patient should be fasting for at least 4 hours before the procedure. This minimizes the likelihood of aspiration during the procedure. A careful history should be obtained to exclude drug allergies, coagulation abnormalities, and any difficulties with swallowing that may identify esophageal pathology. The use of anticoagulation is not in itself a contraindication to TEE, although one may often see a small amount of blood in secretions from patients receiving anticoagulants.

Any dentures or oral prostheses should be removed. In addition, it should be determined that the patient has adequate transportation home should he receive sedation that would make the operation of an automobile inadvisable.

All patients undergoing TEE at our institution have an IV line inserted. The purpose of this IV line, typically an 18-gauge antecubital vein catheter kept open by dextrose in water, is threefold. First, this is the site for IV sedation should that be required. Second, most individuals undergo an injection of ultrasound contrast agent to exclude intracardiac shunts.

Third, in the unlikely event of a complication, immediate IV access is ensured. Although the tendency in some individuals with poor vascular access is to proceed without an IV line, we strongly recommend that this not be done. Unfortunately, this portion of the procedure may prolong the overall time of the procedure substantially in individuals with poor venous access.

Laboratory Equipment Essential for the Performance of TEE

Most cardiologists who are performing TEE are equipping their current outpatient laboratory so that they can perform both surface and transesophageal imaging in the same suite. Probably most important to the safe and successful performance of TEE in awake patients is the oximeter. Continuous measurement of oxygen saturation is strongly recommended, particularly in some patients with lung disease or left ventricular systolic dysfunction. It is particularly reassuring to the team performing the procedure to see a constant adequate oxygen saturation at a time when the patient may appear dusky and may be producing upper airway sounds that suggest compromised ventilation. In addition, if IV sedation is used, monitoring of oxygen saturation is particularly helpful in ensuring that the patient is not becoming oversedated and hypoventilatory. It is our opinion that oximetry is absolutely essential to the performance of TEE in awake patients.

It is important that adequate suction equipment be available throughout the procedure and that an individual assist who can use the suction catheter to avoid aspiration of oral contents. Often, the patient can be instructed to hold the suction catheter and use it as necessary on himself.

We have an automated blood pressure monitoring device that determines systemic blood pressure at a regular interval. This unit is combined with the oximeter and, in an automatic mode, is a helpful adjunct to other monitoring equipment.

Of course, electrocardiographic monitoring is present constantly on the ultrasound machine. It is important that an adequate lead be obtained at the outset and that the leads be applied firmly to the patient so that contact is maintained.

Since an echocardiographic contrast study is performed in most patients, we have available a three-way stopcock with two 10- to 12-cc syringes, one of which is filled with bacterostatic water for the purpose of injecting echo contrast. The water is agitated by injecting between the two syringes through the stopcock. The stopcock is then applied via a large-bore needle to the side port of the IV tubing, and the IV injection is given while recording images across the interatrial septum or while viewing appropriate structures to assess for a cardiac shunt.

As with any invasive or semi-invasive procedure, appropriate equipment for cardiopulmonary resuscitation must be made available and maintained in satisfactory working order. Included in this equipment should be oxygen and other medication for the acute treatment not only of cardiac arrest but also of congestive heart failure or pulmonary edema. In addition, because of the small but real possibility of sustained ventricular and supraventricular arrhythmias, appropriate antiarrhythmics should be available. Although the occurrence of these events is extremely unlikely,[11] all measures should be taken to treat any eventuality. In combination with appropriate therapy, personnel involved in the procedure should be familiar with basic cardiopulmonary resuscitation.

Anesthetic/Sedation

During or immediately after insertion of the IV line, we begin the administration of local anesthetic to the mouth and oropharynx. A number of topical anesthetics are available, including Cetacaine, lidocaine (Xylocaine) spray, and other topical anesthetics in either spray or viscous form. We have found that an aerosolized application is the most effective. Others however, have combined viscous lidocaine with a fruit-flavored solution that is gargled and then swallowed. The application is repeated several times until the patient notices that the tongue has "become thick" and until such time that the person performing the procedure is able to insert a finger or tongue depressor into the back of the throat without eliciting a significant gag reflex. Sometimes five or six applications of topical anesthetic are necessary.

Probably the most important component in making the experience tolerable to the patient is that of the sedation provided by calming the patient, and developing a good working relationship with that patient. In general, this is much easier in the older patient. Younger individuals tend to be more anxious about the procedure and are more likely to ultimately receive IV sedation. The person performing the procedure as well as the assistant should be encouraged to describe all of the components of the study as they are being done and to reassure the individual that the sensations he may be experiencing are typical for this procedure. It is particularly useful to explain to the patient exactly how he will feel at various points of the procedure, including during insertion, during probe manipulation, and after the study.

In our experience, approximately 90% of studies can be performed in the outpatient setting without any IV sedation. This does not hold true for hospitalized individuals; they may be awake at the time of the study but are more likely to be ill and apprehensive.[12]

Many individuals performing TEE administer IV midazolam hydrochloride (Versed, Roche), typically in doses less than 5 mg. This agent decreases anxiety, provides amnesia to a certain extent, and produces sedation. Sedation occurs in the first several minutes after injection, with the drug remaining active for up to several hours after the procedure. Other agents that have been used include IV opiates such as meperidine and fentanyl. The diminution of the gag reflex with these agents may be greater than with others. Another advantage of these agents is their reversibility by IV naloxone HCl (Narcan, DuPont Multi-Source Products). It is anticipated, however, that an antagonist for Versed, "Reversed," should be available in the not too distant future.

The risk of complications from TEE is extremely low,[13] and much of that risk is related to the use of IV sedation. In addition, when IV sedation is given, facilities and personnel for holding and monitoring the patient after the study must be available. For these two reasons, we have tried, whenever possible, not to give IV sedation. We, in fact, use the inducement of being able to leave the laboratory immediately after completion of the study as a means of convincing the patient not to receive IV sedation. As mentioned previously, if a good relationship is established between the patient and physician and the procedure is carried out in a systematic, orderly manner, there is usually no reason to give IV sedation. Some laboratories give IV sedation routinely. Because of our experiences and the fact that much of the risk is related to sedation, we recommend that it be used as needed and sparingly.

Drying Agents

In order to decrease salivary secretions, glycopyrrolate (Robinul, A.H. Robbins) can be administered. This IV agent given in a standard dose of 0.2 mg at least 5 minutes before the endoscopy will frequently result in decreased secretions. One may see an increase in heart rate in those individuals with high resting vagal tone. Because of its anticholinergic effects, this agent should be used with caution, especially in individuals with conditions such as glaucoma. From our experience, the procedure can be made more difficult because of the intense drying that can take place in some patients. This makes manipulation of the transducer more difficult and has resulted in frequent episodes of dysphagia after the procedure. For that reason, we have stopped using this agent. The continued application of a suction catheter in the mouth of the patient should be adequate to effectively deal with excessive secretions.

Antibiotic Prophylaxis

This issue is discussed more thoroughly in Chapter 3. In general, we have not used antibiotic prophylaxis in individuals undergoing TEE. For those very high risk individuals, i.e., those with a mechanical valve or complex congenital heart disease, we have used aqueous penicillin G, 1 million units IV administered 5 minutes before the procedure. It is the impression of the director of our microbiology laboratory, after observing the procedure, that most of the risk for invasion by bacteria into the bloodstream would occur because of trauma in the oropharynx, unlike an upper gastrointestinal endoscopic procedure where biopsy of esophageal and gastric mucosa may induce mucosal trauma in the lower portion of the upper gastrointestinal tract. For that reason, it was felt that penicillin would provide adequate coverage for upper pharyngeal organisms, most of which are not resistant to penicillin. On the other hand, we have not provided antibiotic prophylaxis for those penicillin-allergic individuals. This issue remains unsettled, although recent studies are suggesting that the decision be individualized.[14–16]

Recovery of Patients After TEE

There have been a number of deaths related to the use of midazolam in doses approaching 5 mg while endoscopy is being performed. Any individuals receiving IV sedation must be monitored for a period of time after the procedure to ensure that no complications occur. Frequently, facilities for outpatient surgical procedures can be made available for recovery of these individuals. For individuals not receiving IV sedation, the only postprocedure requirements are waiting 30 to 60 minutes before drinking or eating. The patient should be cautioned about the time required for the local anesthetic effect to dissipate.

Care of the Transesophageal Probe

With transesophageal probes costing tens of thousands of dollars, it is important that meticulous care be taken in handling and cleaning, etc. We have, at our institution, used a disposable sheath in virtually all cases. This sheath is available through medical suppliers, as well as several of the ultrasound manufacturers. Not only does the sheath protect the exterior of the transducer, but also the insertion of a large quantity of transmission gel into the sheath may actually enhance coupling with the esophageal wall in some cases. In addition, with this barrier there is reason to expect that standard cleansing in antimicrobial solution such as Cidex-7 (Surgikos, Inc., Arlington, Tex) can be limited to 10 minutes and still allow for sufficient protection of the patient. After cleansing, the probe should be stored in such a manner that it is not coiled but rather kept in an unflexed position. Limiting the number of individuals who handle the transducer will clearly extend the life of the probe since handling by inexperienced individuals appears to be the most likely cause of damage to the probe.

Probe Insertion

The technique of probe manipulation for precise image acquisition is discussed at length in Chapter 2. Proper insertion of the probe is particularly important since the initial placement is typically the most painful portion of the procedure.[17] With the patient in the left lateral decubitus position to avoid aspiration, the neck is flexed and the mouth opened wide. The patient will tend to withdraw from the probe by extending the neck, which should be avoided since this tends to direct the probe anteriorly toward the trachea. Some individuals use both the index and middle fingers of either hand to direct the probe over the back of the tongue toward the cricopharangeal muscle. The method of using two fingers to direct the probe is particularly useful in sedated, partially unconscious patients such as those in the gastrointestinal endoscopy suite. However, in an unsedated patient, the presence of this portion of the hand and the probe can often be quite uncomfortable. For this reason, we sometimes insert the probe to the back of the tongue and then position the bite block in place. We then advance the probe by using only the index finger, which is inserted along the lateral aspect of the tongue, to maintain the midline position of the probe. This has an advantage over the other technique because it is less uncomfortable to the awake patient and reduces the risk of being bitten. As the probe passes posterior to the cricopharangeal muscle, the patient is asked to swallow. As the patient swallows and the cricopharangeal muscle relaxes, one will feel the sensation of the probe being "pulled" into the esophagus. At this time, the endoscopic probe should be fully inserted into the gastric fundus. This level, approximately 40 to 50 cm from the incisor teeth, should be obtained initially. It is best to give the patient a moment to become accustomed to the probe while at the same time reassuring the patient and applying more "verbal sedation," thereby maintaining the sense of calm that is very helpful.

With regard to insertion of the probe, it is important never to force the probe. After being certain of the midline location of the probe, it is readily apparent to the physician that the patient is swallowing. It is only at this time that the probe should be advanced, and it should pass with minimal pressure. If the probe cannot be passed after repeated attempts, consideration should be given to termination of the study or consultation with a gastroenterologist. There are cases in which an endoscopic probe has been inserted into an esophageal diverticulum; here undue force could have resulted in catastrophic complications.

We strongly advocate that all procedures be performed in a systematic manner. Having inserted the probe fully into the gastric fundus, we then begin recording on videotape immediately. The videocassette recorder (VCR) is left in the record mode throughout the entire study. In addition, the audio portion is recorded so that the operator or other observers can make comments concerning images obtained throughout the study. This is particularly helpful for subsequent review. After the probe is inserted to the full depth, the procedure is then carried out primarily by withdrawing the probe and rotating or flexing it as needed to obtain the views as described in Chapter 2. In general, we recommend that an entire study be obtained and that the tendency to "go for the money" be avoided. We can cite numerous examples where important aspects of the study were completely forgotten because the operator was focused only on the abnormality for which the study was performed. Further justification for performing the entire procedure in a systematic manner is provided by the multicenter survey by Daniel et al., which pointed out that far fewer than 1% of studies were terminated early.[13]

The entire awake study can frequently be performed in 8 to 15 minutes, depending on the extent of cardiac abnormalities and whether or not single-plane or biplane imaging is performed. Most video recorders have a timer that allows for easy monitoring of procedure duration. It is unlikely that much additional information can be obtained after 15 minutes by an experienced individual, and it is very likely that the discomfort of the patient would exceed any potential benefits beyond this time period.

It has been our experience that the majority of information obtained from TEE comes from two-dimensional images, i.e., paravalvular abscess, vegetations, thrombi, and ventricular function to name a few. Of course, very important information is derived from color flow, especially in defining regurgitant jets and intracardiac shunts. In general, however, two-dimensional images contain the most information. It is also our experience that individuals beginning in TEE tend to overuse color Doppler and record too little two-dimensional information. Given the time constraints involved in an awake-patient study, it is important to keep this fact in mind and not become too caught up with the evaluation of color jets and forget to obtain key two-dimensional images.

It is important to communicate with the patient throughout the procedure whether the information is being obtained and how the physician perceives that the study is progressing. Much verbal sedation can also be provided by personnel assisting with the procedure.

PROCEDURE COST AND CHARGES

The range of charges for the technical and professional components of TEE performed in the awake patient varies substantially across the United States. An informal poll taken of noninvasive laboratories in several regions in 1991 revealed total costs varying from $650 to $1,200, some of which did not include hospital/technical components. As mentioned previously, the cost borne by the patient can vary a great deal, especially depending on whether the procedure is performed in an existing endoscopy suite where charges for endoscopy suite personnel and space use may be added on to basic costs for the cardiologist and ultrasound equipment and technologist. Currently, a CPT (Current Procedural Terminology) code (93312) exists, and reimbursement through various third-party payers for outpatient studies is quite variable.

Likewise, reimbursement for TEE performed as a component of monitoring in the intraoperative setting is quite variable. Some institutions have reasonable success in reimbursement for intraoperative monitoring, while others have had this service denied because it was deemed to be a portion of the anesthesiology monitoring fee. This reimbursement varies widely according to geographic areas, and there is active discussion concerning a uniform reimbursement policy toward both studies in awake patients and intraoperative monitoring. As this procedure becomes more universally used both in the outpatient and intraoperative setting, one can anticipate a uniform fee schedule and reimbursement level to appear.

INDICATIONS FOR TEE

The chapters in this volume cover the various indications for TEE in both awake and unconscious patients, whether in the echocardiography laboratory or in the operating room. Table 1–1 lists common indications for TEE. Obviously, in the awake patient the frequency of these indications will vary substantially depending on the referral source. Our institution cares for a large proportion of individuals

TABLE 1–1.
Indications for Transesophageal Echocardiography

TEE in the Awake Patient/Outpatient	TEE in the Unconscious/ Intraoperative Patient
Native valvular disease	Monitoring of ischemia
Bacterial endocarditis	Intraoperative assessment of valve repair
Vegetation	
Paravalvular disease	
Prosthetic valvular disease	Intracardiac air during neurosurgery
Mitral valve	
Aortic valve	
Suboptimal transthoracic images	Monitoring volume/ hemodynamics
Aortic disease	Critical care evaluation
Acute traumatic dissection	
Atheromatous plaque	Intracoronary contrast agents
Aortic thrombus	
Congenital heart disease	
Source of cardiac embolism	
Paracardiac disease	
Potential applications in ischemic heart disease	
In conjunction with stress	
Atrial pacing	
Dobutamine	
Adenosine	
Coronary artery anatomy	
Origin of vessel	
Doppler assessment of vascular tone	

with native and prosthetic valve disease. As a consequence, approximately 25% to 35% of our studies are done for this reason. Other centers may see only 10% to 15% of individuals undergoing TEE because of valvular disease, while up to 40% are studied to evaluate for possible sources of embolism (see Chapter 4). Because the technology continues to evolve (see Chapter 12), the indications for and clinical applications of TEE are not firmly established. For instance, the relative importance of left atrial spontaneous contrast, patent foramen ovale, interatrial septal aneurysm, and atheromatous aortic plaques as markers for cardioembolic risk are only now being more fully appreciated. Only time will determine the ultimate utility of this relatively new technology.

Certainly, the use of TEE in patients who cannot be imaged adequately by surface echo because of a poor acoustic window will remain a small but definite subgroup. Caution must be taken, however, to apply this semi-invasive technique appropriately. For instance, one would be hard-pressed to justify the performance of TEE to assess for a benign condition such as mitral valve prolapse simply because the surface echo was suboptimal. Even though criteria for the detection of mitral valve prolapse by TEE may exist, we recommend that the study not be performed solely for this reason.

SUMMARY

This chapter introduces the topic of TEE and its performance, particularly in the outpatient, awake individual. Criteria for training of physicians in performing the endoscopy required as well as interpretation of esophageal images are discussed. The personnel and equipment required to carry out outpatient TEE are introduced, and the techniques of anesthesia/sedation as well as probe insertion are discussed. Finally, indications for TEE, particularly in the outpatient, are reviewed.

REFERENCES

1. Frazin L, Talano J, Stephanides L, et al: Esophageal echocardiography. *Circulation* 1976; 54:102–108.
2. Matsuzaki M, Matsuda Y, Ikee Y, et al: Esophageal echocardiographic left ventricular anterolateral wall motion in normal subjects and patients with coronary artery disease. *Circulation* 1981; 63:1085–1092.
3. Matsuzaki M, Ikee Y, Yorozu T, et al: Clinical application of esophageal echocardiography to the mitral valve prolapse syndrome. *Proc Jpn J Med Ultrason* 1977; 31:89–90.
4. Matusumoto M, Hanrath P, Kremer P, et al: Evaluation of left ventricular performance during supine exercise by transesophageal M-mode echocardiography in normal subjects. *Br Heart J* 1982; 48:61–66.
5. Hisanaga K, Hisanaga A, Nagata K, et al: A new transesophageal real-time two-dimensional echocardiographic system using a flexible tube and its clinical application. *Proc Jpn J Med Ultrasonogr* 1977; 32:43–44.
6. Schlüter M, Langenstein B, Poister J, et al: Transesophageal cross-sectional echocardiography with a phased array transducer system: Technique and initial clinical results. *Br Heart J* 1982; 48:67–72.
7. Schlüter M, Hinrichs A, Thier W, et al: Transesophageal two-dimensional echocardiography: Comparison of ultrasonic and anatomic sections. *Am J Cardiol* 1984; 53:1173–1178.
8. Matsumoto M, Oka Y, Strom J, et al: Application of transesophageal echocardiography to continuous intraoperative monitoring of left ventricular performance. *Am J Cardiol* 1980; 46:95–105.
9. Seward JB, Khandheria B, Oh J, et al: Transesophageal echocardiography: Technique, anatomic correlations, implementation, and clinical applications. *Mayo Clin Proc* 1988; 63:649–680.
10. Fleischer DE, Goldstein FA: Transesophageal echocardiography: What the gastroenterologist thinks a cardiologist should know about endoscopy. *J Am Soc Echocardiogr* 1990; 3:428–434.
11. Geibel A, Kasper W, Behroz A, et al: Risk of transesophageal echocardiography in awake patients with cardiac diseases. *Am J Cardiol* 1988; 62:337–339.
12. Oh JK, Seward J, Khandheria B, et al: Transesophageal echocardiography in critically ill patients. *Am J Cardiol* 1990; 66:1492–1495.
13. Daniel WG, Erbel R, Kasper W, et al: Safety of transesophageal echocardiography: A multicenter survey of 10,419 examinations. *Circulation* 1991; 83:817–821.
14. Steckelberg JM, Khandheria B, Anhalt J, et al: Prospective evaluation of the risk of bacteremia associated with transesophageal echocardiography. *Circulation* 1991; 84:177–180.
15. Voüler H, Schröder K, Gast D, et al: Does the incidence of positive blood cultures during transesophageal echocardiography necessitate antibiotic prophylaxis? *Circulation* 1990; 82(suppl 3):244.
16. Chan KL, Cheung P, Wong S, et al: Transesophageal echocardiography and bacteremia. *Circulation* 1990; 82(suppl 3):244.
17. Dittrich HC: Undergoing transesophageal studies: A cardiologist's perspective. *Clin Cardiol* 1991; 14:501–503.

Chapter 2

Examination Technique, Anatomy, and Image Orientation

Ramesh C. Bansal, M.D.

Transesophageal echocardiography (TEE) represents an exciting development and major advance in the field of cardiovascular ultrasound. Since the first use of transesophageal M-mode echocardiography, reported in 1976,[1] many developments have taken place. Initial attempts were limited because of M-mode imaging, but further applications were defined with the introduction of two-dimensional imaging in the late 1970s and early 1980s.[2-4] Advances in probe design and ultrasonic transducer technology and the unique clinical applications for TEE stimulated further interest in the field. These developments have substantially increased the use of TEE in cardiology practice to the point that this new procedure is now considered an extension of the complete transthoracic echocardiographic examination.

The initial TEE probe had a single phased-array transducer mounted at the tip of a flexible gastroscope-like device (monoplane or uniplane probe). This monoplane transesophageal probe with a horizontal (transverse) ultrasonic sectioning plane allowed assessment of cardiac anatomy by using the short-axis and four-channel tomographic views. More recently, a biplane transesophageal probe has become available.[5] This probe has a second transducer mounted at the tip in such a manner that the sectioning ultrasonic beam is oriented in the longitudinal plane, or parallel to the shaft of the probe. This particular transducer allows assessment of cardiac anatomy by using the long-axis tomographic views of the heart. These biplane probes are therefore capable of providing nearly orthogonal tomographic views equivalent to the short and long axis of the heart.

This chapter describes in detail the standard TEE examination, including image orientation and standard images obtained from both the transverse and horizontal (biplane) image planes.

EQUIPMENT AND PROBE DESIGN

A TEE probe is interfaced with an echocardiographic machine to obtain the two-dimensional, M-mode pulsed Doppler and color flow echocardiographic information from the esophagus. Some of the newer probes also have steerable continuous-wave Doppler capability. In most monoplane transesophageal probes, a single phased-array ultrasound transducer is mounted at the tip of a conventional, flexible gastroscope without fiberoptics and suction capabilities. This transducer is mounted in such a manner that it allows a 90-degree horizontal or transverse tomographic plane of section that is at a right angle to the shaft of the probe.

Hewlett-Packard (Andover, Mass) manufactures a monoplane transesophageal probe (Echoscope model 21362A) with 64 phased-array imaging crystals incorporated into the tip of a flexible gastroscope-like device, and this transducer has a carrier frequency of 5.0 MHz. This probe is 100 cm long and has a shaft diameter of 10 mm, tip width of 14 mm, and tip length of 27 mm. Two rotary-controlled knobs, located at the base of the probe, provide 90 degrees of forward (anteflexion) and backward (retroflexion) and approximately 70 degrees of lateral mobility of the flexible tip (Fig 2–1). The smaller outer knob controls the lateral mobility of the tip. The clockwise rotation of this outer knob produces right lateral flexion, and the counterclockwise rotation produces the left lateral flexion of the flexible tip of the scope. The larger inner rotary knob controls the anteroposterior mobility of the flexible tip. Clockwise rotation of this knob produces anteflexion, and counterclockwise rotation produces retroflexion of the flexible tip. A thermistor monitors the probe temperature and automatically shuts down when the esophageal temperature exceeds 42° C to avoid thermal mucosal injury and electrical hazards. In a febrile patient, however, this feature may prevent complete examination because of repeated shutdown of the imaging due to high core temperature.

The Aloka Corporation (Tokyo) manufactures a uniplane probe that employs a 48-element transverse-plane scanning phased-array transducer operating at a frequency of 5.0 MHz. This probe is 100 cm long and has a shaft diameter of 9 mm, tip width of 12 mm, and tip length of 19 mm. In 1989, Omoto et al.[5] developed the first biplane transesophageal probe in collaboration with the biomedical engineering department of the Aloka Corporation. The Aloka biplane probe is also 100 cm long and has a shaft diameter of 9 mm and tip width of 13.5 mm, but the tip length is increased to 29.5 mm (Fig 2–2). The tip length is increased to accommodate the two transducers, each containing 32 elements and operating at a frequency of 5.0 MHz. The distal transducer provides a transverse-plane section and is labeled 1, and the more proximal transducer allows ultrasonic examination in the longitudinal plane and is labeled transducer 2 (see Fig 2–2). The centers of these two transducers are separated by 1.0 cm. Two electronic cables exit the base handle of the scope and connect to the two transducer ports on the Aloka-870 ultrasound equipment. The Aloka Corporation also supplies a monoplane pediatric transesophageal probe with a horizontal scanning transducer containing 24 elements and operating at a frequency of 5.0 MHz (Fig 2–3). The length of the pediatric echoscope is 70

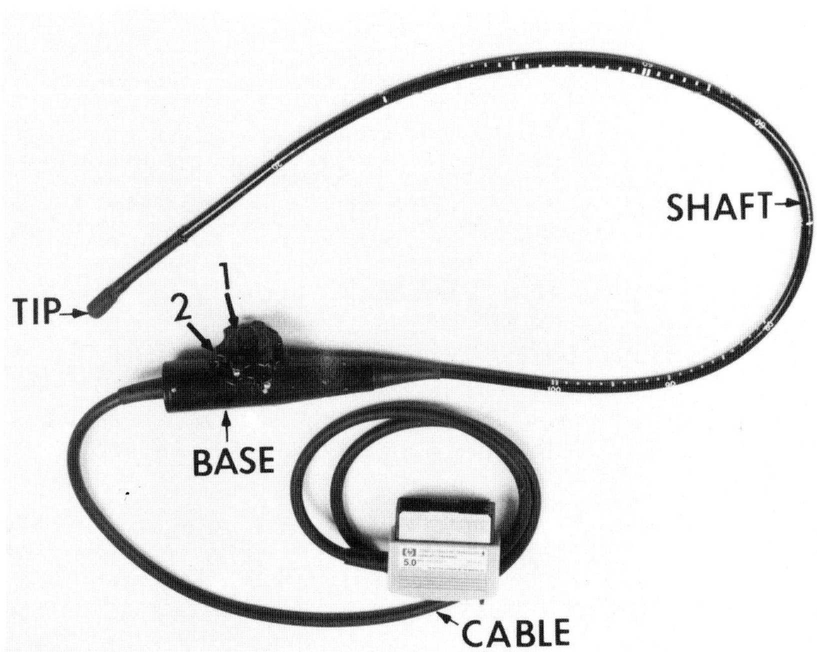

FIG 2–1.
Monoplane TEE probe available with Hewlett-Packard ultrasound equipment (Andover, Mass). This probe has a 64-element, phased-array transducer in the flexible tip that provides a horizontal scanning plane. Two rotary knobs located on the base handle control the mobility of the tip. The smaller outer knob labeled *no. 1* controls the lateral, and the larger inner knob labeled *no. 2* controls the anteroposterior mobility of the flexible tip. The electronic cable exits the base handle and is connected to the transducer port of the ultrasound equipment.

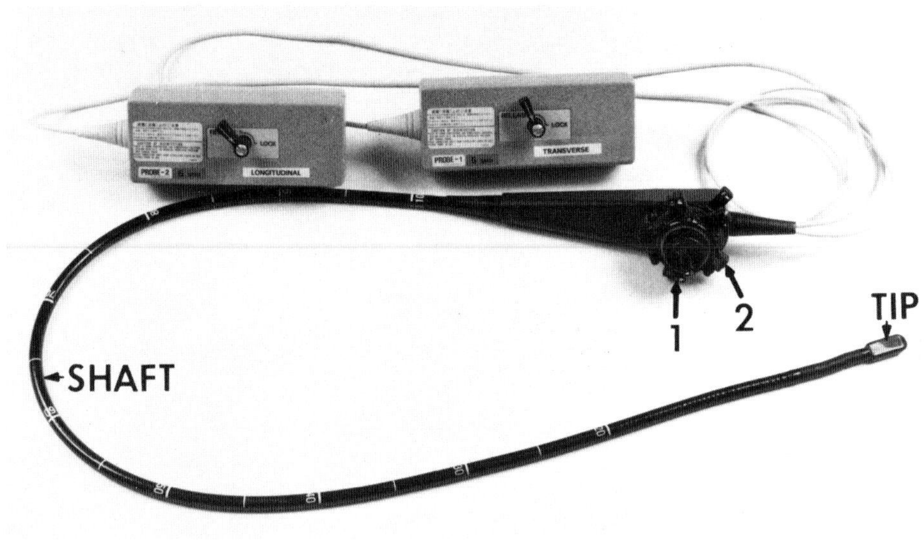

FIG 2–2.
Biplane TEE probe available with Aloka ultrasound equipment (Tokyo). The smaller outer rotary control knob *(no. 1)* controls the lateral, and the inner larger rotary control knob *(no. 2)* controls the anteroposterior mobility of the flexible tip. The flexible tip has two transducers, each containing 32 phased-array elements. Two electronic cables exit the base handle. The distal transducer on the tip connects to probe no. 1 on the Aloka-870 ultrasound equipment and provides a horizontal or transverse plane of section; the more proximally located transducer connects to probe no. 2 on the ultrasound equipment and provides a longitudinal ultrasonic sectioning plane. (From Bansal RC, et al: *J Am Soc Echocardiogr* 1990; 3:348–366. Used by permission.)

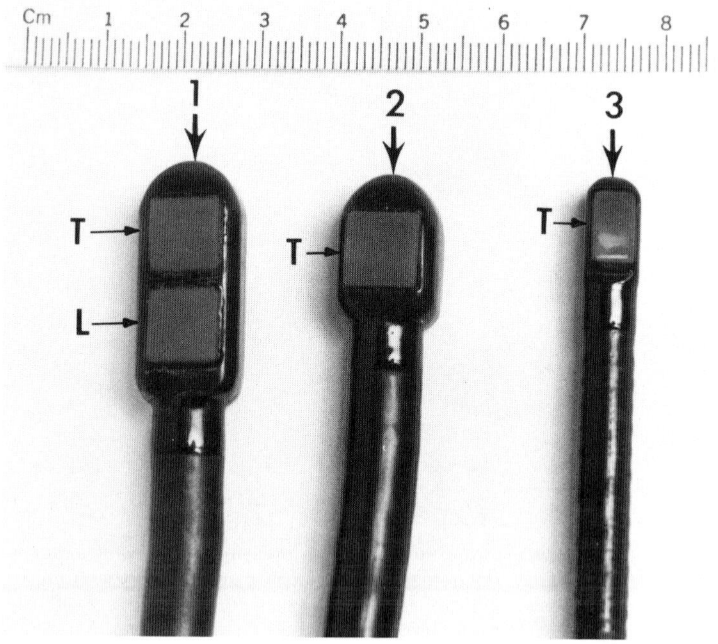

FIG 2–3.
Comparison of the tip size and configuration of biplane *(no. 1)*, uniplane *(no. 2)*, and pediatric *(no. 3)* TEE probes. The transducer labeled *T* provides a transverse echocardiographic sectioning plane; the transducer labeled *L* provides a longitudinal echocardiographic sectioning plane. (From Bansal RC, et al: *J Am Soc Echocardiogr* 1990; 3:348–366. Used by permission.)

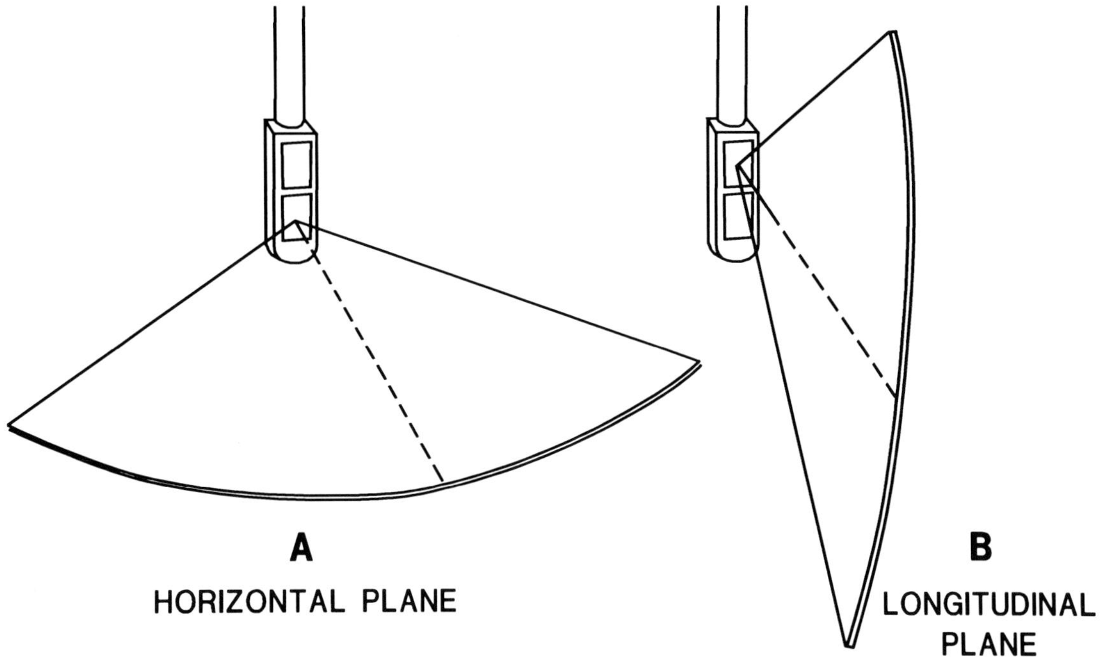

FIG 2–4.
Illustration of the horizontal (transverse) **(A)** and longitudinal **(B)** scanning planes originating from the two transducers of a biplane TEE probe. These sectioning planes are nearly orthogonal to each other.

to 100 cm, and it has a shaft diameter of 6.8 mm, maximum tip width of 7 mm, and tip length of 14 mm. Figure 2–3 compares the tip size and configuration of the Aloka uniplane, biplane, and pediatric transesophageal echoscopes.

Advanced Technology Laboratory (ATL, Bellevue, Wash) also supplies a biplane probe; it is 100 cm long and has a shaft diameter of 10 mm, tip width of 14 mm, and tip length of 34 mm. Each transducer contains 48 elements and operates at a

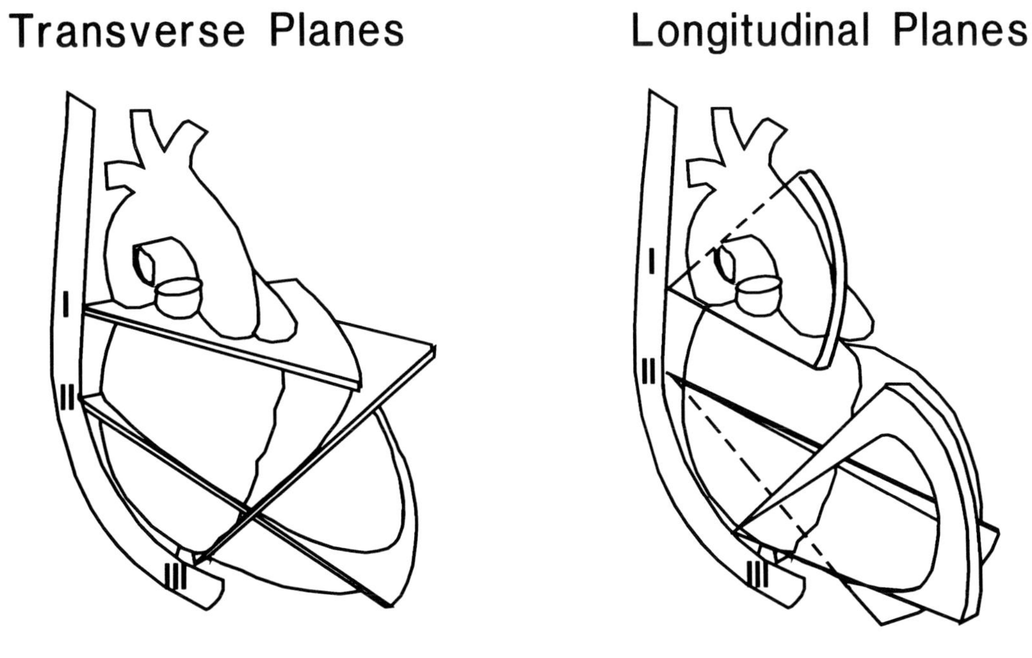

FIG 2–5.
The three basic transesophageal positions for complete examination of the heart with the transverse or horizontal *(left)* and the longitudinal *(right)* scanning transducers. *Position III* provides the transgastric views, midesophageal *position II* provides the four- and two-chamber views, and the basal *position I* shows the various short- and long-axis images of the basal cardiovascular structures.

TABLE 2–1.
Biplane Transesophageal Echocardiographic Views*

View	Transverse Plane†	Longitudinal Plane†
Heart		
Transgastric position views (35 to 40 cm)	1. Short-axis view of the LV at the level of the papillary muscles	1. Transgastric two-chamber view (LA, MV, LV)
	2. Short-axis view of the LV at the level of the mitral valve	2. Transgastric long-axis view (LA, MV, LV, AO)
Midesophageal (four-chamber) position views (30 cm)	1. Four-chamber view	1. Midesophageal two-chamber view (LA, MV, LV)
	2. Five-chamber view	2. Two-chamber and LAA view
	3. RV inflow and CS view	
Basal views (25 to 30 cm)	1. Short-axis view at the aortic valve, RVOT, and atrial septum	1. LV inflow and LUPV view
	2. Coronary arteries	2. RVOT and MPA long-axis view
	3. LAA	3. Ascending aortic long-axis view
	4. Short-axis view of the SVC and ascending aorta	4. SVC and atrial septal long-axis view
	5. Pulmonary veins	5. RUPV view
	6. Main pulmonary artery	6. LVOT long-axis view
		7. Aortic valve short-axis view
Descending thoracic aorta and arch	1. Descending thoracic aorta in the short-axis view	1. Descending thoracic aorta in the long-axis view
	2. Arch in the long-axis view	2. Arch in the short-axis view with brachiocephalic branches

*Adapted from Bansal RC, et al: *J Am Soc Echocardiogr* 1990; 3:348–366.
†AO = ascending aorta; CS = coronary sinus; LA = left atrium; LAA = left atrial appendage; IVC = inferior vena cava; LUPV = left upper pulmonary vein; LV = left ventricle; MPA = main pulmonary artery; MV = mitral valve; RUPV = right upper pulmonary vein; RVOT = right ventricular outflow tract; SVC = superior vena cava.

frequency of 5.0 MHz. The distal transducer provides imaging in the horizontal plane, and the more proximal transducer images the longitudinal plane. Clockwise rotation of the outer smaller rotary knob, located on the base handle, produces right lateral flexion, and counterclockwise rotation produces left lateral flexion of approximately 70 degrees. Clockwise rotation of the larger inner rotary knob produces anteflexion of more than 90 degrees, and counterclockwise rotation produces retroflexion of up to 90 degrees. The anteroposterior flexion of the tip is frequently utilized during both monoplane and biplane TEE examination. However, the utility of right or left lateral flexion is minimal and limited to

FIG 2–6.
Composite of various TEE views from the three primary positions with use of the transverse-plane scanning uniplane transducer. **A** and **B,** transgastric views obtained from transesophageal position III at the level of the left ventricular papillary muscles and mitral valve orifice *(MVO)*, respectively. **C–E,** TEE views obtained from the midesophageal position through the four-chamber plane, left ventricular outflow tract *(LVOT)*, and long axis of the coronary sinus, respectively. **F–H,** the three representative views obtained at the base of the heart at the level of the aortic valve *(AV)*, left atrial appendage *(LAA)*, and the main pulmonary artery *(MPA)*, respectively. In the directional map, *A* = anterior; *I* = inferior; *L* = left; *P* = posterior; *R* = right; *S* = superior. *AA* = ascending aorta; *AL* = anterior leaflet of the mitral valve; *AO* = aorta; *APM* = anterolateral papillary muscle; *AW* = anterior wall of the left ventricle; *CS* = coronary sinus; *IAS* = interatrial septum; *IW* = inferior wall; *L* = left coronary cusp; *LA* = left atrium; *LV* = left ventricle; *MV* = mitral valve; *N* = noncoronary aortic cusp; *PL* = posterior leaflet of the mitral valve; *PPM* = posteromedial papillary muscle; *PW* = posterior wall of the left ventricle; *R* = right coronary cusp of the aortic valve; *RA* = right atrium; *RPA* = right pulmonary artery; *RV* = right ventricle; RVOT = right ventricular outflow tract; VS = ventricular septum. (From Bansal RC, et al: *J Am Soc Echocardiogr* 1990; 3:348–366.)

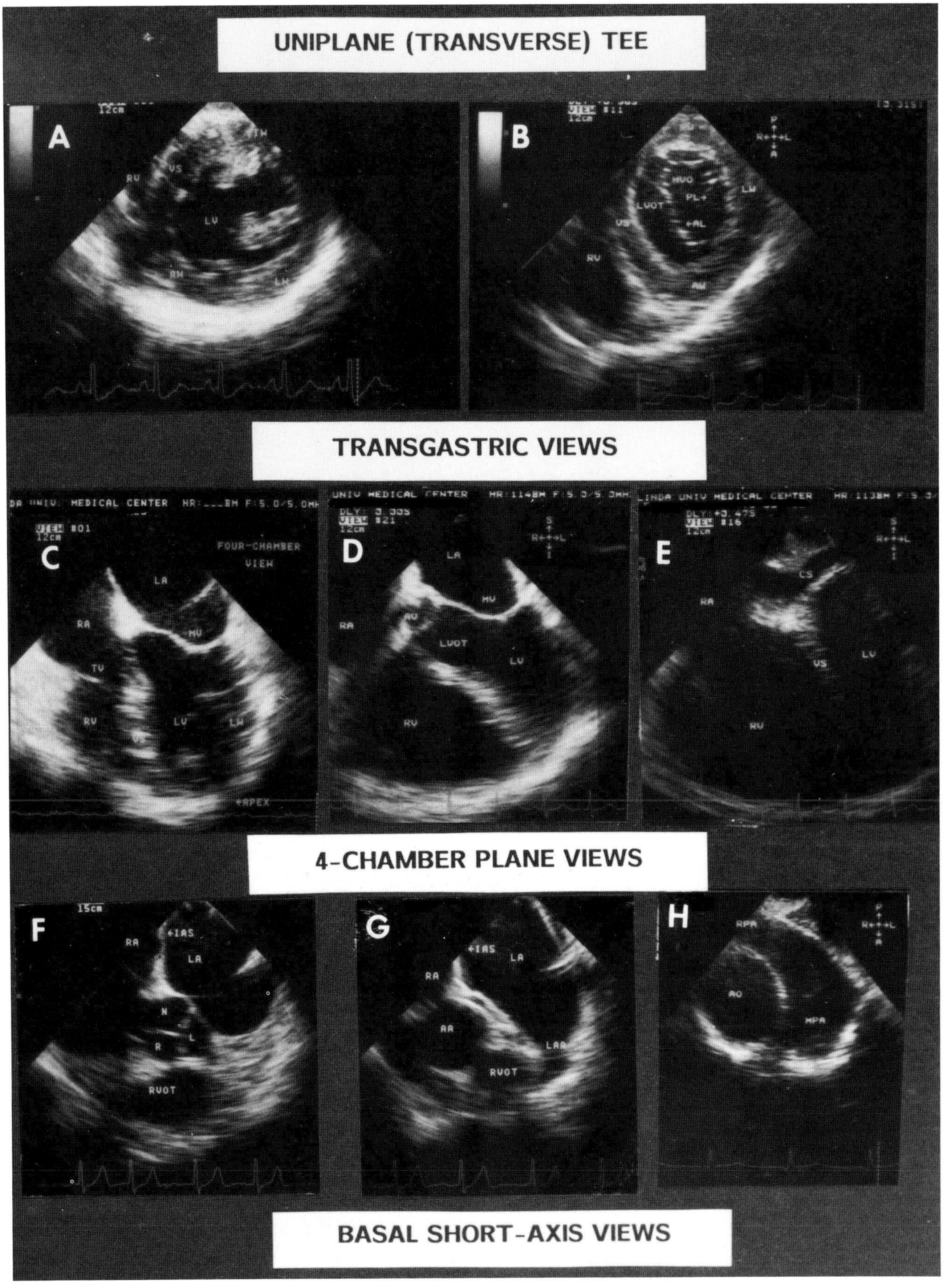
UNIPLANE (TRANSVERSE) TEE
A
RV
VS
LV
LW
B
MVO
LVOT
PL
AL
LW
VS
RV
TRANSGASTRIC VIEWS
C
FOUR-CHAMBER VIEW
LA
RA
MV
TV
RV
LV
LW
VS
APEX
D
LA
MV
RA
LVOT
LV
RV
E
CS
RA
VS
LV
RV
4-CHAMBER PLANE VIEWS
F
RA
IAS
LA
N
R
L
RVOT
G
IAS
LA
RA
RVOT
LAA
H
RPA
AO
MPA
BASAL SHORT-AXIS VIEWS

the transesophageal examination of longitudinal scanning planes.

Hewlett-Packard (Andover, Mass) has recently introduced a biplane TEE probe with a steerable continuous-wave Doppler examination capability in both scanning planes. Acuson Corporation (Mountain View, Calif) has also introduced a biplane probe with steerable Doppler and dual-frequency capabilities on both transducers.

IMAGE ORIENTATION

A complete discussion of facilities, equipment, patient preparation, and esophageal intubation is presented in Chapter 1. After positioning the echoscope in the esophagus, a comprehensive transesophageal examination of the heart and aorta should first be performed. This is followed by a goal-directed examination for detailed assessment of lesions or pathology suspected by clinical and transthoracic echocardiographic studies. Two sectioning planes of a biplane probe are shown in Figure 2–4. The three primary transesophageal transducer positions and planes of sections for biplane TEE examination are shown in Figure 2–5. Table 2–1 summarizes the various biplane transesophageal tomographic sections of the heart and aorta.

BIPLANE TRANSESOPHAGEAL EXAMINATION OF THE HEART

Anatomy and Image Orientation With the Transverse Scanning Transducer

Transesophageal imaging of the heart with a biplane probe is generally begun by imaging with the distal transducer, which provides tomographic views of the heart through the short-axis and four-chamber planes.[6–8] As mentioned previously, the transverse plane is the plane imaged with monoplane transducers. In the preset mode of the instrument, the transverse-plane images are presented in such a manner that the posterior structures located

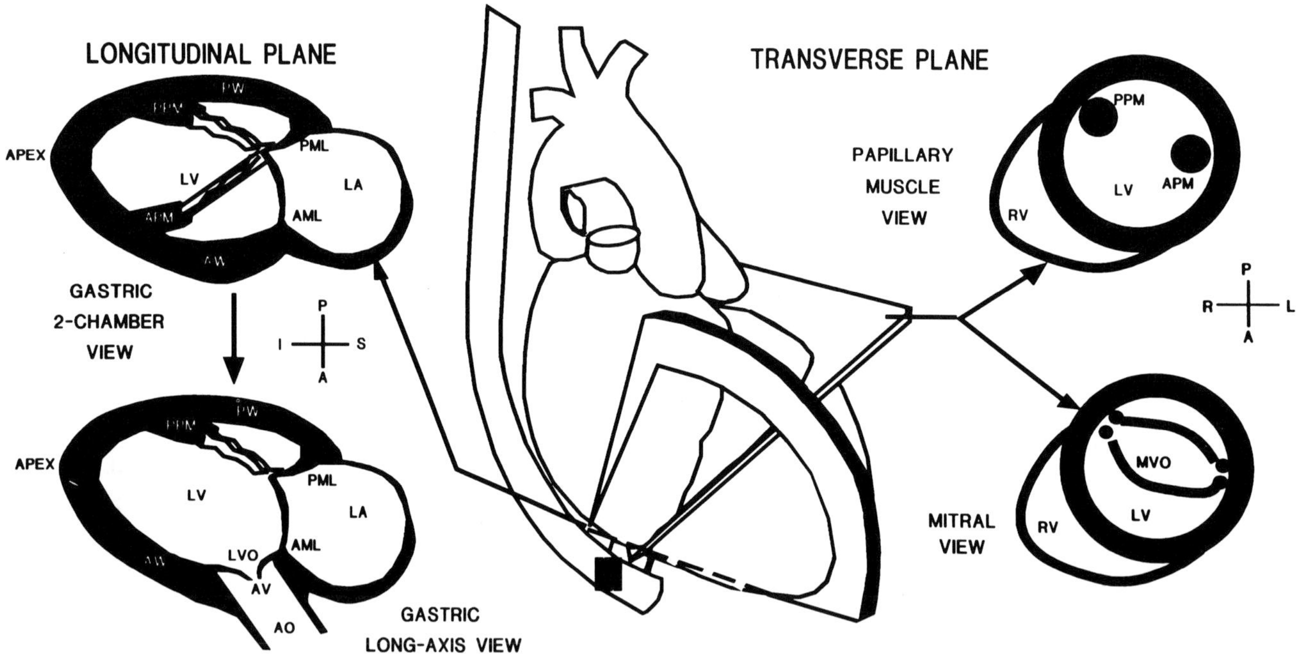

FIG 2–7.

Biplane TEE planes and views from the transgastric position III. The *right side* of the diagram shows the views obtained with the transverse plane probe at the level of the papillary muscles and at the level of the mitral valve. A transgastric two-chamber view obtained with the use of a longitudinal plane probe is displayed in the *upper left panel*. The *lower left panel* shows the transgastric long-axis view, which is obtained by slight rightward flexion and anteflexion of the tip of the probe. In the directional map, *A* = anterior; *I* = inferior; *L* = left; *P* = posterior; *R* = right; *S* = superior. *AML* = lateral segment of the anterior mitral leaflet; *AO* = ascending aorta; *APM* = anterior papillary muscle; *AV* = aortic valve; *AW* = anterior wall of the left ventricle; *LA* = left atrium; *LV* = left ventricle; *LVO* = left ventricular outflow tract; *MVO* = mitral valve orifice; *PML* = medial scallop of the posterior mitral leaflet; *PPM* = posteromedial papillary muscle; *PW* = posterior wall of the left ventricle; *RV* = right ventricle. (Adapted from Bansal RC, et al: *J Am Soc Echocardiogr* 1990; 3:348–366.)

near the transducer appear at the top and the anterior structures located farthest from the transducer appear at the bottom of the video screen. The left-sided structures are displayed to the viewer's right and the right-sided structures to the viewer's left.

Transgastric Short-Axis Views

The tip of the endoscope is advanced in neutral position with unlocked wheels into the fundus of the stomach. The distance of the tip of the scope from the incisor teeth is generally between 35 to 40 cm (see Fig 2–5, position III). The tip is anteflexed and progressively withdrawn to obtain the transgastric short-axis views of the heart at the level of the apex, left ventricular papillary muscles, and the mitral valve orifice (Figs 2–6,A and B; 2–7; and 2–8,A). The left ventricle is displayed to the viewer's right and the right ventricle to the viewer's left. Posterior structures are viewed at the top of the video screen and the anterior structures at the bottom. Transgastric left ventricular short-axis views are utilized for evaluation of myocardial ischemia and global left ventricular function.

Midesophageal Four-Chamber Views

The echoscope is withdrawn to approximately 30 to 35 cm from the incisors (see Fig 2–5, position II), and the tip is slightly anteflexed or retroflexed to obtain the various four-chamber tomographic views of the heart (Figs 2–6,C–E; 2–9; and 2–10,A). The four-chamber views are displayed with the apex oriented downward. Both atria are on the top, the left ventricle to the viewer's right, and the right ventricle to the viewer's left on the video screen. From the four-chamber recording position, progressive anteflexion of the tip will display the left ventricular outflow tract and the long axis of the aortic valve and aorta (see Fig 2–6,D), similar to the transthoracic apical five-chamber view. Slight advancement and extreme retroflexion of the tip from the four-chamber recording position will display the inflow tract of the right ventricle and long axis of the coronary sinus (see Fig 2–6,E). Midesophageal tomographic sections from the various four-chamber planes allow assessment of the atria, atrial septum, ventricular septum, ventricles, internal crux of the heart, both atrioventricular valves with their support structures, and the left ventricular outflow tract. The anterolateral papillary muscle is generally visualized on the lateral wall of the left ventricle from the midesophageal five-chamber view. Color flow imaging and pulsed Doppler interrogation can be performed from the four-chamber position to evaluate normal and

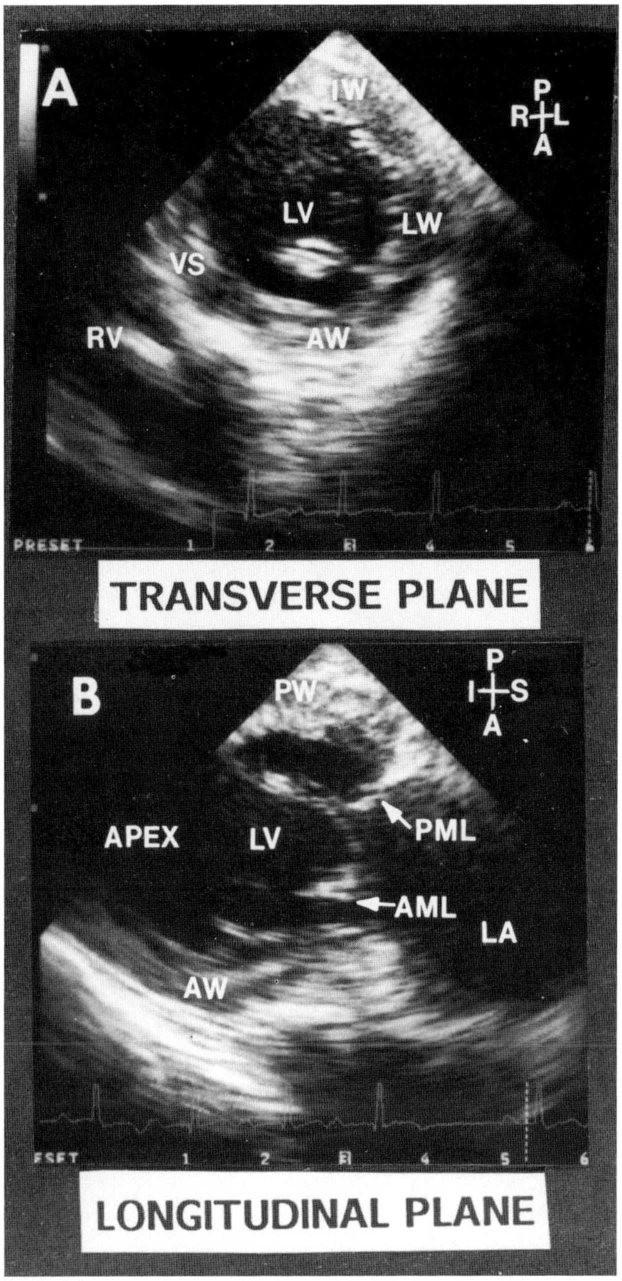

FIG 2–8.

Biplane TEE views from transgastric position III. **A,** the left ventricular cross-sectional view obtained with the transverse scanning probe. **B,** from this starting transverse-plane view, a transgastric two-chamber view is obtained by switching to the longitudinal-plane probe. This view displays the posterior structures to the *top* of the video screen, anterior structures to the *bottom*, superior structures to the viewer's *right* side, and inferior structures to the viewer's *left* side. In the directional map, *A* = anterior; *I* = inferior; *L* = left; *P* = posterior; *R* = right; *S* = superior. *AML* = anterior mitral leaflet; *AW* = anterior wall of the left ventricle; *IW* = inferior wall of the left ventricle; *LA* = left atrium; *LV* = left ventricle; *LW* = lateral wall of the left ventricle; *PW* = posterior wall of the left ventricle; *RV* = right ventricle; *VS* = ventricular septum. (Adapted from Bansal RC, et al: *J Am Soc Echocardiogr* 1990; 3:348–366.)

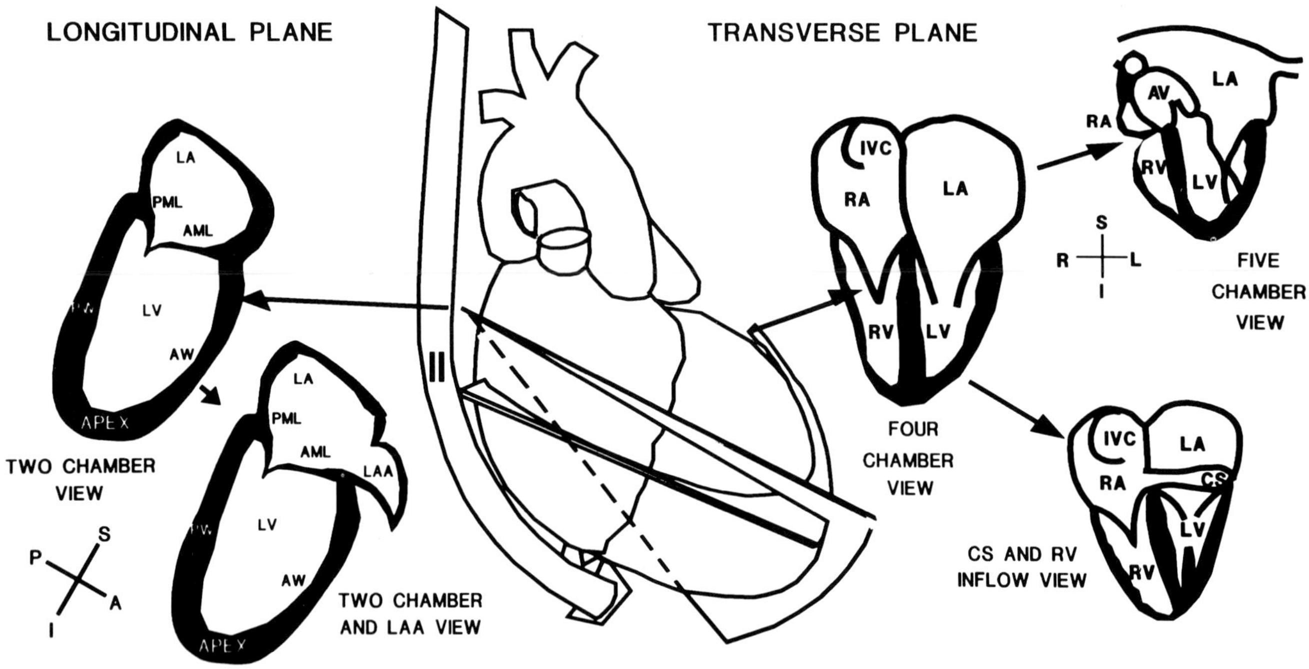

FIG 2–9.
Biplane TEE planes and views at the midesophageal position II. The *right side* of the diagram shows the views obtained with the use of the transverse scanning plane including four-chamber, five-chamber, and coronary sinus *(CS)* views. The *upper left panel* shows the midesophageal two-chamber view obtained with the longitudinal scanning transducer. From this recording position, slight leftward or counterclockwise rotation of the shaft of the probe will also demonstrate the left atrial appendage *(LAA)* as shown in the *lower left panel*. In the directional map, *A* = anterior; *I* = inferior; *L* = left; *P* = posterior; *R* = right; *S* = superior. *AML* = lateral segment of the anterior mitral leaflet; *AV* = aortic valve; *AW* = anterior wall of the left ventricle; *IVC* = inferior vena cava; *LA* = left atrium; *LV* = left ventricle; *PML* = middle scallop of the posterior mitral leaflet; *PW* = posterior wall of the left ventricle; *RA* = right atrium; *RV* = right ventricle. (Adapted from Bansal RC, et al: *J Am Soc Echocardiogr* 1990; 3:348–366.)

abnormal mitral flow patterns. Steerable continuous-wave Doppler can also be used to record the high-velocity jets of mitral stenosis and regurgitation. The apical five-chamber view is useful for evaluation of the left ventricular outflow tract in patients with discrete subaortic stenosis and hypertrophic obstructive cardiomyopathy with systolic anterior motion of the mitral valve. Color flow examination of the left ventricular outflow tract is useful in evaluating the presence and severity of aortic regurgitation. Steerable continuous-wave Doppler techniques may be useful in the assessment of high-velocity systolic and diastolic jets related to aortic obstruction or regurgitation, respectively.

Basal Short-Axis Views

After completion of the four-chamber plane sections, the tip of the echoscope is slightly withdrawn to the base of the heart at approximately 25 to 30 cm from the incisors (see Fig 2–5, position I) to obtain the various basal short-axis views (Figs 2–6,F–H and 2–11). All the short-axis views display the anterior structures at the bottom of the video screen, posterior structures at the top, and left-sided structures to the viewer's right. By slow and gradual withdrawal and progressive anteflexion of the tip of the scope, a short-axis scan of the basal cardiac structures will be obtained, including tomographic views at the level of the aortic valve, coronary arteries, left atrial appendage, right ventricular outflow tract, superior vena cava, and left and right upper pulmonary veins and pulmonary arteries. Anatomic abnormalities of these structures can be evaluated by using two-dimensional imaging. Flow patterns can be assessed by using color flow imaging and pulsed Doppler techniques.

Anatomy and Image Orientation With the Longitudinal Scanning Transducer

The proximal transducer of the biplane transesophageal probe generates long-axis images of the cardiovascular structures from each of the three transesophageal positions.[7, 8] The transducer control switch on the echocardiographic machine determines which of the two transducers is active. It

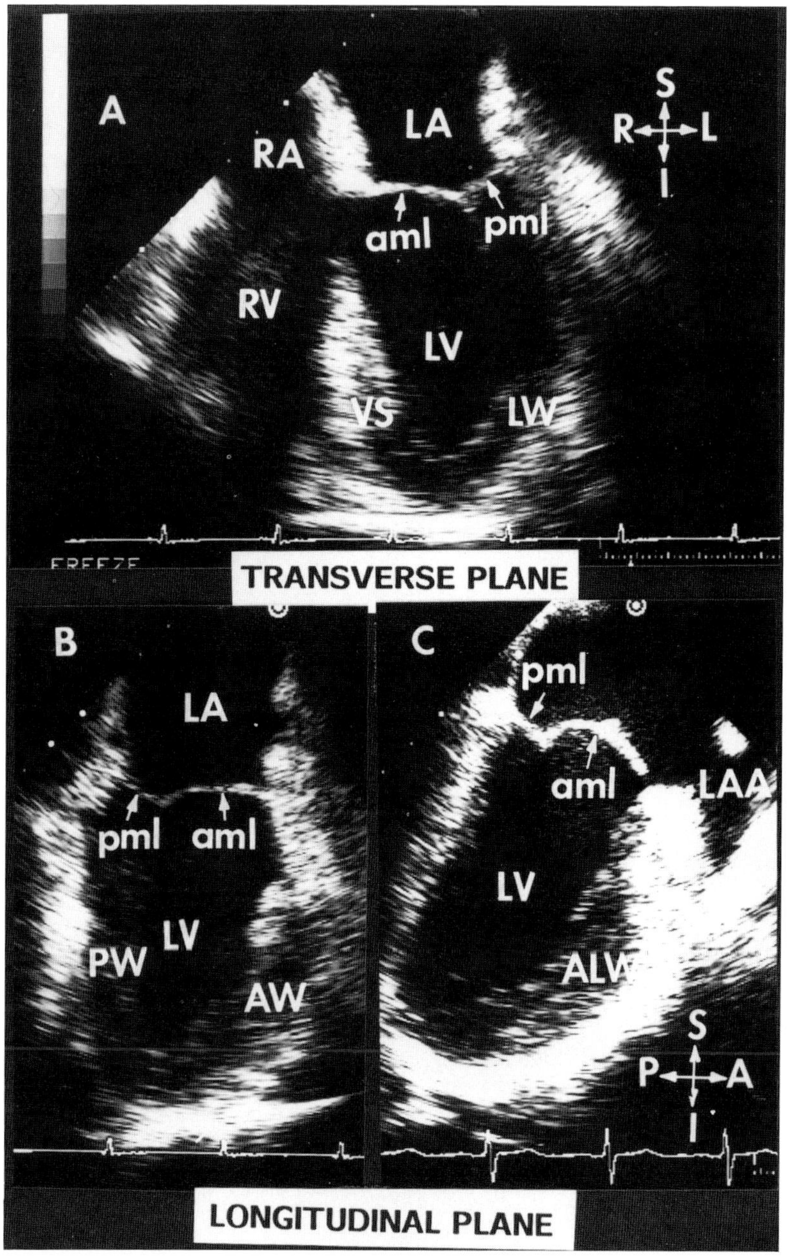

FIG 2–10.

Biplane TEE views from the midesophageal position II. **A,** typical four-chamber view obtained from the midesophageal position with use of the transverse scanning probe. **B,** from this starting transverse-plane view, a midesophageal two-chamber view is obtained by switching to the longitudinal-plane probe. **C,** slight leftward rotation of the tip helps in visualization of the left atrial appendage *(LAA)*. In the directional map, *A* = anterior; *I* = inferior; *L* = left; *P* = posterior; *R* = right; *S* = superior. *aml* = anterior mitral leaflet; *AW* = anterior wall of the left ventricle; *ALW* = anterolateral wall of the left ventricle; *LA* = left atrium; *LV* = left ventricle; *LW* = lateral wall of the left ventricle; *pml* = posterior mitral leaflet; *PW* = posterior wall of the left ventricle; *RA* = right atrium; *RV* = right ventricle; *VS* = ventricular septum.

should be noted that all of the longitudinal-plane images are presented similar to the views that would be seen by an operator sitting on the right side of a supine patient and looking at the cross-sectioned heart from the patient's right side. In the preset mode of the echocardiographic instrument, these tomographic views obtained by the longitudinal scanning transducer display the posterior structures, either to the top of the video screen or to the viewer's left; the anterior structures, either to the bottom of

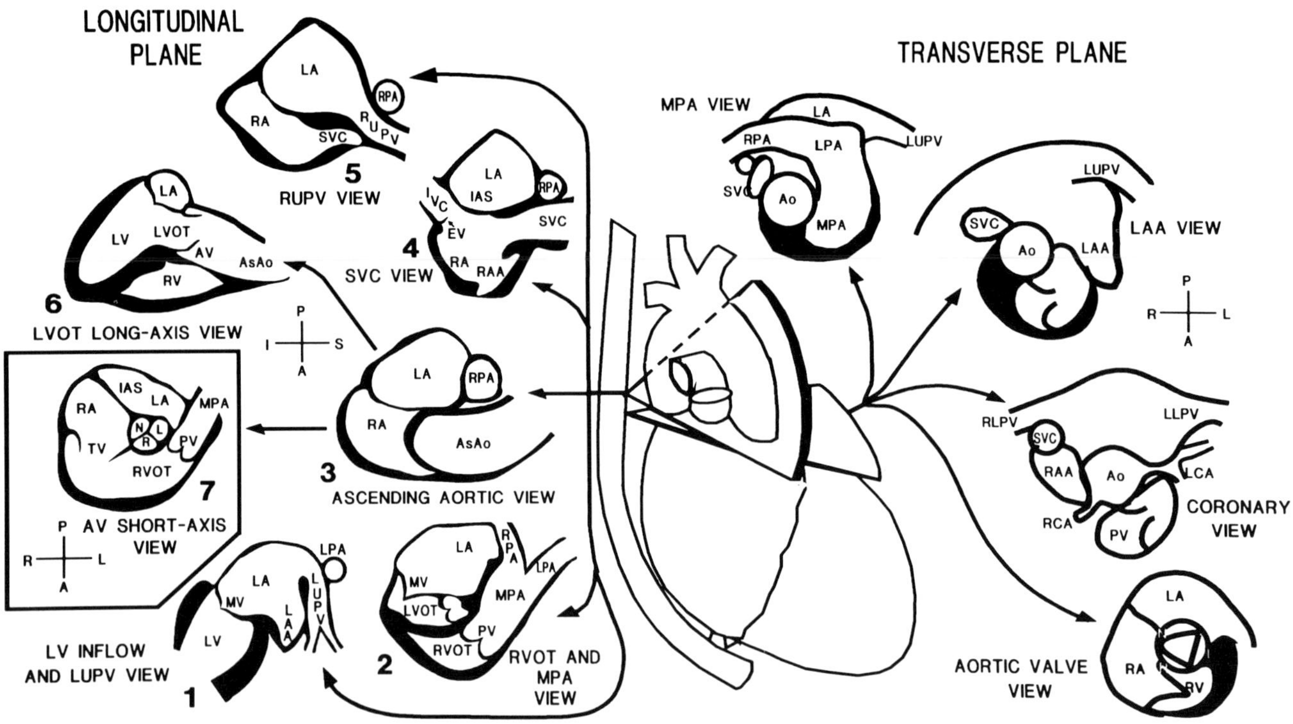

FIG 2–11.

Biplane TEE planes and views from the base of the heart at position I. The *right side* of the diagram illustrates the various short-axis views obtained by use of the transverse-plane transducer with gradual withdrawal and progressive anteflexion of the probe. The *left portion* displays the views obtained by using the longitudinal-plane probe. A longitudinal basal scan is obtained as the transducer tip is rotated left to right. The most leftward view is that of left ventricular *(LV)* inflow and left upper pulmonary vein *(LUPV)*, or view *no. 1*. As the tip is rotated rightward, it sequentially displays the right ventricular outflow tract *(RVOT)* and the main pulmonary artery *(MPA)*, followed by the ascending aorta *(AsAo)*, superior vena cava *(SVC)*, and right upper pulmonary vein *(RUPV)*, or views *2 to 5*. From the ascending aortic view, the left ventricular outflow tract *(LVOT)* long-axis view can be obtained (view *no. 6*). A single short-axis view at the level of the aortic valve can also be generated by using the longitudinal-plane probe (view *no. 7*). In the directional map, *A* = anterior; *I* = inferior; *L* = left; *P* = posterior; *R* = right; *S* = superior. *Ao* = aorta; *AV* = aortic valve; *EV* = eustachian valve; *IAS* = interatrial septum; *L* = left coronary aortic cusp; *LA* = left atrium; *LAA* = left atrial appendage; *LCA* = left coronary artery; *LLPV* = left lower pulmonary vein; *LPA* = left pulmonary artery; *LV* = left ventricle; *MV* = mitral valve; *N* = noncoronary aortic cusp; *PV* = pulmonary valve; *R* = right coronary aortic cusp; *RA* = right atrium; *RAA* = right atrial appendage; *RCA* = right coronary artery; *RLPV* = right lower pulmonary vein; *RPA* = right pulmonary artery; *RV* = right ventricle; *RVOT* = right ventricular outflow tract; *SVC* = superior vena cava; *TV* = tricuspid valve.

the video screen or to the viewer's right; and the superior structures, either to the viewer's right or to the top of the screen.

Transgastric Two-Chamber View

From the transgastric position (see Fig 2–5, position III, and Fig 2–7), after the left ventricular short-axis view is obtained by using the transverse-plane scanning transducer, the imaging is switched to the longitudinal-plane transducer by using the appropriate selection switch on the machine. A longitudinal scan plane from this position provides a transgastric two-chamber view and permits evaluation of the left atrium, medial scallop of the posterior mitral leaflet, lateral segment of the anterior mitral leaflet, and the left ventricle. The posterior left ventricular wall is displayed at the top of the video screen, the anterior wall at the bottom, the apex to the left, and the left atrium to the viewer's right (see Figure 2–8,B). Asynergy of the left ventricular posterior and anterior walls and apex can be evaluated. A transgastric long-axis view can sometimes be obtained by slight right lateral flexion and anteflexion of the tip (see Fig 2–7). This view may allow continuous-wave Doppler examination of the left ventricular outflow tract.

Midesophageal Two-Chamber View

After imaging from the transgastric position is completed, the transducer tip is withdrawn to the midesophageal level to approximately 30 cm from the incisors (see Fig 2–9, position II). The transverse-plane probe allows sectioning through the four-chamber plane of the heart. After this view is obtained, the imaging is switched to the longitudinal plane, and a midesophageal two-chamber view of the heart is obtained (see Figs 2–9 and 2–10,B). This view displays the left ventricular posterior wall to the viewer's left, the left ventricular anterior wall to the viewer's right, the left atrium at the top, and the left ventricular apex at the bottom of the video screen. From this recording position, slight leftward or counterclockwise rotation of the shaft of the probe provides visualization of the left atrial appendage along with the left atrial cavity and the left ventricle (Fig 2–10,C). These views allow assessment of the left atrial appendage, left atrial cavity, middle scallop of the posterior mitral leaflet, the lateral segment of the anterior mitral leaflet, and wall motion abnormalities of the left ventricular posterior, anterior, and apical segments.

Basal Longitudinal-Plane Views

The transducer tip is withdrawn to the upper portion of the esophagus at about 25 cm from the incisors (see Fig 2–11). First, a basal short-axis scan is performed by using the transverse-plane transducer, and then the imaging is switched to the longitudinal scanning plane. Five longitudinal-plane views are obtained at the base of the heart by rotation of the scope from the left to the right side of the heart (see Figs 2–11 to 2–15). We generally obtain the short-axis view of the aortic valve or ascending aorta by using the transverse-plane transducer and then switch the imaging to the longitudinal plane. This maneuver would generally display the ascending aorta in its long axis (see Fig 2–11, view 3). Clockwise or rightward rotation of the shaft of the probe from this recording position will sequentially display the superior vena cava and atrial septal view (see Fig 2–11, view 4), followed by the right upper pulmonary vein view (see Fig 2–11, view 5). Counterclockwise or leftward rotation of the probe from the longitudinal ascending aortic view will sequentially display the right ventricular outflow tract view (see Fig 2–11, view 2) followed by the left ventricular inflow and left upper pulmonary vein view (see Fig 2–11, view 1). All of these longitudinal-plane views display the posterior structures to the top of the video screen and the superior structures to the viewer's right.

Left Ventricular Inflow and Left Upper Pulmonary Vein View.—When the base of the heart is imaged from the upper esophageal position at about 25 cm from the incisors, the sectioning plane of the longitudinal transducer can be directed to the extreme left to obtain a view of the left ventricular inflow tract and the left upper pulmonary vein. The left pulmonary artery, left upper pulmonary vein, and left atrial appendage are displayed anteriorly (Figs 2–11, view 1, and 2–12,E). This tomographic section allows assessment of these structures and the left ventricular inflow tract. Occasionally, both the left upper and lower pulmonary veins can be simultaneously visualized by combined maneuvers of counterclockwise rotation and left lateral flexion of the tip.

Right Ventricular Outflow Tract and Main Pulmonary Artery Long-Axis View.—Slight clockwise or rightward rotation of the probe from the left ventricular inflow tract view will produce a view of the right ventricular outflow tract, pulmonic valve, main pulmonary artery, and both branches (Figs 2–11, view 2; 2–12,D; and 2–13). This view displays the left atrium posteriorly and the right ventricular outflow tract anteriorly. The left ventricular outflow tract is also well seen. This view is well suited for assessment of abnormalities of the right ventricular outflow tract and pulmonary arteries.

Ascending Aortic Long-Axis View.—Further clockwise or rightward rotation of the shaft of the scope results in visualization of the long axis of the proximal portion of the ascending aorta (see Figs 2–11, view 3, and 2–12,C). If one starts with transverse-plane imaging and obtains the short-axis view of the aortic valve first and then switches the imaging to the longitudinal plane, the ascending aortic long-axis view is generally visualized (Fig 2–14). Slight medial or lateral rotation of the scope is required to align the longitudinal sectioning plane to the long axis of the ascending aorta. Depending on the position and orientation of the aortic annulus and ascending aorta, different degrees of oblique views of the aortic cusps are obtained. In this view, the left atrium is visualized posteriorly, the right ventricular outflow tract anteriorly, and the ascending aorta to the viewer's right. The short axis of the right pulmonary artery is displayed in the posterosuperior location. The fossa ovalis region of the atrial septum is well visualized, and shunting across a patent foramen ovale can be evaluated by using echo-contrast techniques.

Superior Vena Cava and Atrial Septal Long-Axis View.—Additional clockwise or rightward rotation of the scope will generate an image of the

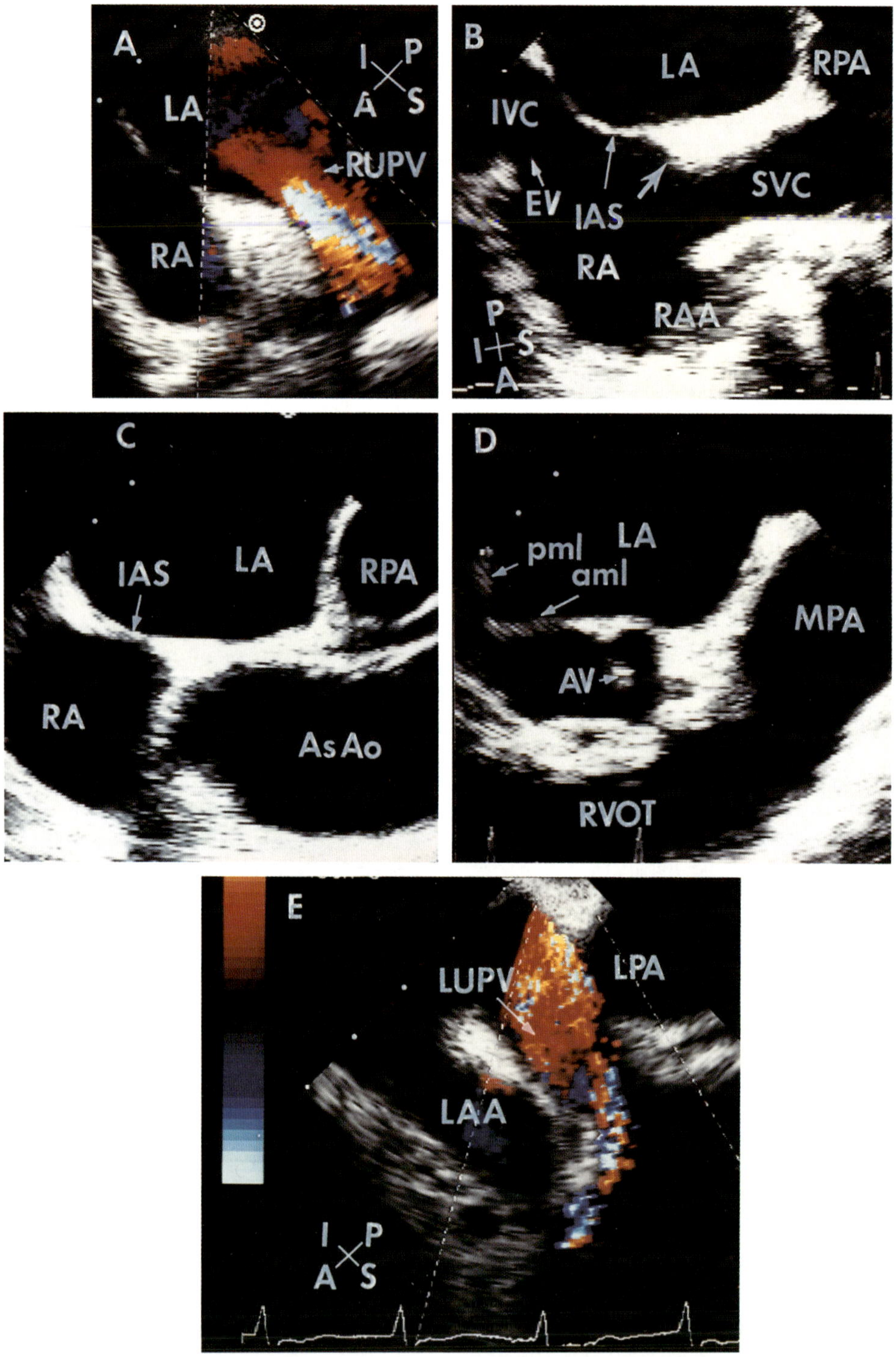

FIG 2–12.
This figure is a composite of five basal longitudinal-plane views from position I. **A,** the right upper pulmonary vein *(RUPV)* view is obtained by the most rightward position of the scanning plane. **B,** the superior vena cava *(SVC)* and atrial septal *(IAS)* view is obtained by slight leftward or counterclockwise rotation of the probe from the RUPV view. **C,** the ascending aortic *(AsAo)* view is obtained by further leftward rotation of the probe. **D,** a view of the right ventricular outflow tract *(RVOT)* and main pulmonary artery *(MPA)* is obtained by further leftward rotation of the probe. **E,** a left upper pulmonary vein *(LUPV)* view is obtained by the most leftward position of the probe. In the directional map, *A* = anterior; *I* = inferior; *P* = posterior; *S* = superior. *aml* = anterior mitral leaflet; *AV* = aortic valve; *EV* = eustachian valve; *IVC* = inferior vena cava; *LA* = left atrium; *LAA* = left atrial appendage; *LPA* = left pulmonary artery; *pml* = posterior mitral leaflet; *RA* = right atrium; *RAA* = right atrial appendage; *RPA* = right pulmonary artery.

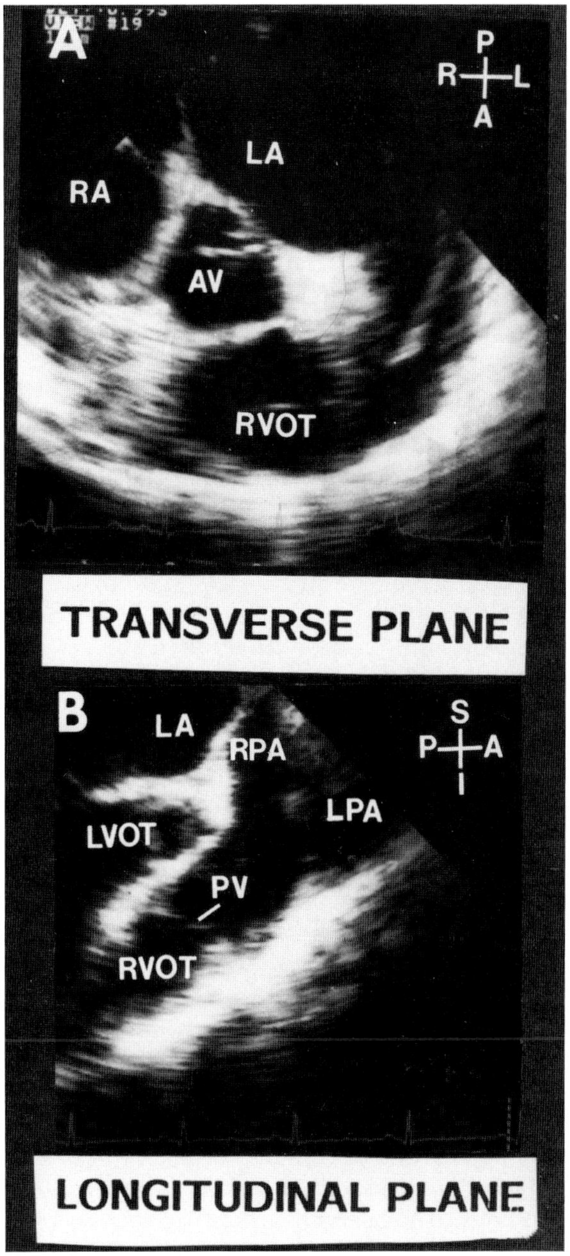

FIG 2–13.
Biplane TEE views at the base of the heart from position I at the level of the right ventricular outflow tract *(RVOT)* and pulmonary artery. **A,** a typical transverse or horizontal section of the heart at the level of the aortic valve *(AV)* and RVOT is obtained with the transverse-plane probe. **B,** after the transverse section shown in **A** is obtained the imaging is switched to the longitudinal scanning transducer, and the shaft of the probe is rotated counterclockwise, or leftward, to obtain this view of the RVOT. In the directional map, *A* = anterior; *I* = inferior; *L* = left; *P* = posterior; *R* = right; *S* = superior. *AV* = aortic valve; *LA* = left atrium; *LPA* = left pulmonary artery; *LVOT* = left ventricular outflow tract; *MPA* = main pulmonary artery; *MV* = mitral valve; *PV* = pulmonary valve; *RPA* = right pulmonary artery. (Adapted from Bansal RC, et al: *J Am Soc Echocardiogr* 1990; 3:348–366.)

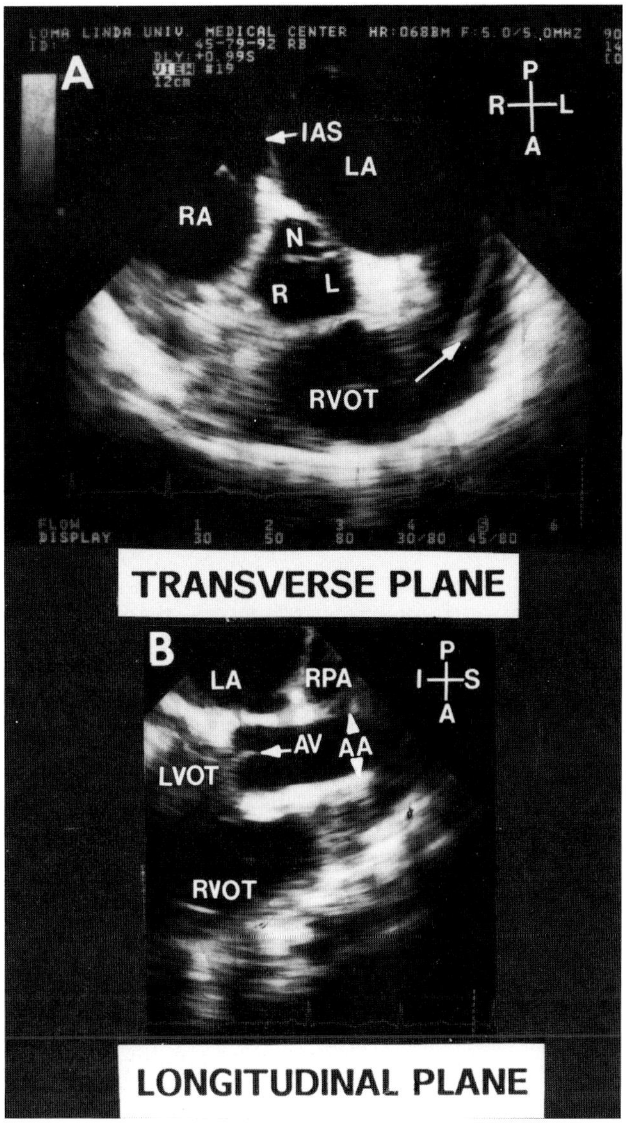

FIG 2–14.
Biplane TEE views from the base of the heart at position I. **A,** cross-sectional view obtained at the level of the aortic valve *(AV)* with use of the transverse scanning transducer. The *arrow* shows the catheter coursing through the right ventricular outflow tract *(RVOT)* into the pulmonary artery. **B,** a long-axis view of the ascending aorta *(AA)* is obtained by slight clockwise rotation of the shaft after switching to the longitudinal-plane probe. In the directional map, *A* = anterior; *I* = inferior; *L* = left; *P* = posterior; *R* = right; *S* = superior. *IAS* = interatrial septum; *L* = left coronary aortic cusp; *LA* = left atrium; *LVOT* = left ventricular outflow tract; *N* = noncoronary aortic cusp; *R* = right coronary aortic cusp; *RA* = right atrium; *RPA* = right pulmonary artery. (Adapted from Bansal RC, et al: *J Am Soc Echocardiogr* 1990; 3:348–366.)

long axis of the superior vena cava and atrial septum (see Figs 2–11, view 4, and 2–12,B). This view displays the left atrium posteriorly, right atrium anteriorly, superior vena cava to the viewer's right, and inferior vena cava to the left. Posterosuperior to the superior vena cava, the right pulmonary artery is transected in its short axis. The entire atrial septum is well visualized, and this view is particularly suited for delineation of sinus venosus atrial septal defects. The right atrium and its appendage are also well seen anteriorly. Slight advancement of the scope displays an image of the long axis of the inferior vena cava, the junction of the inferior vena cava to the right atrium, and the eustachian valve (see Fig 2–12,B). Color flow imaging and pulsed Doppler techniques can be utilized to study the normal and abnormal caval flow patterns. An alternate method to obtain the superior vena cava and atrial septum long-axis view is to first start imaging in the transverse plane to obtain the short axis of the superior vena cava and then bring this structure to the middle of the video screen by clockwise rotation of the probe and then switch imaging to the longitudinal-plane transducer (Fig 2–15). This type of maneuver is very helpful for beginners in this field to understand the biplane anatomy.

Right Upper Pulmonary Vein View.—Still further clockwise or rightward rotation of the tip of the scope will align the longitudinal plane along the long axis of the right upper pulmonary vein. Slight withdrawal of the tip of the scope is required to obtain the long-axis view of the right pulmonary vein, which is seen to enter the posteriorly situated left atrium at approximately the 5 o'clock position (see Figs 2–11, view 5, and 2–12,A). The right pulmonary artery in its short axis is located superior to the right upper pulmonary vein. Further clockwise rotation and slight advancement of the tip may sometimes visualize the right lower pulmonary vein. Occasionally, both right upper and lower pulmonary veins can be simultaneously visualized by the combined maneuvers of clockwise rotation and rightward lateral flexion of the tip.

Left Ventricular Outflow Tract Long-Axis View.—After recording the ascending aortic long-axis view, the tip of the scope is slightly flexed left laterally by counterclockwise rotation of the outer smaller knob on the base handle of the scope. Additionally, slight rightward or clockwise rotation of the tip of the scope is required to optimize this long-axis view of the left ventricular outflow tract (Figs 2–11, view 6, and 2–16).

Aortic Valve Short-Axis View by Using the Longitudinal Plane.—Longitudinal-plane imaging at the base of the heart allows visualization of most of the structures along their long axes. However, if one starts with the ascending aortic long-axis view and utilizes the combined maneuver of clockwise or rightward flexion and counterclockwise or leftward rotation of the tip, a basal short-axis view of the aortic valve is obtained. In this tomographic view, the aortic valve is displayed in the center, the left and right atria posteriorly, and the right ventricular outflow tract anteriorly. The tricuspid valve is seen to the viewer's left and the pulmonary valve to the viewer's right (Figs 2–11, view 7, and 2–17). This view is similar to the parasternal short-axis view at the level of the aortic valve and should be ideal for transesophageal continuous-wave Doppler assessment of tricuspid regurgitation jets.

BIPLANE TRANSESOPHAGEAL EXAMINATION OF THE THORACIC AORTA AND ARCH

The esophagus courses through the chest from the pharnyx to the stomach with slight side-to-side and anterior-to-posterior deviations. The relationship between these two structures is covered in great detail in Chapter 7, "Aortic Disease." Because of the changing relationships of the esophagus to the aorta and the lack of definite internal anatomic landmarks, precise anterioposterior and right-left orientations of the descending thoracic aorta and the TEE views are difficult. Therefore, in order to determine the site of observed aortic disease, the depth of the transducer tip from the incisors is recorded throughout withdrawal.

Anatomy and Image Orientation for Study of the Ascending and Descending Thoracic Aortas

TEE assessment of the aorta is begun by examination of the aortic root (sinuses) and ascending aorta. The probe is advanced down to approximately 30 cm from the incisors, and the transducer faces anteriorly and is below the tracheal carina. The aortic valve is identified in cross section with the transverse-plane scanning probe. A scan of the proximal

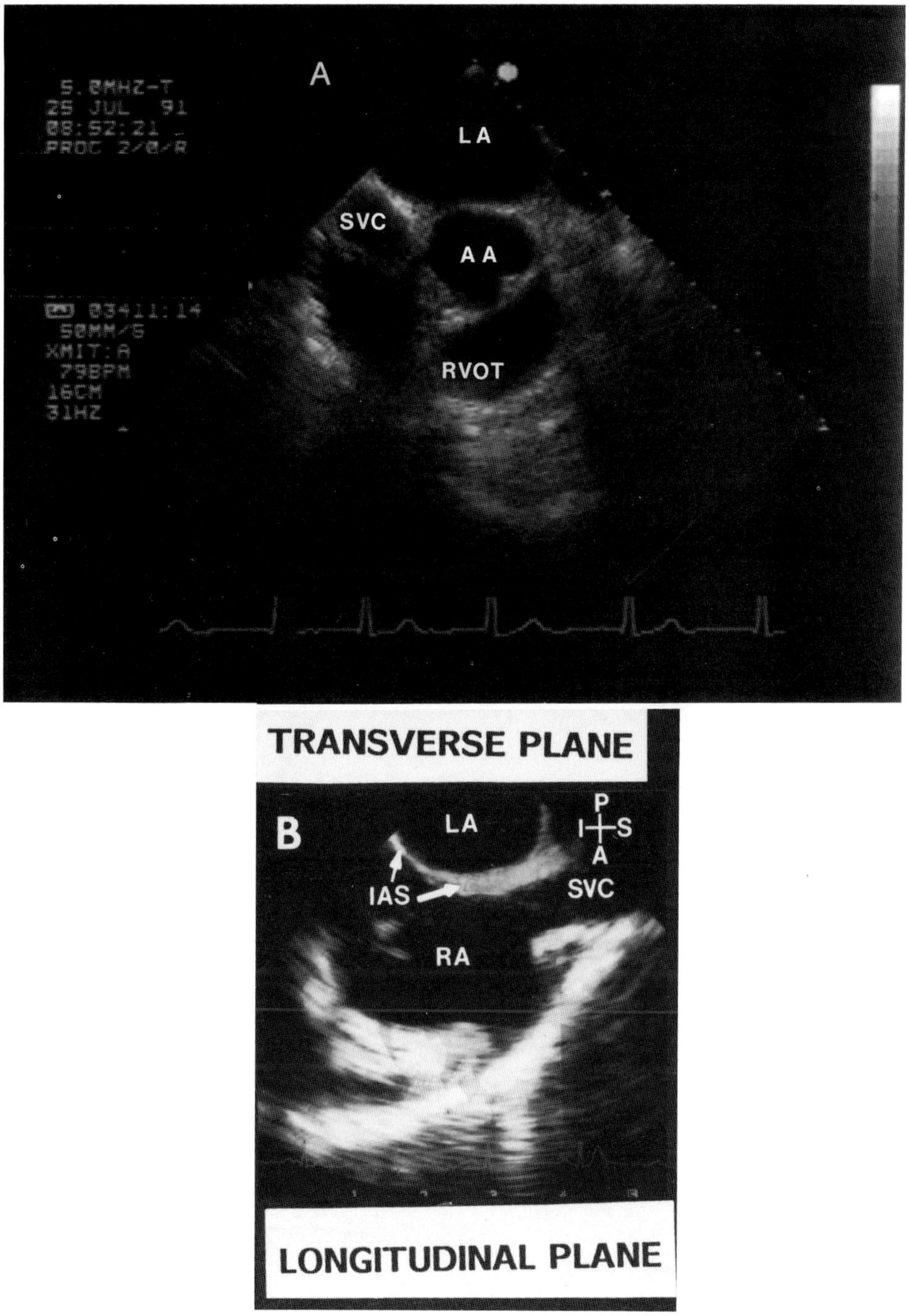

FIG 2–15.
Biplane TEE views obtained from the base of the heart at position I at the level of the ascending aorta *(AA)*, superior vena cava *(SVC)*, and interatrial septum *(IAS)*. **A,** a transverse section of the heart at the base is obtained through the SVC and AA by use of the transverse scanning probe. **B,** by switching to the longitudinal-plane scanning probe, a long-axis view of the SVC and the entire IAS is obtained. The thick portion of the IAS adjacent to the SVC where sinus venosus atrial septal defects are located is very well seen *(thick arrow)*. The thin portion of the IAS *(thin arrow)*, representing the fossa ovalis where ostium secundum defects are located, is also well visualized. In the directional map, *A* = anterior; *I* = inferior; *L* = left; *P* = posterior; *R* = right; *S* = superior. *AV* = aortic valve; *LA* = left atrium; *RA* = right atrium; *RVOT* = right ventricular outflow tract. (Adapted from Bansal RC, et al: *J Am Soc Echocardiogr* 1990; 3:348–366.)

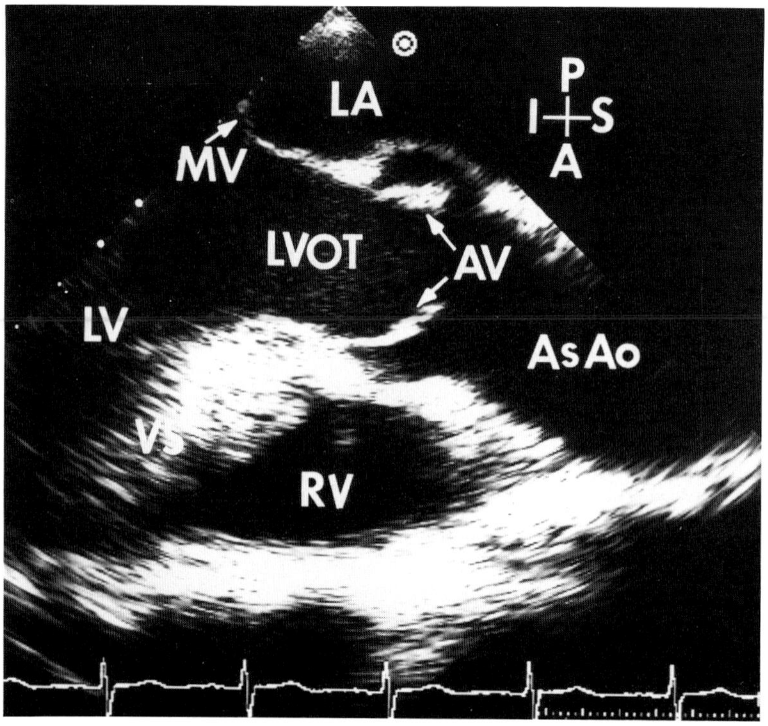

FIG 2–16.
Left ventricular outflow tract *(LVOT)* long-axis view obtained by using the longitudinal-plane scanning probe at the base of the heart at position I. In the directional map, *A* = anterior; *I* = inferior; *P* = posterior; *S* = superior. *AV* = aortic valve; *AsAo* = ascending aorta; *LA* = left atrium; *LV* = left ventricle; *MV* = mitral valve; *RV* = right ventricle; *VS* = ventricular septum.

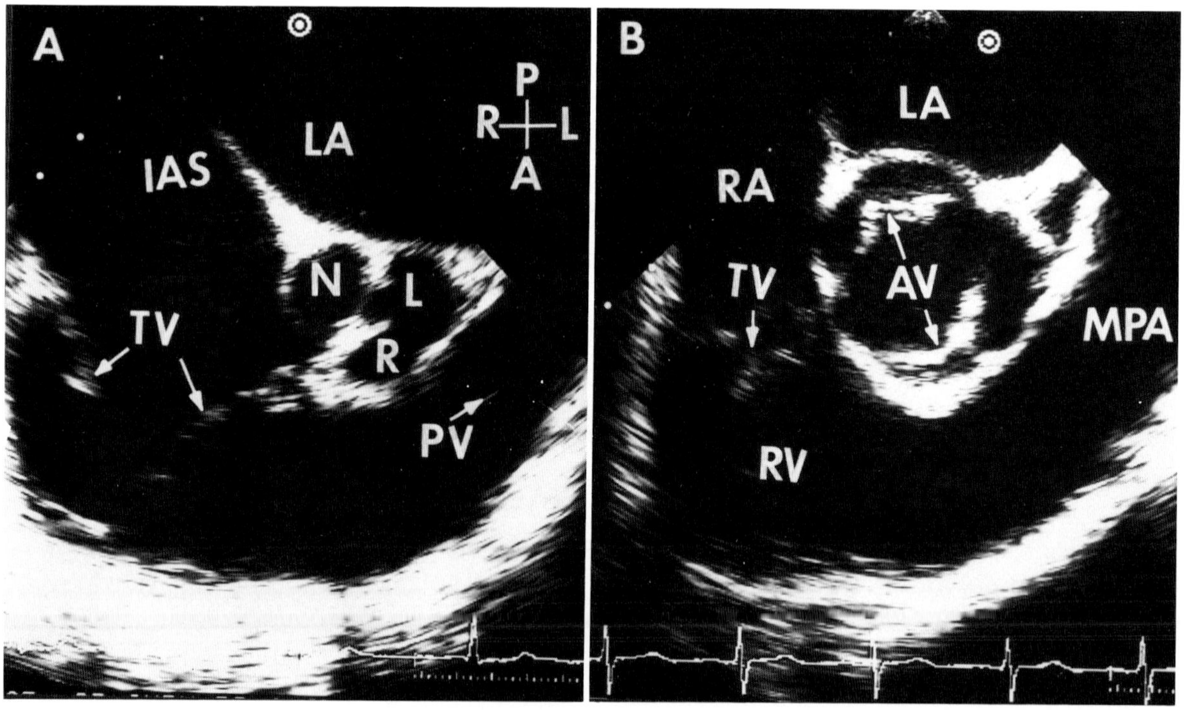

FIG 2–17.
Aortic valve *(AV)* short-axis view obtained by using the longitudinal-plane probe at the base from transesophageal position I. **A,** basal aortic valve short-axis view from a patient with three leaflets. **B,** short-axis aortic valve view from a patient with a bicuspid valve. In the directional map, *A* = anterior; *L* = left; *P* = posterior; *R* = right. *IAS* = interatrial septum; *L* = left coronary aortic cusp; *LA* = left atrium; *MPA* = main pulmonary artery; *N* = noncoronary aortic cusp; *PV* = pulmonary valve; *R* = right coronary aortic cusp; *RA* = right atrium; *RV* = right ventricle; *TV* = tricuspid valve.

portion of the ascending aorta in cross section at different levels can be obtained by slow withdrawal of the transducer tip up to the level of the pulmonary artery bifurcation (Figs 2–18 and 2–19,A–C). Extreme anteflexion of the tip of the transverse-plane scanning probe can display the proximal aspect of the ascending aorta and valve in the long-axis view (see Figs 2–18 and 2–19,D). The distal ascending aorta above the level of the right pulmonary artery, however, cannot be visualized by the transverse-plane scanning uniplane probe because of the interposition of the main-stem bronchi and trachea between the upper portion of the ascending aorta and the esophagus. The longitudinal-plane scanning transducer at this level, however, provides visualization of the majority of the ascending aortic segment (see Figs 2–18 and 2–19,E). After visualization of the ascending aorta, the shaft of the echoscope is rotated slightly counterclockwise or leftward to visualize the cross section of the midthoracic descending aorta by use of the transverse-plane scanning transducer (see Figs 2–18 and 2–19,F). The scope is then gradually advanced into the stomach (about 45 to 50 cm from the incisors) while keeping the aorta in view. As the probe is advanced, more counterclockwise or posterior rotation is needed to keep the aorta in view because the esophagus lies anterior to the aorta at the level of the diaphragm. Slight anteflexion of the tip of the echoscope provides better contact of the transducer with the esophagus. The scope

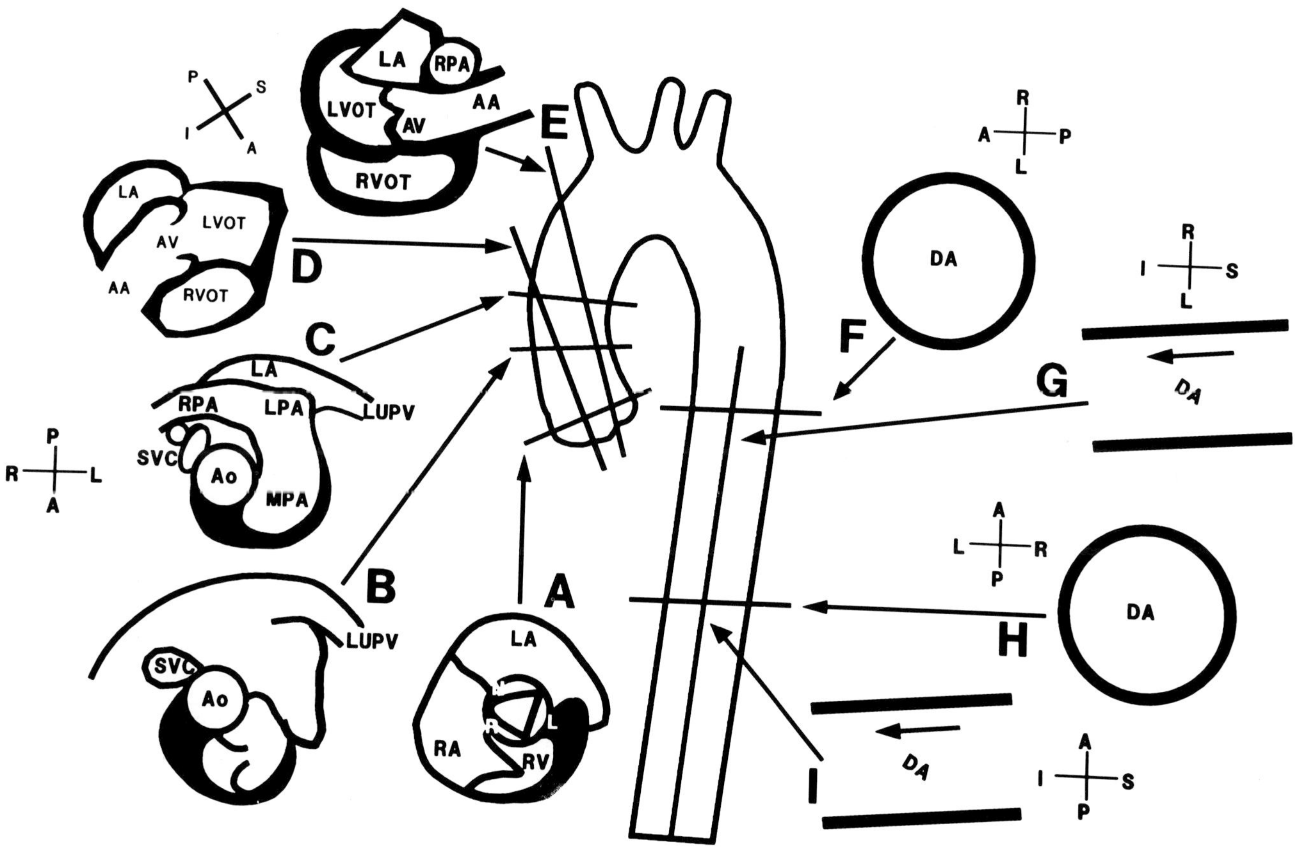

FIG 2–18.
A schematic of various planes and views of the ascending (*left side* of the diagram) and descending thoracic aorta (*right side* of the diagram) with use of the biplane transesophageal probe. Freeze frames of the transesophageal views through these planes are shown in Figure 2–19. **A–C,** short-axis views of the ascending aorta at different levels are obtained by using the transverse-plane probe. **D,** a long-axis view of the ascending aorta *(AA)* is obtained by using the transverse-plane probe with marked anteflexion of the tip. **E,** the longitudinal-plane ascending aortic long-axis view. **F** and **H,** views of the upper and lower portions of the descending aorta with the transverse-plane probe. **G** and **I,** longitudinal plane views of the upper and lower descending thoracic aorta. In the directional map, *A* = anterior; *I* = inferior; *L* = left; *P* = posterior; *R* = right; *S* = superior. *AA* = ascending aorta; *Ao* = aorta; *AV* = aortic valve; *DA* = descending thoracic aorta; *L* = left coronary aortic cusp; *LA* = left atrium; *LPA* = left pulmonary artery; *LVOT* = left ventricular outflow tract; *MPA* = main pulmonary artery; *N* = noncoronary aortic cusp; *R* = right coronary aortic cusp; *RA* = right atrium; *RPA* = right pulmonary artery; *RVOT* = right ventricular outflow tract. (Adapted from Bansal RC, et al: *J Am Soc Echocardiogr* 1990; 3:348–366.)

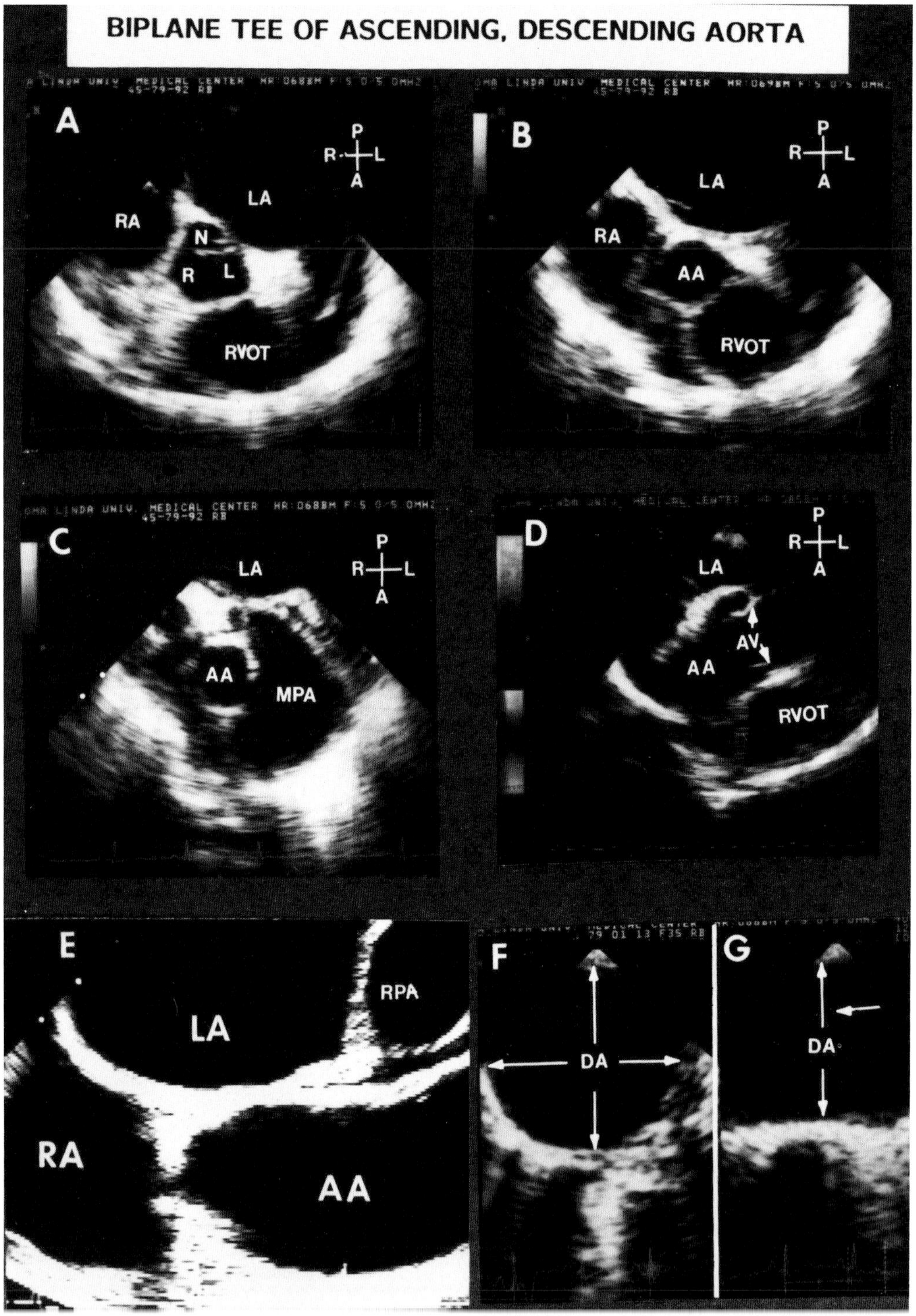

FIG 2–19.

A composite of various transesophageal views of the ascending aorta *(AA)* and descending thoracic aorta *(DA)* with use of the biplane TEE probe. **A,** a view of the aorta at the level of the aortic sinuses is obtained by use of the transverse-plane scanning probe. **B,** a cross-sectional view of the tubular portion of the AA above the level of the sinuses is obtained by withdrawing the probe slightly. **C,** a view of the middle portion of AA at the level of the main pulmonary artery *(MPA)* is obtained by further withdrawal of the probe. **D,** extreme anteflexion of the probe provides a long-axis view of the AA by use of the transverse scanning probe. **E,** a much better view of the entire AA is obtained more consistently with use of the longitudinal-plane scanning probe. **F,** a cross-sectional view of the DA is obtained by use of the transverse-plane scanning probe. **G,** the DA in its long-axis view with use of the longitudinal-plane scanning probe. In the directional map, *A* = anterior; *I* = inferior; *L* = left; *P* = posterior; *R* = right; *S* = superior. *AV* = aortic valve; *L* = left coronary aortic cusp; *LA* = left atrium; *N* = noncoronary aortic cusp; *R* = right coronary aortic cusp; *RA* = right atrium; *RPA* = right pulmonary artery; *RVOT* = right ventricular outflow tract. (From Bansal RC, et al: *J Am Soc Echocardiogr* 1990; 3:348–366. Used by permission.)

is gradually withdrawn in 5-cm increments while the aorta is kept in view to examine the upper abdominal and entire descending thoracic aorta in cross sections. The mid and distal abdominal aorta cannot be seen because of difficulty in maintaining good contact of the esophageal transducer with the mucosa of the stomach. Long-axis views of the descending thoracic aorta can be recorded at any level by switching to the longitudinal-plane scanning transducer (see Figs 2–18 and 2–19,G). In the upper portion of the chest, the esophagus is situated along the right lateral margin of the descending aorta, and the orientation of the short-axis view obtained by scanning with the transverse-plane probe will be such that the right margin of the descending aorta will be at the top, the left margin at the bottom, the posterior wall to the viewer's right, and the anterior wall to the viewer's left (see Fig 2–18,F). While imaging in the longitudinal plane from this position, the right wall of the aorta will be at the top and the left wall at the bottom of the video screen (see Fig 2–18,G). The image orientation of the short-axis view of the descending thoracic aorta in its lower portion (more than 30 to 35 cm from the incisors) is such that the anterior wall is displayed at the top of the screen, the posterior wall at the bottom, the left margin to the viewer's left, and the right margin of the aorta to the viewer's right. Images of the vertebral bodies and intervertebral disks are posterior to the posterior aortic wall (see Fig 2–18,H). When the longitudinal plane is imaged from this position, the anterior wall of the aorta is at the top and the posterior wall at the bottom of the video screen (see Fig 2–18,I).

Anatomy and Image Orientation for Study of the Aortic Arch

The arch can be imaged by slowly withdrawing the probe to about 18 to 20 cm. As the tip of the echoscope approaches the posterior portion of the pharynx, the gag and cough reflexes will increase and cause discomfort to the patient, which prevents prolonged imaging in this position. Because the aortic arch lies slightly anterior to the esophagus, the operator, while withdrawing the scope from the midthoracic aorta, should rotate the probe slightly clockwise, or to the patient's right. The transverse-plane scanning probe displays a long-axis view of the arch with the ascending portion to the viewer's left and descending portion to the viewer's right side of the video screen (Figs 2–20 and 2–21,A).

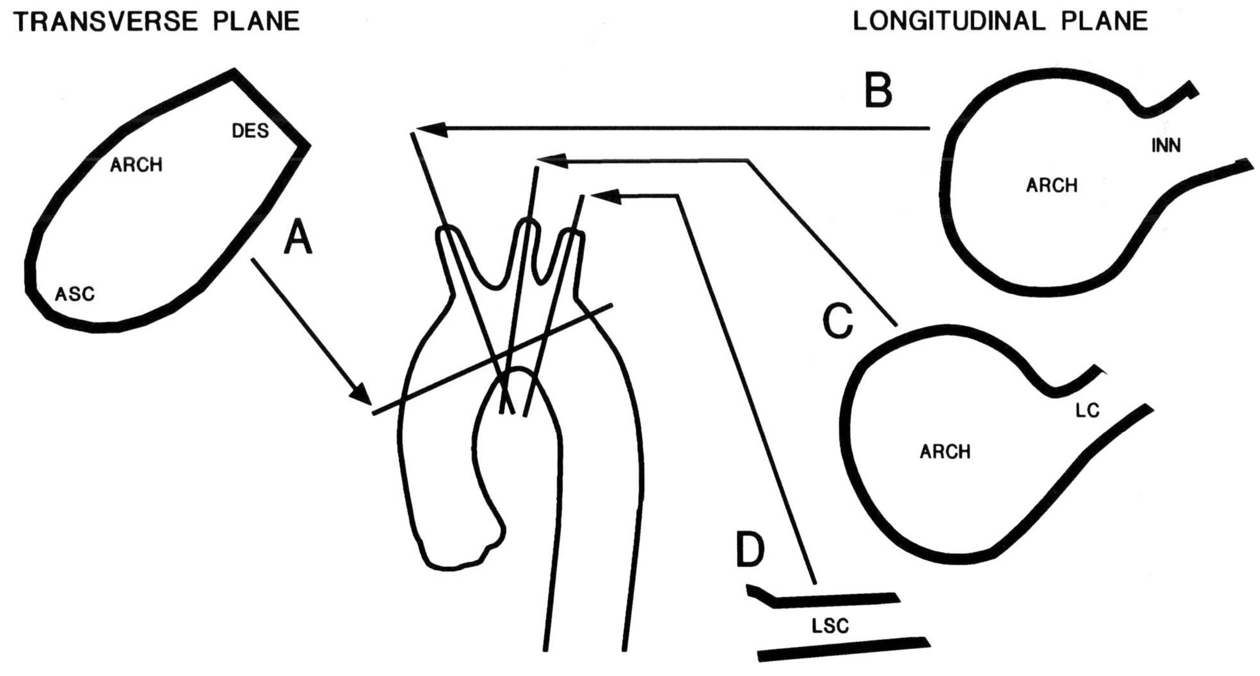

FIG 2–20.
Schematic of planes and views of the aortic arch with use of the biplane transesophageal probe. **A,** this schematic of the aortic arch in its long-axis view was obtained with the transverse-plane scanning probe. **B,** Longitudinal-plane scanning showing the long-axis of the right innominate artery *(INN)*. **C,** Longitudinal-plane scanning showing the left carotid artery *(LC)*. **D,** the long axis of the left subclavian artery *(LSC)* is less frequently visualized. *ASC* = ascending portion of arch; DES = descending portion of the arch. (Adapted from Bansal RC, et al: *J Am Soc Echocardiogr* 1990; 3:348–366.)

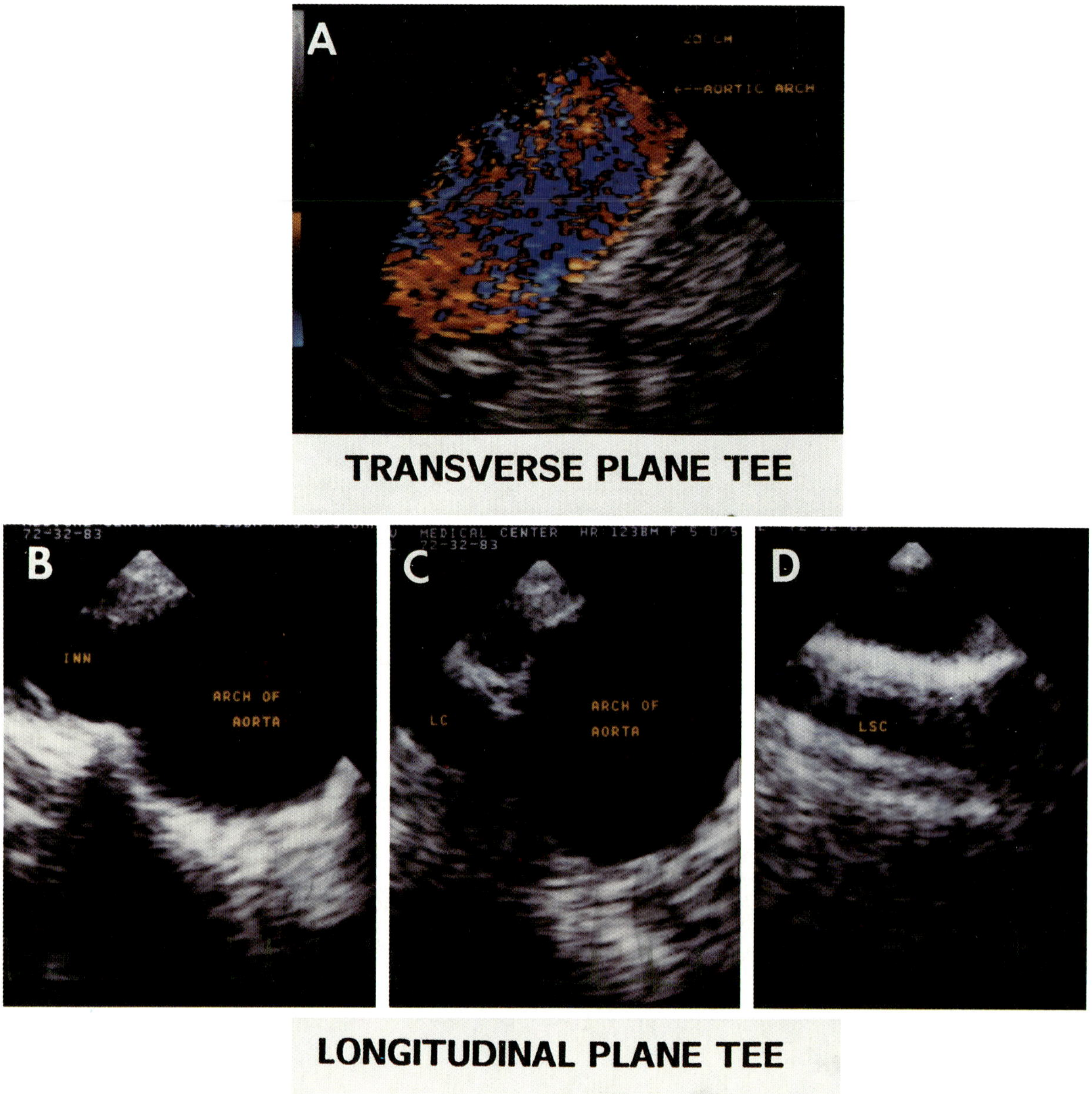

FIG 2–21.
Biplane TEE views of the aortic arch. **A,** the aortic arch in its long axis with color flow imaging by using the transverse-plane scanning probe and imaging at about 20 cm from the incisors. **B,** long axis of the right innominate artery *(INN)* and the short axis of the arch by using the longitudinal-plane scanning probe. **C,** long axis of the left carotid artery *(LC)* and the short axis of the arch by using the longitudinal-plane scanning probe. **D,** the long axis of the left subclavian artery is less frequently visualized with the longitudinal-plane probe. The orientation shown in **B, C,** and **D** is obtained by use of the right-to-left electronic reorientation switch. (Adapted from Bansal RC, et al: *J Am Soc Echocardiogr* 1990; 3:348–366.)

The left common carotid artery and the proximal portion of the left subclavian artery may also be displayed in the short axes when the probe is withdrawn superior to the aortic arch. The right innominate artery cannot be seen because of the air-filled trachea. From the aortic arch position, by switching to the longitudinal-plane scanning transducer, the short axis of the arch with one of the brachiocephalic vessels in its long axis (commonly the left carotid or right innominate artery) is often recorded. By combined maneuvers of side-to-side rotation and angulation of the tip of the transducer, the right innominate and left carotid arteries can frequently be seen. The left subclavian artery is less frequently visualized in its long axis (see Figs 2–20 and 2–21,B–D).

IDENTIFICATION OF SPECIFIC CARDIAC STRUCTURES

In our experience and that of others, the biplane transducers have significantly expanded the diagnostic capability of TEE.[7–12] This type of examination provides multiple tomographic views in two orthogonal planes for more complete assessment of different cardiac structures.

Left Atrial Appendage

The left atrial appendage, a site of clot formation in patients with large fibrillating atria, and rheumatic and prosthetic mitral valve disease are well seen when using biplane TEE. The left atrial appendage is visualized as a triangular outpouching of the left atrium and is seen from the transverse-plane view of the left atrium at the level of the appendage (see Fig 2–6,G) and the midesophageal two-chamber view of the left heart (see Fig 2–10,C). Muscular ridges or pectinate muscles within the left atrial appendage are generally well seen and should not be confused with thrombi. The entrance of the left upper pulmonary vein and the left atrial appendage into the main atrial cavity is separated by a distinct ridgelike infolding of the wall and should not be confused with a pathologic mass (see Fig 3–3).

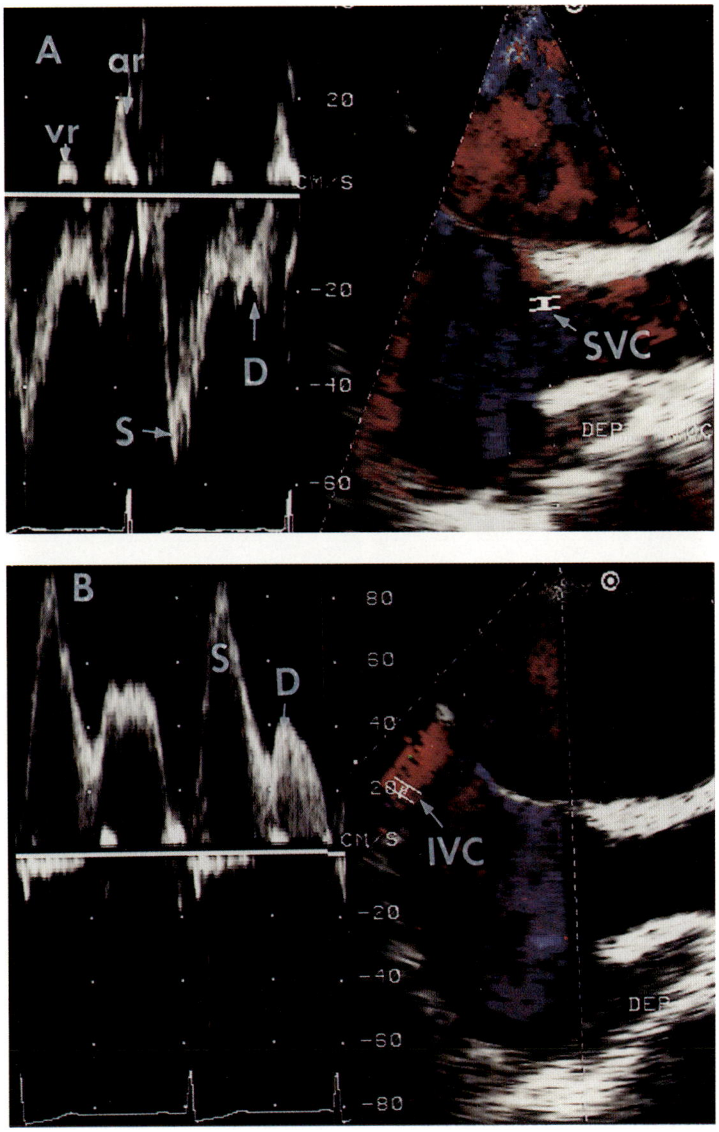

FIG 2–22.
Pulsed Doppler interrogation of superior **(A)** and inferior vena cava *(IVC)* **(B)** flows from the longitudinal-plane superior vena caval *(SVC)* basal view. The systolic peak *(S)* is slightly larger than the diastolic *(D)* peak. Slight degrees of reversed flow in systole *(vr)* and following atrial contraction *(ar)* are demonstrated in the SVC flow.

Right Atrial Appendage

The right atrial appendage appears as a triangular outpouching of the anterior right atrial wall and is best seen by using the longitudinal-plane view at the level of the superior vena cava and atrial septum (see Fig 2–12,B).

Superior and Inferior Vena Cava

Caval connections to the right atrium are best demonstrated by using the basal longitudinal-plane view at the level of the superior vena cava (see Fig 2–12,B). Color flow and pulsed Doppler techniques allow interrogation of their flow patterns (Fig 2–22).

Pulmonary Veins

Both left and right upper pulmonary veins can be visualized by using the basal transverse- and longitudinal-plane views (Fig 2–23). The right lower pulmonary vein can also be frequently seen. Color flow imaging and Doppler techniques allow a demonstration of the pulmonary venous flow patterns (Fig 2–23,B and C).

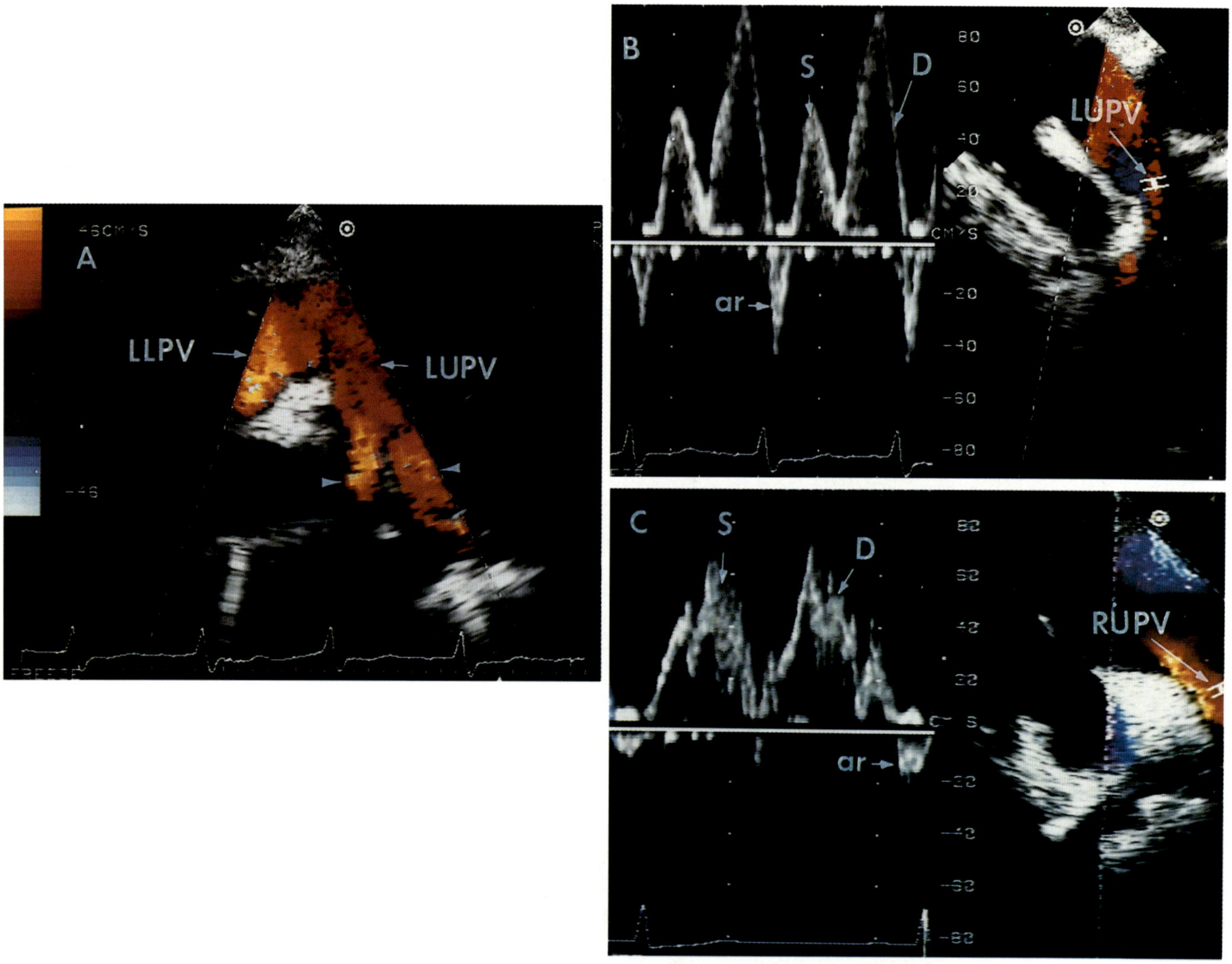

FIG 2–23.
Two-dimensional imaging: color and pulsed Doppler interrogation of pulmonary veins. **A,** both the left upper *(LUPV)* and left lower *(LLPV)* pulmonary veins can be visualized by using the longitudinal-plane transducer while imaging at the base of the heart. This freeze frame taken in systole shows the red color flow velocities representing flow into the left atrium. Between the *arrowheads* two tributaries of the left upper pulmonary vein are noted. **B,** imaging of the LUPV by using the longitudinal-plane probe and pulsed Doppler interrogation of its flow. Note the smaller systolic *(S)* and the larger diastolic *(D)* peaks on the spectral display. Mild reversal of flow is noted following atrial contraction *(ar)*. **C,** imaging of the right upper pulmonary vein *(RUPV)* by using the longitudinal-plane scanning transducer at the base of the heart. Pulsed Doppler interrogation shows systolic *(S)* and diastolic *(D)* filling waves. A slight degree of reversed flow is noted following atrial contraction *(ar)*.

Atrial Septum

The entire atrial septum can be evaluated by a combination of transverse-plane midesophageal four-chamber (see Fig 2–10,A), longitudinal-plane ascending aortic (see Fig 2–12,C), and superior vena caval views (see Fig 2–12,B). A patent foramen ovale and right-to-left shunting are best evaluated by using echo-contrast studies while imaging in the longitudinal plane at the level of the ascending aorta and/or superior vena cava. An ostium secundum atrial septal defect located in the fossa ovalis region can be seen from four-chamber and longitudinal-plane views. A sinus venosus atrial septal defect in the upper muscular portion of the atrial septum is seen immediately beneath the superior vena cava from the longitudinal-plane view (see Figs 2–12,B and 2–15,B).

Mitral Valve

Biplane TEE permits a detailed and complete evaluation of the various components of the mitral valve apparatus (left atrial cavity and wall, mitral annulus, leaflets and different scallops, commissures, chordae tendineae, papillary muscles, and left ventricular walls). TEE permits an evaluation of both segments of the anterior mitral leaflet (lateral and medial) and all three scallops of the posterior mitral leaflet (medial, middle, and lateral) by use of a combination of transgastric short-axis and two-chamber views and four-chamber, five-chamber, and two-chamber views from the midesophageal position (Fig 2–24). The transgastric short-axis views demonstrate the entire mitral valve and its opening in the short axis, and it is possible to evaluate both segments of the anterior leaflet and all three scallops of the posterior leaflet. The transgastric two-chamber view allows evaluation of the medial scallop of the posterior leaflet and lateral segment of the anterior leaflet. A transesophageal four-chamber view with a slight posterior tilt generally allows assessment of the medial segment of the anterior leaflet and the middle scallop of the posterior leaflet. A four-chamber view with slight anterior tilt would generally help in evaluating the lateral segment of the anterior leaflet and lateral scallop of the posterior leaflet. A two-chamber view from the midesophageal position usually displays the lateral segment of the anterior leaflet and medial or middle scallop of the posterior mitral leaflet. With this approach, more precise localization of the anatomic fault responsible for mitral

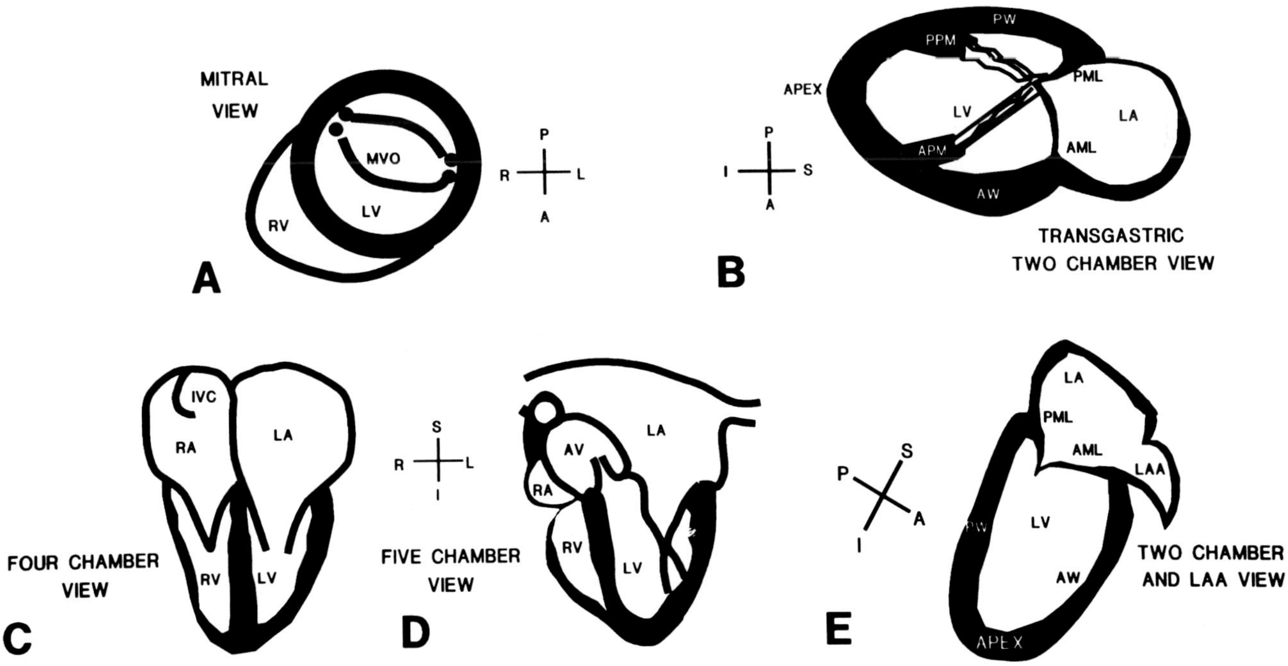

FIG 2–24.
Schematic illustration of the various biplane views for examination of the mitral valve apparatus. Refer to the text for a description. In the directional map, *A* = anterior; *I* = inferior; *L* = left; *P* = posterior; *R* = right; *S* = superior. *AML* = anterior mitral leaflet; *AV* = aortic valve; *APM* = anterior papillary muscle; *AW* = anterior wall; *IVC* = inferior vena cava; *LA* = left atrium; *LAA* = left atrial appendage; *LV* = left ventricle; *MVO* = mitral valve orifice; *PML* = posterior mitral leaflet; *PPM* = posterior papillary muscle; *PW* = posterior wall; *RA* = right atrium; *RV* = right ventricle. (Adapted from Bansal RC, et al: *J Am Soc Echocardiogr* 1990; 3:348–366.)

regurgitation, including endocarditis, perforation, mitral valve aneurysm, and ruptured chordae tendinae with flail leaflet, is feasible. The information regarding the type, cause, and degree of structural abnormality of the various components of the mitral valve apparatus is extremely valuable for predicting the feasibility of mitral valve repair. Biplane orthogonal transesophageal views allow visual reconstruction of the three-dimensional distribution of the area of mitral regurgitation and may permit more accurate quantitative assessment (see Chapter 5). Normal (Fig 2–25) and abnormal mitral flows can be interrogated by using color flow imaging and pulsed Doppler methods. Biplane views allow better evaluation of the mitral annulus and are superior in precise localization and quantitation of perivalvular leaks in patients with prosthetic mitral valves (see Fig 9–6).

Tricuspid Valve

The tricuspid valve and tricuspid regurgitation can be evaluated by using the transverse-plane right ventricular inflow view (see Fig 2–6,E), the midesophageal four-chamber view (see Fig 2–6,C), and the longitudinal-plane basal short-axis view at the level of the aortic valve (see Fig 2–17). The longitudinal-plane view will also allow continuous-wave Doppler interrogation of the tricuspid regurgitation jet.

Aortic Valve

Congenital and acquired abnormalities of the aortic valve can be assessed by utilizing the transverse-plane midesophageal five-chamber and basal short-axis view at the level of the aortic valve (see Fig 2–6,D and F) and the longitudinal-plane basal aortic valve short-axis view (see Fig 2–17). The left ventricular outflow tract can be imaged from the transverse-plane midesophageal five-chamber and longitudinal-plane ascending aortic views. By utilizing these views, pathology of the aortic valve and left ventricular outflow tract can be assessed. The number of aortic valve cusps can be determined (see Fig 2–17). Normal flows of the left ventricular outflow tract and ascending aorta can be interrogated by using color flow imaging and pulsed Doppler techniques (Fig 2–26). The severity of aortic regurgitation can be assessed by using color flow imaging. Continuous-wave Doppler interrogation using steerable Doppler techniques may be useful in assessing the severity of left ventricular outflow tract obstruction. Systolic anterior motion of the anterior mitral leaflet and discrete subaortic stenosis can be assessed by using these left ventricular outflow tract views.

Pulmonary Valve, Pulmonary Arteries, and Right Ventricular Outflow Tract

These structures can be evaluated by using transverse-plane basal short-axis and longitudinal-plane long-axis views of the outflow tract, pulmonary valve, and main pulmonary artery and its branches (see Figs 2–6,H; 2–12,D; and 2–13). The presence and severity of obstructive lesions of the outflow tract, pulmonary valve, and pulmonary arteries can be assessed. Congenital shunt lesions between the aorta and pulmonary arteries can be evaluated by using color flow imaging.

Coronary Arteries

The proximal segments of the coronary arteries can be evaluated by using the transverse-plane view just above the aortic valve and the longitudinal-plane basal short-axis view of the aorta at the level of the valve (see Figs 2–6,F, 2–11, and 2–17).

Coronary Sinus

This structure is best visualized by using the transverse-plane right ventricular inflow tract view from the midesophageal position (see Fig 2–6,E).

Left Ventricle

Left ventricular wall motion can be better assessed by using the transverse-plane transgastric short-axis view at the level of the papillary muscles and the longitudinal-plane transgastric and midesophageal two-chamber views. This combinedapproach provides better assessment and localization of myocardial ischemia to different segments of the left ventricle (Fig 2–27).

SUMMARY

This chapter presents standard transesophageal images from both the transverse and longitudinal planes and in so doing identifies landmarks and structures that can be identified from these views. The manipulation of the probe that is required to obtain these views is discussed in detail and, in combi-

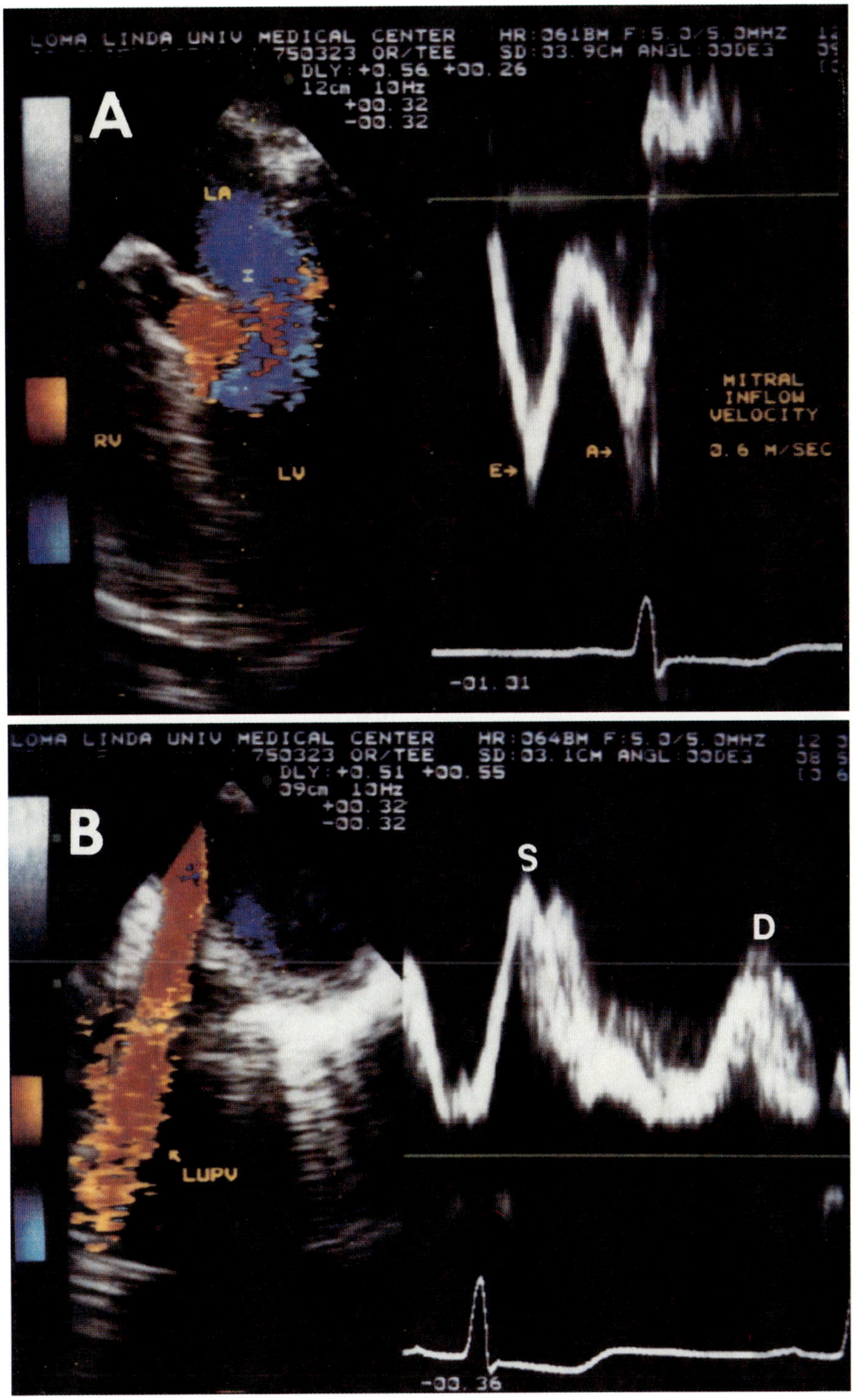

FIG 2–25.

Color flow imaging and pulsed Doppler interrogation of the mitral valve flow **(A)** and left upper pulmonary vein *(LUPV)* flow **(B).** The left half of **A** shows the transesophageal four-chamber view and the color flow imaging across the mitral valve. The right half of **A** shows the typical pulsed Doppler-derived mitral flow with a peak in early diastole *(E)* and another peak following atrial contraction *(A).* The flow is displayed below the zero line since it is away from the transducer. Left upper pulmonary venous flow in red is shown on the left half of **B.** The right half of **B** shows the positive pulsed Doppler pulmonary venous flow with a larger peak in systole *(S)* and a smaller peak in diastole *(D).* LA = left atrium; LV = left ventricle; RV = right ventricle.

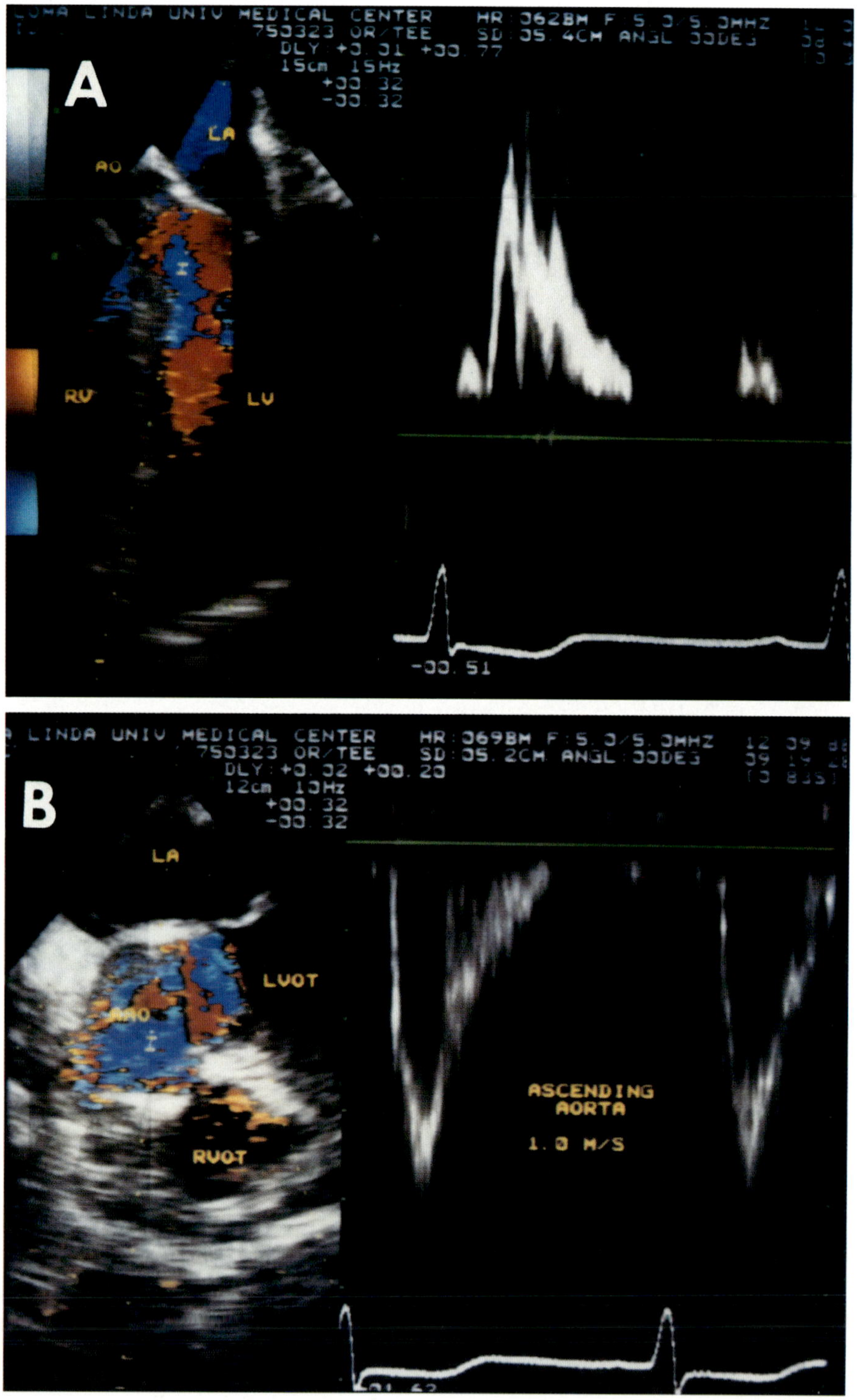

FIG 2–26.
Color flow mapping and pulsed Doppler interrogation of the left ventricular outflow tract **(A)** and ascending aorta **(B)** from the transesophageal views. The left half of **A** shows the five-chambered view from the midesophageal position with color flow imaging in the left ventricular outflow tract. The right half of **A** shows the positive pulsed Doppler flow during systole displayed above the zero line. Each calibration mark is 0.25 m/sec. The left half of **B** shows the color flow image in the ascending aorta *(AAo)* during systole. The pulsed Doppler interrogation of this flow shows a systolic velocity of 1.0 m/sec displayed below the zero line on the right half of **B.** *AO* = aorta; *LA* = left atrium; *LV* = left ventricle; *LVOT* = left ventricular outflow tract; *RV* = right ventricle; *RVOT* = right ventricular outflow tract.

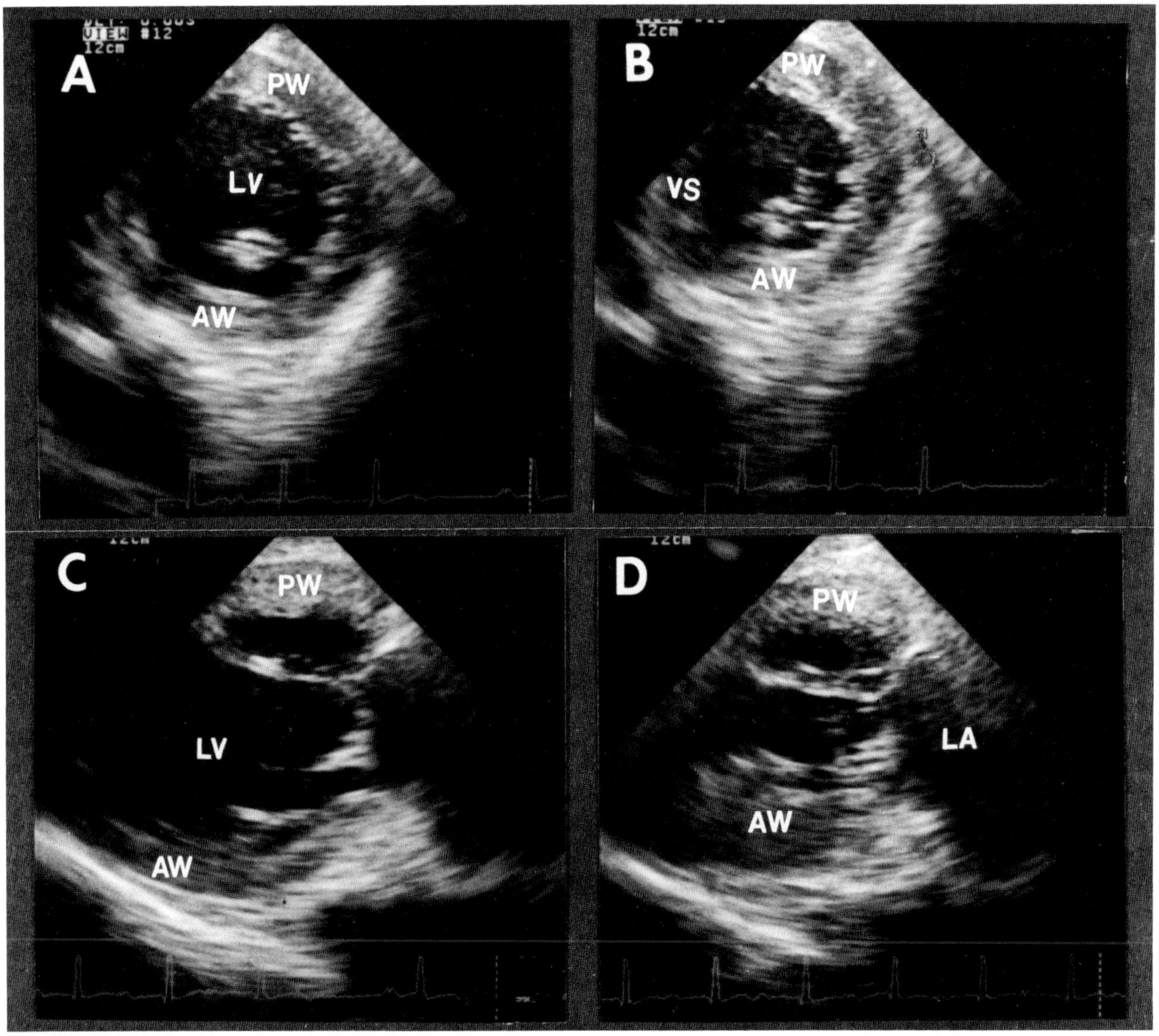

FIG 2–27.
Transgastric transverse short-axis view of the left ventricle *(LV)* at the level of the papillary muscles (diastolic frame **[A]** and systolic frame **[B]**) and gastric longitudinal two-chamber view (diastolic frame **[C]** and systolic frame **[D]**) from a patient with acute posterior wall *(PW)* myocardial infarction. Systolic frames show good excursion and marked thickening of the anterior wall *(AW)* but no motion or thickening of the PW. *LA* = left atrium; *VS* = ventricular septum. (From Bansal RC, et al: *J Am Soc Echocardiogr* 1990; 3:348–366. Used by permission.)

nation with the images shown, should provide a systematic approach to obtaining biplane TEE images.

Acknowledgment

I express my gratitude to Louise Ceccarelli and Bob Knabenbauer for the artwork, to Jerry Daly and other members of the Media Services for assistance with photography, and to Brenda Mayne for typing and preparation of the manuscript.

REFERENCES

1. Frazin L, Talano JV, Stephanides L, et al: Esophageal echocardiography. *Circulation* 1976; 54:102–108.
2. Hanrath P, Kremer P, Langenstein BA, et al: Transösophageale Echokardiographie: ein neues Verfahren zur dynamischen Ventrikelfunktions-analyse. *Dtsch Med Wochenschr* 1981; 106:523–525.
3. Schlüter M, Langenstein BA, Poister J, et al: Transesophageal cross-sectional echocardiography with a phased array transducer system: Technique and initial clinical results. *Br Heart J* 1982; 48:67–72.
4. Schlüter M, Hinrichs A, Thier W, et al: Transesoph-

ageal two-dimensional echocardiography: Comparison of ultrasonic and anatomic sections. *Am J Cardiol* 1984; 53:1173–1178.

5. Omoto R, Kyo S, Matsumura M, et al: Biplane color transesophageal Doppler echocardiography (color TEE): Its advantages and limitations. *Int J Card Imaging* 1989; 4:57–58.
6. Seward JB, Khandheria BK, Oh JK, et al: Transesophageal echocardiography: Technique, anatomic correlations, implementation and clinical applications. *Mayo Clin Proc* 1988; 63:649–680.
7. Seward JB, Khandheria BK, Edwards WD, et al: Biplanar transesophageal echocardiography: Anatomic correlations, image orientation, and clinical applications. *Mayo Clin Proc* 1990; 65:1193–1213.
8. Bansal RC, Shakudo M, Shah PM: Biplane transesophageal echocardiography: Technique, image orientation, and preliminary experience in 131 patients. *J Am Soc Echocardiogr* 1990; 3:348–366.
9. Stümper O, Fraser AG, Ho SY, et al: Transesophageal echocardiography in the longitudinal axis: Correlation between anatomy and images and its clinical implications. *Br Heart J* 1990; 64:282–288.
10. Cohen, GI, Chan KL, Walley VM: Anatomic correlations of the long-axis views in biplane transesophageal echocardiography. *Am J Cardiol* 1990; 66:1007–1010.
11. Nanda NC, Pinheiro L, Sanyal RS, et al: Transesophageal biplane echocardiographic imaging: Technique, planes, and clinical usefulness. *Echocardiography* 1990; 7:771–778.
12. Cohen GI, Chan KL: Biplane transesophageal echocardiography: Clinical applications of the long-axis plane. *J Am Soc Echocardiogr* 1991; 4:155–163.

Chapter 3

Problems and Pitfalls

Daniel G. Blanchard, M.D.

Howard C. Dittrich, M.D.

In the past several years, the use of transesophageal echocardiography (TEE) has increased dramatically. When compared with transthoracic echocardiography, the transesophageal technique has provided superior images and resolution of most cardiac structures, but this enhanced detail, along with the multiple and sometimes confusing transesophageal imaging planes, has caused various uncertainties in TEE interpretation. Also, the semi-invasive nature of TEE has raised concerns over complications and patient discomfort. Finally, the use of TEE in less familiar territory (e.g., the operating room) has occasionally made routine imaging difficult and time constrained. This chapter addresses technical problems and diagnostic "pitfalls" unique to TEE.

RISKS ASSOCIATED WITH TEE

Risks to the Patient

A review of the last decade's experience indicates that TEE is, in general, a remarkably safe procedure associated with relatively few complications. Several risks are present, however, and depend on operator skill, patient selection, and underlying disease states. In conscious patients, TEE almost always causes some degree of discomfort, especially at the time of probe insertion. In several North American centers, this discomfort is treated with intravenous sedation and analgesia such as midazolam, diazepam, droperidol, and meperidine. Unfortunately, this increases the chance of respiratory difficulties and aspiration[1] and probably represents the greatest overall source of risk to the patient. In the large European series, most procedures in ambulatory subjects have been performed with local (pharyngeal) anesthesia only; with this approach, most patients have had minimal discomfort. At our institution, we prefer local anesthetic alone, if possible, and use intravenous sedation only if it is apparent after the physician's initial evaluation that sedation will be necessary or if the patient cannot tolerate passage of the TEE probe. We also limit the procedural time to 15 minutes whenever feasible to minimize discomfort and the risk of aspiration.

Although the potential for oral and esophageal damage caused by TEE certainly exists, catastrophic complications are exceedingly rare,[2] and several series[3–5] have documented low (<1%) complication rates. Probe insertion and flexion may occasionally cause high intraesophageal pressures[6] and have resulted in a Mallory-Weiss tear in one case;[7] esophageal perforation, however, has not been reported.

The risk of pharyngeal and esophageal damage during TEE has been compared with that of gastroscopy, with a perforation risk of 1 in 3,000.[8] This risk may be somewhat elevated because of the blind insertion approach in TEE and relative operator inexperience, but this increase is offset by the reluctance to use TEE when known esophageal disease is present. A preliminary report of a North American center's experience noted major complications in 0.5% of 2,070 consecutive TEE procedures and a total mortality of 0.04%.[9] In a multicenter survey of over 10,000 TEE examinations,[2] only 1 death occurred (mortality rate, 0.0098%); this resulted from fatal esophageal bleeding in a patient with lung cancer and esophageal infiltration. To avoid complications, careful probe insertion is necessary. The probe should never be forced down the esophagus, especially when the patient is unconscious or unable to react. Because probe placement is "blind," transtracheal advancement is possible, although quite rare. A recent report[10] demonstrated that transtracheal and transesophageal echocardiographic images in a dog model were unnervingly similar. The authors concluded that "the triad of resistance to probe advancement at approximately 30 cm from the incisors, unusual image orientation or quality, and patient decompensation (cyanosis or oxygen desaturation) should suggest endotracheal TEE probe placement."

If esophageal disease is suspected, a screening barium radiographic study or esophagoscopy is indicated. TEE is relatively (if not absolutely) contraindicated in cases of esophageal carcinoma, varices, fistulas, diverticula, strictures, and bleeding, as well as in patients with past mediastinal irradiation.[11] To avoid the risk of emesis and aspiration, patients should have nothing by mouth for at least 4 to 6 hours prior to probe insertion, and suction must be immediately available during the procedure.

Complications not directly related to the esophagus can also occur. Various investigators have reported hypertension, vagal reactions, respiratory distress, atrioventricular block, atrial and ventricular tachyarrhythmias, bronchospasm, hypoxia, hypotension, and angina pectoris associated with TEE.[2, 3, 11, 12] Although these occur in a small minority of cases, blood pressure and oxygen saturation must be monitored throughout the procedure. The risk of complications may be slightly higher in critically ill patients.[13] We have used intravenous sedation with careful monitoring more frequently in the intensive care unit setting, and this has resulted in improved patient acceptance and hemodynamic stability.

Endocarditis from transient probe-related bacteremia is a potentially disastrous complication, and the issue of antibiotic prophylaxis for TEE has been controversial. While the American Heart Association guidelines do recommend antibiotic prophylaxis for patients at risk during upper endoscopy with biopsy, upper endoscopy without biopsy is considered to be a very low or no-risk procedure.[14] Although a prospective study of 24 patients undergoing TEE noted positive blood cultures in 4 (17%) after the procedure,[15] no patient developed endocarditis, and only one case report to date[16] has documented a temporal relation between TEE and a case of endocarditis. In a series of 100 patients, only 2 had positive blood cultures, and both of these grew bacteria that were considered contaminants.[2] Three separate studies have reported positive postprocedure blood cultures in 1.4% to 4% of a total of 289 patients undergoing TEE.[17–19] The majority of isolates were coagulase-negative staphylococci or anaerobes, and all were considered to be contaminants. During follow-up, no patients with positive blood cultures developed signs of infection. In the largest survey of patients, no cases of endocarditis occurred.[2] Because of this, most authorities do not recommend routine antibiotic prophylaxis for low-risk patients. In high-risk individuals (for example, those with prosthetic cardiac valves or severe rheumatic valvular disease), there is no consensus, and many centers use prophylactic antibiotics in these patients.

Finally, there is a remote risk of introducing pathogens into the patient via the TEE probe, including bacteria, protozoa, and viruses. Fortunately, no cases of such transmission have been reported. To prevent this, the probe should be thoroughly cleaned and treated with an effective antiviral agent (e.g., Cidex-7, 2% glutaraldehyde solution [Surgikos, Johnson & Johnson, Arlington, Tex]) before each use. In addition, latex sheaths are available to further reduce contamination. These sheaths occasionally tear, however, and routine disinfection of the probe between cases is still necessary.

Risks to the Echocardiographic Probe

TEE probes are a major expense, and several precautions are necessary to avoid malfunction. First, a bite block should be used unless the patient is edentulous, whether he is conscious or not. Besides stopping the unsedated patient from biting the shaft of the probe, it also prevents inadvertent damage by movement of the probe back and forth across the anesthetized patient's teeth. Also, the probe's flexion knobs should be in the unlocked position during storage to prolong the lifetime of the flexion mechanism and cables. Finally, when used intraoperatively, the echocardiography machine should be turned off or the probe disconnected during periods of inactivity to prevent the probe from overheating.

DIAGNOSTIC AND IMAGING PITFALLS

Cardiac Chambers and Structure

Although TEE usually provides superior definition of the myocardium and intracardiac structures, the imaging planes are not always comparable to those used in transthoracic echocardiography. For example, the transgastric/short-axis view is usually not truly perpendicular to the long axis of the heart inasmuch as the body of the anterolateral papillary muscle and the chordal structures of the posteromedial papillary muscle are often visualized at the same time (see Fig 2–8,A). Because of anatomic variability between the stomach and heart, significant foreshortening and skewing may occur and cause inaccurate assessment of regional wall motion, particularly of the interventricular septum. In addition, if left atrial or right ventricular enlargement is present (e.g., with severe mitral stenosis), the left ventricle may be shifted away from the stomach, and a satisfactory short-axis view may be unobtainable.

This same type of problem with foreshortening can occur in the transesophageal four-chamber view. Typically, this imaging plane does not include the true apex of the heart, and retroflexion of the probe to better assess the apex can cause inadequate tissue contact and image dropout. Again, significant left atrial enlargement can make adequate views of the left ventricle and apex difficult or impossible. Biplane TEE is often helpful in this respect but still does not guarantee complete visualization, and apical defects or thrombi can frequently be missed. For these reasons, quantitative assessment of left ventricular size and volume by TEE is likely to be inaccurate. Recent preliminary data suggest, however, that left ventricular ejection fraction measurements by TEE do correlate well with values derived from transthoracic images.[20]

Right-sided cardiac structures are usually well defined by TEE, but several potential problems exist. Right ventricular function and flow characteristics are often best determined in the four-chamber view. If prosthetic valves are present in the mitral, aortic, or tricuspid positions, acoustic shadowing across the right ventricle can obscure the echo image and make meaningful interpretation impossible. In this case, views of the right ventricle from the short-axis position may aid in the assessment of function, but accurate Doppler interrogation of inflow and outflow will not be feasible.

The right atrium contains two structures that may be inaccurately diagnosed as abnormalities. A prominent eustachian valve is a common finding on transthoracic echocardiography; on transesophageal views, this may appear as a bright right atrial density and can be misdiagnosed as a mass. However, slow movement of the probe back and forth will demonstrate that the "mass" is actually a ridge of tissue that slopes into the base of the right atrium. Similarly, as the TEE probe is positioned to view the high right atrium, another bright and sometimes round density appears (Fig 3–1,A). This represents the tissue reflection at the junction of the right atrium and superior vena cava, and careful probe withdrawal will confirm that the density joins with and is a part of the proximal portion of the superior vena cava (Fig 3–1,B).

There are also several diagnostic "pitfalls" in the area of the left atrium. One of the most useful applications of TEE is detailed imaging of the left atrial appendage, but familiarity with its anatomy is essential. In the normal state, small ridges of pectinate muscle are visible in the appendage. These ridges are spaced regularly along the atrial wall, are noncalcified and of consistent echo density, and move concordantly with the appendage wall (see Fig 2–6,G and 2–10,C). In addition, the muscular ridges are generally small and never completely fill the appendage in its widest diameter. In contrast, appendage clots may have irregular or rounded borders, are occasionally calcified and of variable echo density, and when mobile, move discordantly with the atrial wall (see Fig 4–9). Nonmobile and laminar thrombi will obscure the regular pattern of pectinate ridges and may completely fill the lumen of the appendage.

The appendage must be distinguished from the left upper pulmonary vein, which lies just posterior and lateral to the left atrium. This is usually not difficult because the pulmonary vein has no pectinate ridges and demonstrates characteristic biphasic forward flow on pulsed-wave Doppler interrogation. Biplane TEE is very helpful in this area since the appendage and left upper pulmonary vein are generally well imaged in the longitudinal plane (see Fig 2–12,E).

When the left atrium is enlarged, it is usually not difficult to identify the appendage. If the left atrium is normal or only mildly enlarged, optimal anatomic imaging planes are essential to prevent artifacts. In the transverse TEE plane, the appendage is generally best imaged at the level of the coronary arteries. At this level, the proximal portion of the right ventricular outflow tract (but not the pulmonic valve) should be visible (Fig 3–2,A). If the probe is pulled back beyond this point and if fluid is present in the oblique sinus and around the appendage, an image of a false appendage may appear. The most superior portion, or "roof," of the true appendage may then simulate a left atrial mass or thrombus (Fig 3–2,B).

Another "pseudomass" is sometimes seen in the left atrium at the junction of the left upper pulmonary vein. The tissue fold between the atrial wall and the anterior portion of the pulmonary vein occasionally creates the impression of a rounded or oval density because of its increased echo reflectance (Fig 3–3,A). This finding (which we have called the warfarin ridge for the many times this drug was mistakenly given because of the structure) is artifactual and does not represent a mass or thrombus. Depending

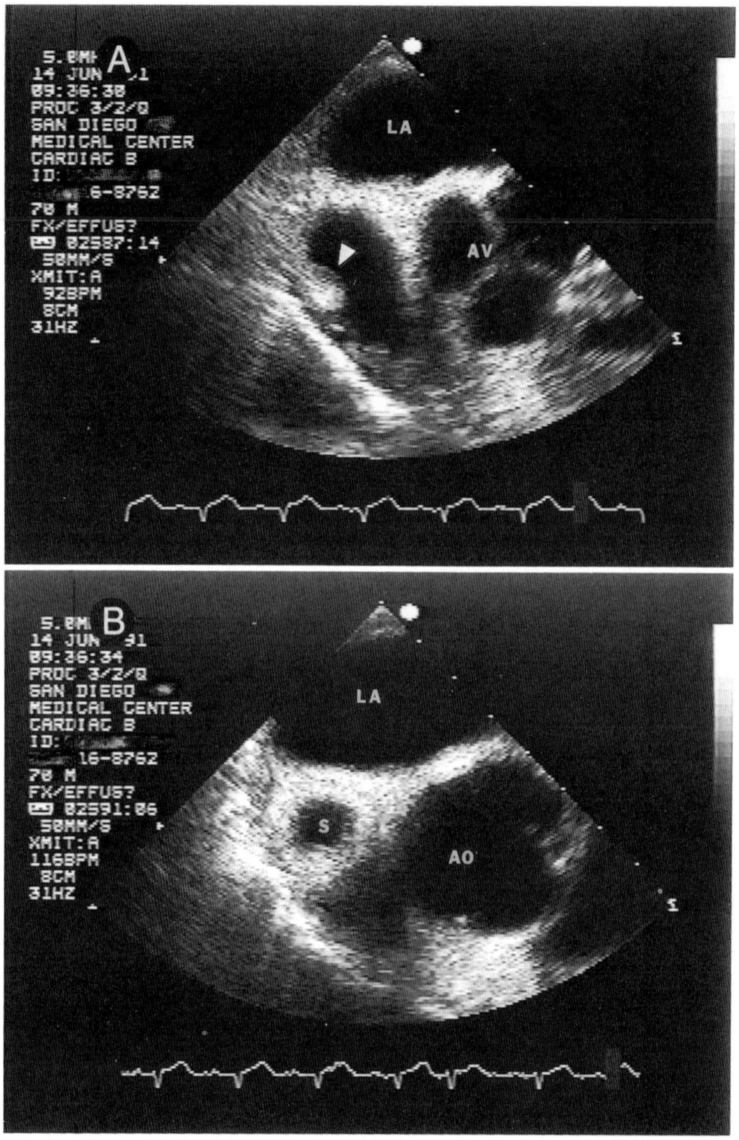

FIG 3–1.
A, "pseudomass" *(arrowhead)* at the lateral border of the right atrium. *LA* = left atrium; *AV* = aortic valve. **B,** slight withdrawal of the TEE probe demonstrates continuity of the "pseudomass" with the wall of the superior vena cava *(S)*. *AO* = aorta.

on the obliquity of the imaging plane, the structure may appear quite large (Fig 3–3,B).

An interesting finding in the left atrium (and occasionally left ventricle) that has attracted recent attention is the presence of spontaneous echo contrast or "smoke." This phenomenon may be due to increased red blood cell or platelet aggregation in areas of relative stasis (see Fig 4–9). One report has described resolution of this finding in a patient after taking a platelet disaggregatory agent (trifluoperazine),[21] but a subsequent study failed to confirm this finding.[22]

Left atrial spontaneous contrast has been associated with an increased thromboembolic risk in patients with mitral valve disease and is detected much more frequently with TEE than with transthoracic echocardiography.[23] Unfortunately, visualization of spontaneous contrast is somewhat operator dependent, and improper gain settings can lead to both false-positive and false-negative results. The examination should be performed in a darkened room (because improper lighting can make spontaneous contrast difficult to detect), with the gain and transmission set to create high contrast between the atrial wall and chamber. If gain settings are too low, spontaneous contrast will be missed; if too high, spurious

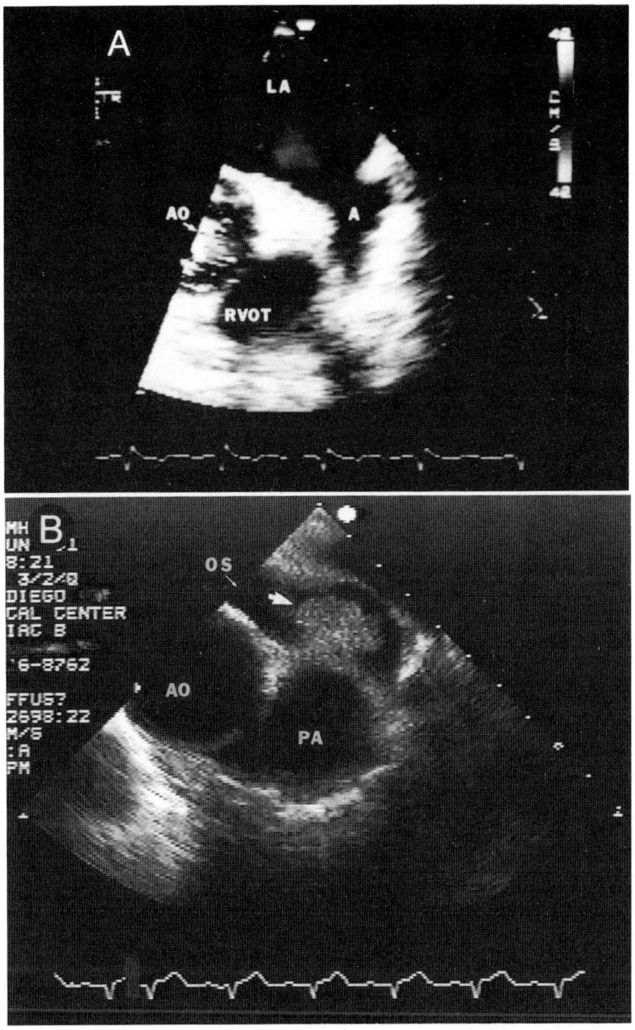

FIG 3–2.
A, Optimal transverse imaging plane for identification of the left atrial appendage. *LA* = left atrium; *A* = left atrial appendage; *AO* = aorta; *RVOT* = right ventricular outflow tract. **B,** incorrect position for imaging the left atrial appendage. The TEE probe has been withdrawn to the plane of the aorta *(AO)* and pulmonary artery *(PA).* Fluid is present in the oblique sinus *(OS),* which mimics the appearance of the left atrial appendage. The roof of the true left atrium *(large arrow)* may be mistaken for an appendage thrombus or mass.

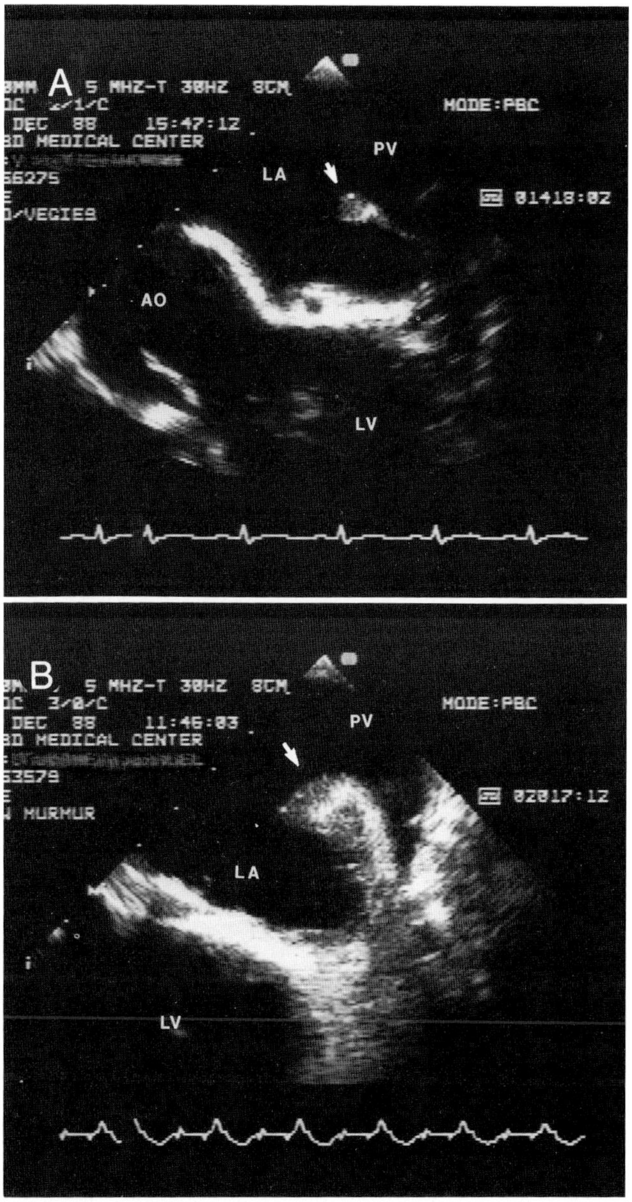

FIG 3–3.
A, the "warfarin ridge" *(arrow)* may simulate a mass at the junction of the left upper pulmonary vein *(PV)* and the left atrium *(LA). AO* = aorta; *LV* = left ventricle. **B,** another example of the warfarin ridge *(arrow),* which appears large in size due to an oblique imaging plane.

contrast may appear. It is sometimes useful to compare the right atrium and pulmonary veins with the left atrium if spontaneous contrast is suspected. It is distinctly unusual to see true spontaneous contrast in all these chambers. Also, spontaneous contrast is rarely present in a completely normal left atrium, and in these situations, the contrast may be artifactual. Finally, true spontaneous contrast is always in motion and appears to "swirl" in the left atrium and appendage. Suspected contrast that does not move is usually spurious.

Cardiac Valves

TEE is well suited to investigate valvular function and pathology, but several potential problems exist. While the mitral valve is usually easy to visualize in its entirety, the tricuspid valve may be more difficult to assess, especially if a single-plane probe is used. All three leaflets of the tricuspid valve are not visible in the four-chamber single-plane view and must be evaluated either in the transgastric short-axis imaging plane or with biplane views; in this manner all tricuspid leaflets can be inspected together in the longitudinal plane through the tricuspid anulus (see Fig 2–17).

The pulmonic valve is poorly visualized by single-plane TEE and may be impossible to image altogether. Biplane views through the right and left ventricular outflow tracts are essential for assessing this valve as well as the main pulmonary artery.

A notable pitfall in TEE interpretation occurs in the area of the aortic valve. Since this valve is imaged obliquely in single-plane views, it is extremely difficult to image all three leaflets equally at the same time. At the level of the right and noncoronary cusps, the left coronary cusp may appear as a mass or vegetation: this appearance can occasionally be quite convincing (Fig 3–4). However, careful motion of the probe back and forth will demonstrate continuity of this "mass" with the left coronary leaflet.

Magnified views of the aortic valve may occasionally demonstrate very small echodensities on the leaflets. In the appropriate clinical setting, these may represent vegetations, especially if associated valvular pathology such as aortic insufficiency is present. These small densities may also be Lambdl's excrescences, which are normal variants and generally not a cause for concern. In general, if these densities are seen on an otherwise normal valve and are present predominantly on the midportions of the aortic cusps, they are probably a normal variant.

The mitral valve is generally well seen with TEE and abnormalities easily identified. If viewed obliquely, however, an appearance similar to vegetation or diffuse thickening can be produced (Fig 3–5,A and B).

TEE often provides excellent delineation of val-

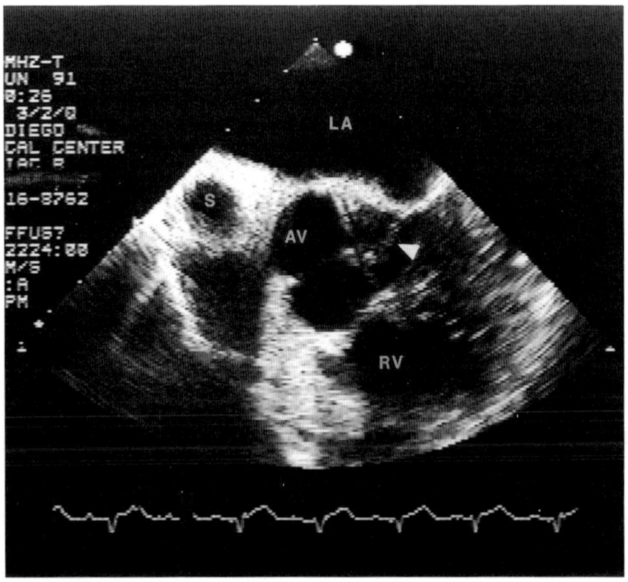

FIG 3–4.
"Pseudomass" *(arrowhead)* on the aortic valve *(AV)*, which is produced by an oblique imaging plane through the left coronary cusp. *RV* = right ventricular outflow tract; *S* = superior vena cava; *LA* = left atrium.

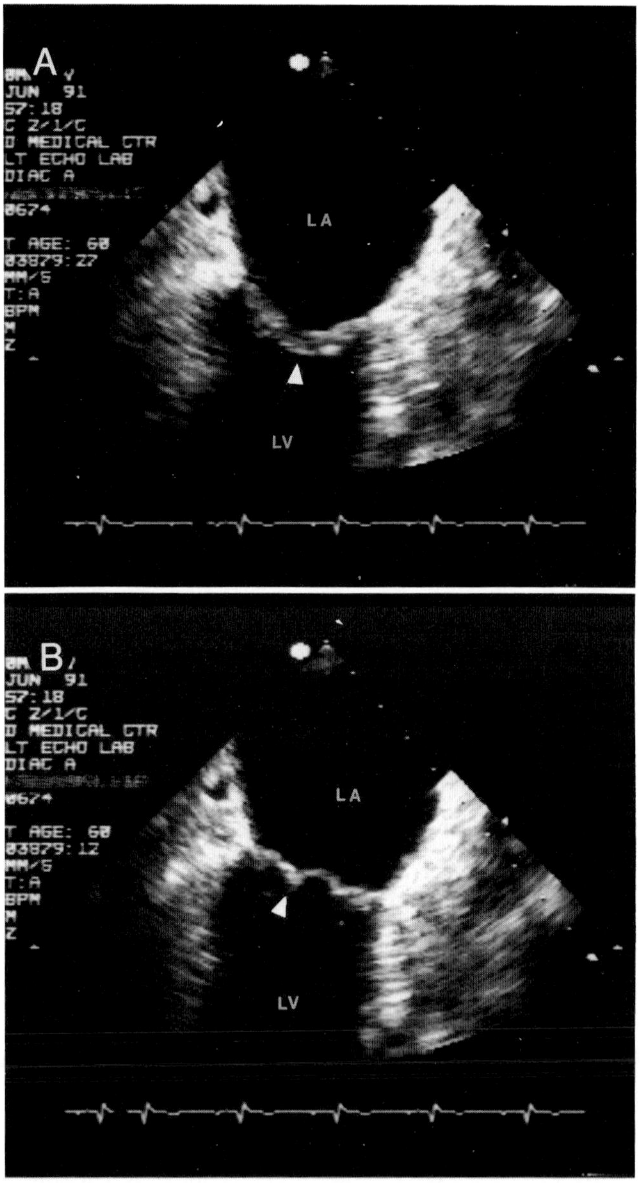

FIG 3–5.
A, oblique (longitudinal) imaging plane through the mitral valve that simulates marked thickening of the mitral leaflets *(arrowhead)*. *LA* = left atrium; *LV* = left ventricle. **B,** less oblique view of the mitral valve in the same patient demonstrates normal mitral leaflets *(arrowhead)*.

vular pathology, but assessment of valvular stenosis and insufficiency is sometimes problematic. For example, many TEE probes currently in use do not have continuous-wave Doppler capability, which is essential for determining the severity of both aortic and mitral stenosis by echocardiography. When a probe with continuous-wave Doppler is used, attention to the angle of incidence is important because the severity of stenosis may be significantly underestimated if the Doppler interrogation beam is not parallel to the jet of blood through the stenotic valve.

TEE is extremely sensitive in detecting valvular regurgitation and, in some cases, may be excessively so. In a group of 20 healthy volunteers, Wittlich and Siemer[24] detected mitral and tricuspid regurgitation by TEE in *all* subjects. The regurgitation was typically seen in early systole as a jet of relatively small area associated with valve closure. A small jet of aortic insufficiency was also noted in 75% of the subjects. This study emphasizes the danger of "overreading" TEE images: trivial valvular insufficiency in early systole is often detected by TEE and should not be interpreted as an abnormal finding.

TEE can be helpful in assessing the severity of valvular regurgitation, especially when transthoracic images are suboptimal or inconclusive. Yoshida et al.[25] found that the maximum mitral regurgitant jet area as detected by biplane TEE correlated well with angiographic criteria for severity of mitral insufficiency. This experience, however, may not be applicable to single-plane TEE because regurgitant jets are sometimes missed or incompletely characterized. In another recent study, Smith and colleagues noted a consistent overestimation of valvular insufficiency by TEE when compared with transthoracic echocardiography.[26] Thus, while TEE is a more sensitive test for valvular insufficiency than standard echocardiography, accurate interpretation of severity is often elusive and requires an assessment of several factors, as discussed in Chapter 5.

The imaging of prosthetic cardiac valves presents many problems (this subject is also discussed in more detail in Chapter 5). TEE is ideal for assessing the atrial aspect of mitral prostheses, but the high reflectance and acoustic shadowing of mechanical valves prevent optimal imaging of the ventricular side, and thrombi and vegetations in this area may be undetected. This is also true of aortic prostheses, and accurate gauging of prosthetic aortic regurgitation is often difficult since the left ventricular outflow tract may be obscured by the mechanical valve.[27] Occasionally, the ventricular aspects of mitral and aortic prostheses can be imaged if the TEE probe can be advanced past the transgastric short-axis position and flexed to obtain a foreshortened four- or five-chamber view. Unfortunately, this is not possible in all cases and may cause discomfort to some patients. The longitudinal plane may sometimes add important information (see Fig 2–14,B).

The Aorta

TEE has proved to be a superb diagnostic tool in dissection, aneurysm, and other abnormalities of the aorta.[28, 29] This application is discussed more extensively in Chapter 7. With a reported sensitivity higher than 90% for diagnosing aortic dissection, TEE is now the diagnostic procedure of choice in many centers. When compared with computerized tomography, TEE has the advantage of not requiring contrast injection; when compared with magnetic resonance scanning, TEE can be performed quickly and in nearly any setting. In addition, TEE can localize an intimal tear and gauge the size of a false lumen. Problems do exist, however. With single-plane probes, one of the most significant limitations is adequate imaging of the aortic arch. While the ascending and descending portions of the aorta are well seen, the arch is often a "blind spot." Fortunately, biplane TEE has helped in this area, and the arch can usually be visualized in the longitudinal plane. Pathology in the arch can still be hidden, however, and additional tests may be necessary to completely define this portion of the aorta.

When a dissection is present, it is important to differentiate the true from the false lumen. If an intimal tear and a color Doppler jet from the true lumen into the false lumen are imaged, there is little question which lumen is which, but these Doppler jets are not always visualized. In general, the false lumen is larger than the true one, although exceptions certainly exist. Also, the false lumen has nonhomogeneous, often aliased color flow patterns and may exhibit areas of spontaneous contrast similar to that seen in the enlarged left atrium with associated mitral valve disease. Flow in the true lumen is usually homogeneous, with nonaliased color patterns during systole. Finally, the false lumen may contain a thrombus, which is rarely seen in the true lumen.

In patients with significant atherosclerotic disease, the aortic wall may be thickened and irregular, and this can be mistaken for dissection with thrombosis by TEE. Several echocardiographic signs will help make the distinction between these two possibilities easier. First, no intimal tears or color jets are present in the aortic wall with atherosclerosis alone.

If the diagnosis is in question, a thorough search for these findings is essential. Second, a thrombus in the false lumen of a dissection is usually of homogeneous echodensity, while a thickened, atherosclerotic aortic wall is of variable density and reflectance. Finally, calcification is almost never present in an acute thrombus. If bright specks of calcification are noted within the aortic wall, atherosclerosis is much more likely than dissection.

Intraoperative TEE

Several problems are encountered during intraoperative transesophageal studies. Excessive lighting is common and can lead to both overdiagnosis and underdiagnosis of abnormalities, including valvular thickening, vegetations, and spontaneous contrast (small bubbles in the right heart are common during rapid intravenous infusions, and left atrial and ventricular bubbles are typically seen during and immediately after open heart surgery; these are generally of little importance and should not be misdiagnosed as "smoke"). Occasionally, electrocardiographic lead placement is improper (or absent), and this makes color Doppler and M-mode images difficult to interpret. Also, the positioning of the patient and the TEE operator is often different from that in the echocardiography laboratory, and manipulation of the probe may be more difficult than usual. Bovie cautery creates a characteristic disturbance of the echo image (Fig 3–6), which makes adequate visualization nearly impossible.

If the TEE probe is used during lengthy surgical cases, it may overheat. Some instruments may then switch to the "auto-cool" mode, and real-time images will be lost until the probe recovers. As stated above, this situation can be avoided by turning off the probe when images are not being monitored or when cautery is being performed (newer ultrasound systems may also employ a manual override option). During certain operations, however, the patient may be hyperthermic or require prolonged TEE imaging. At our institution, we have prevented "auto-cooling" by instilling chilled saline solution into the esophagus of a febrile patient via a nasogastric tube.[30]

Often, the cardiologist must compete for space with the anesthesiology staff, thus making the examination cramped and uncomfortable. Other frequent problems are time constraints and inopportune scheduling. Many TEE studies need to be performed quickly, especially if surgery is urgent. To facilitate rapid TEE evaluation in urgent cases (when a

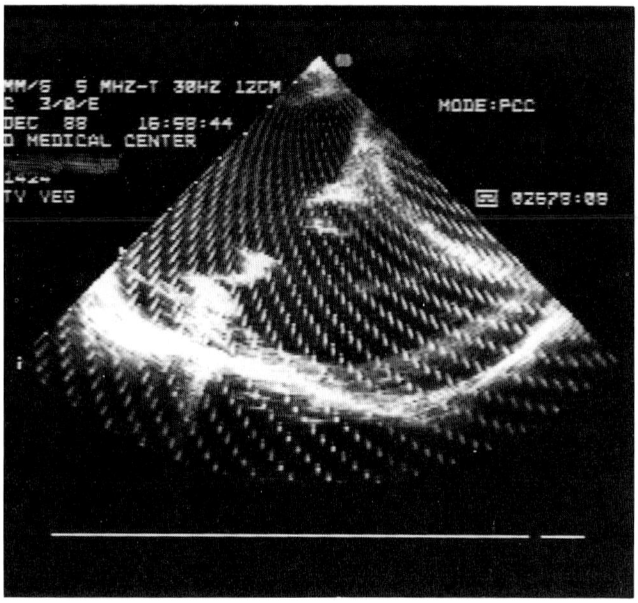

FIG 3–6.
Bovie artifact obscuring the TEE image.

cardiologist may not be available to directly assess the patient during surgery), we have installed audio and video links from the operating room to the echocardiography laboratory.

To keep these problems to a minimum, continuing operator practice and experience is essential. We recommend that all individuals training in TEE spend a good deal of time in the operating room, both to familiarize themselves with the environment and its unique problems as well as to practice probe manipulation and imaging in the unconscious patient.

SUMMARY

The majority of problems encountered during TEE are related to operator inexperience. With time, the operator's familiarity with both probe manipulation and diagnostic pitfalls will grow, and fewer errors will occur. This chapter discusses both problems and the diagnostic "traps" unique to transesophageal imaging. These problems and pitfalls are relatively few and can be overcome by continued practice, careful imaging, and attention to detail.

REFERENCES

1. Miller G: Komplikationen bei der Endoskopie des oberen Gastrintestinaltraktes. *Leber Magen Darm* 1987; 5:299–304.

2. Daniel WG, Erbel R, Kasper W, et al: Safety of transesophageal echocardiography: A multicenter survey of 10,419 examinations. *Circulation* 1991; 83:817–821.
3. Geibel A, Kasper W, Behroz A, et al: Risk of transesophageal echocardiography in awake patients with cardiac diseases. *Am J Cardiol* 1988; 62:337–339.
4. Schlüter M, Hinrichs A, Thier W, et al: Transesophageal two dimensional echocardiography: Comparison of ultrasonic and anatomic sections. *Am J Cardiol* 1984; 53:1173–1178.
5. Erbel R, Boerner N, Steller D, et al: Detection of aortic dissection by transesophageal echocardiography. *Br Heart J* 1987; 58:45–51.
6. Urbanowicz JH, Kernoff RS, Oppenheim G, et al: Transesophageal echocardiography and its potential for esophageal damage. *Anesthesiology* 1990; 72:40–43.
7. Dewhirst W, Stragand JJ, Fleming BM: Mallory-Weiss tear complicating intraoperative transesophageal echocardiography in a patient undergoing aortic valve replacement. *Anesthesiology* 1990; 73:777–778.
8. Silvis SE, Nebel O, Rogers G, et al: Endoscopic complications: Results of the 1974 American Society for Gastrointestinal Endoscopy Survey. *JAMA* 1976; 235:928–930.
9. Khanderia BK, Seward JB, Bailey K, et al: Safety of transesophageal echocardiography: Experience with 2070 consecutive patients (abstract). *J Am Coll Cardiol* 1991; 17:20.
10. Fagan LF, Weiss R, Castello R, et al: Transtracheal placement and imaging with a transesophageal echocardiographic probe. *Am J Cardiol* 1991; 67:909–910.
11. Kuecherer HF, Lee E, Schiller NB: Role of transesophageal echocardiography in diagnosis and management of cardiovascular disease. *Cardiol Clin* 1990; 8:377–388.
12. Lee E, Schiller NB: Transesophageal echocardiography in clinical cardiology, in Marcus ML, Schelbert HR, Skorton DJ, et al (eds): *Cardiac Imaging*. Philadelphia, WB Saunders, 1991.
13. Pearson AC, Castello R, Labovitz AJ: Safety and utility of transesophageal echocardiography in the critically ill patient. *Am Heart J* 1990; 119:1083–1089.
14. Dajani AS, Bisno A, Chung K: Prevention of bacterial endocarditis: Recommendations by the American Heart Association. *JAMA* 1990; 264:2919–2922.
15. Gorge G, Erbel R, Henrichs KJ, et al: Positive blood cultures during transesophageal echocardiography. *Am J Cardiol* 1990; 65:1404–1405.
16. Foster E, Kusumoro FM, Sobol SM, Schiller N: Streptococcal endocarditis temporally related to transesophageal echocardiography. *J Am Soc Echocardiogr* 1990; 3:424–427.
17. Steckelberg JM, et al: Prospective evaluation of the risk of bacteremia associated with transesophageal echocardiography. *Circulation* 1991; 84:177–180.
18. Voller H, Schroder KM, Gast D, et al: Does the incidence of positive blood cultures during transesophageal echocardiography necessitate antibiotic prophylaxis? *Circulation* 1990; 82(suppl 3):244.
19. Chan KL, Cheung P, Wong S, et al: Transesophageal echocardiography (TEE) and bacteremia. *Circulation* 1990; 82(suppl 3):244.
20. Lenhoff SJ, MacPhail B, Smith M, et al: Value and limitations of biplane transesophageal echo in the estimation of left ventricular volumes and ejection fraction (abstract). *J Am Coll Cardiol* 1991; 17:35.
21. Mahony C, Sublett KL, Harrison MR: Resolution of spontaneous contrast with platelet disaggregatory therapy (trifluoperizine). *Am J Cardiol* 1989; 63:1009–1010.
22. Hoffmann R, Lambertz H, Kreis A, et al: Failure of trifluoperizine to resolve spontaneous echo contrast evaluated by transesophageal echocardiography. *Am J Cardiol* 1990; 66:648–649.
23. Daniel WG, Nellessen U, Schroder E, et al: Left atrial spontaneous echocontrast in mitral valve disease: An indicator for an increased thromboembolic risk. *J Am Coll Cardiol* 1988; 11:1204–1211.
24. Wittlich N, Siemer J: Transesophageal color flow mapping in normal subjects (abstract). *Circulation* 1988; 78(suppl 2):297.
25. Yoshida K, Yoshikawa J, Yamaura Y, et al: Assessment of mitral regurgitation by biplane transesophageal color flow mapping. *Circulation* 1990; 82:1121–1126.
26. Smith MD, Harrison MR, Pinton R, et al: Regurgitant jet size by transesophageal compared with transthoracic Doppler color flow imaging. *Circulation* 1991; 83:79–86.
27. Alam M, Serwin J, Rosman H, et al: Transesophageal echocardiographic features of normal and dysfunctioning bioprosthetic valves. *Am Heart J* 1991; 121:1149–1155.
28. Erbel R, Engberding R, Daniel WG, et al: Echocardiography in diagnosis of aortic dissection. *Lancet* 1989; 1:457–461.
29. Mohr-Kahaly S, Erbel R, Rennollet H, et al: Ambulatory follow-up of aortic dissection by transesophageal two-dimensional and color-coded Doppler echocardiography. *Circulation* 1989; 80:24–33.
30. Hunter JJ, Johnson KR, Karagianes TG, et al: Detection of massive pulmonary embolus-in-transit by transesophageal echocardiography: A case report and review of the literature. *Chest* 1991; 100:1210–1214.

PART II

Clinical Applications

Chapter 4

Evaluation of Cardiac Sources of Emboli

Alan Camp, M.D.

Arthur J. Labovitz, M.D.

Cerebrovascular disease is the third leading cause of death in the United States. It accounted for 124,964 fatalities and 660,750 hospitalizations in 1986, the most recent year for which epidemiologic data are available.[1] In addition, cerebrovascular disease is the cause of chronic disability affecting millions of Americans of all ages. Pooled data show that approximately 20% of cerebral ischemic episodes are due to cardiogenic emboli: in the Stroke Data Bank report, 19% of the cerebral infarctions were attributed to cardiac embolic sources, and 45% had an unknown cause.[2] In young patients, some evidence suggests that embolism may be responsible for an even greater proportion of cerebral infarctions.[2] Cardiac embolic sources accounted for approximately one in six ischemic strokes in a recent report of pooled data from the Cerebral Embolism Task Force.[3]

The role of transthoracic (TTE) and transesophageal echocardiography (TEE) in evaluating patients with cerebral ischemic events for cardiac structural abnormalities responsible for embolization has been assessed in numerous studies. In view of the high percentage of cerebral ischemic events due to emboli, the results with TTE have been disappointing. In one study only 1 patient from a group of 65 had a potential etiologic abnormality diagnosed by TTE that was not diagnosed by the history, physical examination, or electrocardiography.[4] TEE, however, has proved to be much more helpful in the evaluation of patients with suspected cardiac embolism. In a recent study performed in our laboratory,[5] 57% of patients with cerebral ischemic events had potential etiologic abnormalities diagnosed by TEE as compared with 15% by TTE.

In light of these encouraging findings and similar results from other investigators, examination of patients with unexplained cerebral ischemia or embolic events has become the most common indication for TEE and has accounted for between 15% and 40% of all TEE procedures performed (Fig 4–1). Advantages of TEE for evaluating patients with suspected cardiac embolic sources as compared with TTE include improved overall image quality and the ability to image regions not seen well by TTE including the left atrial appendage, atrial septum, aortic arch, and the proximal aspect of the ascending aorta. This chapter discusses the special techniques involved in the TEE examination of patients with suspected cardiac embolic sources, the individual cardiac abnormalities that can be identified by TEE and their significance, and the TEE evaluation of intracardiac devices that may be responsible for arterial embolization.

The cardiac conditions that are definitely or potentially associated with cardiogenic emboli are

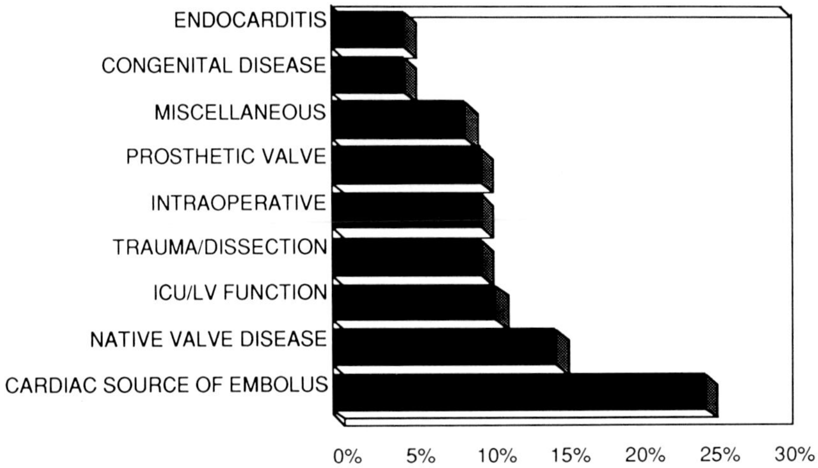

FIG 4–1.
Indications for performance of TEE examinations at St. Louis University Medical Center through April 1991.

listed in Table 4–1. The exact percentages of cardiac emboli due to each listed cause are not known. Atrial fibrillation and left ventricular thrombi are clearly associated with numerous cardiogenic emboli. The clinical significance and prognostic value of some of the other abnormalities listed in Table 4–1 that are diagnosed by TEE, however, remain uncertain. Also, many patients have cerebrovascular disease in addition to one or more cardiac findings, and this complicates the determination of a causative abnormality. Overall, TEE provides an excellent means for either initial diagnosis or confirmation of the diagnosis of the structural abnormalities listed.

PROCEDURAL CONSIDERATIONS IN THE EVALUATION OF CARDIOGENIC EMBOLI

The recommended procedures for general TEE evaluation are described in Chapter 1. There are some additional procedures and concerns that apply specifically to patients with recent cerebral ischemic events.

Blood Pressure Control

In patients with recent cerebral ischemia, careful monitoring of blood pressure before, during, and following the procedure is important. In our laboratory, we use an automatic blood pressure cuff that is programmed to take and display the blood pressure every minute. This alerts the operator to hypertension associated with patient discomfort or apprehension or to hypotension that may be associated with the use of intravenous medications. Intravenous access is maintained throughout the procedure for rapid administration of intravenous fluids or medications.

Local Anesthesia

The administration of effective local anesthesia is of particular importance in patients with cerebral ischemia. Excessive gagging or retching associated with the introduction of the TEE probe can cause hypertension and potentially exacerbate cerebral ischemia. We use multiple applications of an aerosol anesthetic agent to ensure adequate anesthesia. Alternatively, gargling or swallowing viscous lidocaine solution can be effective for patients who are able to swallow without risk of aspiration.

Sedation

In our laboratory, most patients receive some type of sedation with intravenous medications prior to the TEE procedure. In patients with recent cerebral ischemia, particularly those with changing or evolving deficits, the use of small amounts of short-acting sedatives is recommended. Because the overall sedative effect of short-acting benzodiazepines or narcotics can be difficult to predict, it is recommended that small doses be used initially, for example, 0.5 mg of intravenous midazolam. By using small incremental dosages for intravenous sedation, patient discomfort can be minimized, and uncertainty about new or evolving neurologic deficits can be avoided.

TABLE 4–1.
Conditions Associated With Cardiogenic Emboli

- Rhythm disturbances
  - Atrial fibrillation
  - Sick sinus syndrome
- Structural abnormalities
  - Left ventricular wall motion abnormalities with possible left ventricular thrombus
    - Ischemic causes
      - Acute myocardial infarction
      - Akinetic infarcted segments
      - Aneurysms
      - Pseudoaneurysms
    - Nonischemic cardiomyopathies
      - Amyloid
      - Idiopathic
      - Peripartum
      - Myocardial contusion
      - Viral
      - Alcohol
      - Rheumatic
      - Doxorubicin induced
      - Neuromuscular disorders
      - Chagas' disease
  - Atrial abnormalities
    - Atrial septal aneurysm
    - Atrial thrombus
    - Myxoma
  - Valvular abnormalities
    - Mitral valve prolapse
    - Mitral stenosis
    - Mitral annular calcification
    - Infective or noninfective endocarditis
    - Inflammatory valvulitis
    - Calcific aortic stenosis
  - Pathways for paradoxical emboli
    - Atrial septal defect
    - Patent foramen ovale
    - Ventricular septal defect
    - Anomalous systemic venous return
    - Pulmonary arteriovenous fistulas
  - Other causes of cardiac thrombi or masses
    - Primary or metastatic cardiac tumors
    - Myeloproliferative disorders
    - Systemic lupus
    - Hypercoagulable state
  - Mechanical devices within the heart
    - Prosthetic valves
    - Pacemaker leads
    - Ventricular assist devices
  - Other
    - Atherosclerotic aortic debris
    - Spontaneous contrast

Other Considerations

Many of the patients being evaluated for potential cardiac sources of emboli have persistent neurologic deficits at the time of TEE examination. Such deficits require the use of a feeding tube or nasogastric tube for routine patient care. Unfortunately, the presence of a feeding tube or nasogastric tube can complicate the performance of the TEE procedure. In general, it has been our practice to remove the feeding or nasogastric tube if images are suboptimal to ensure adequate contact with the esophageal wall. Due to the absence of a gag reflex in many patients and altered mental status, the clinician must be careful to avoid inadvertent and unrecognized endotracheal intubation.[6] The use of a pulse oximeter may be helpful if the level of consciousness is markedly impaired. In addition, the use of local anesthesia and intravenous sedation may increase the chances of aspiration if care is not taken.

Examination Technique

It is important to image the entire left atrial chamber including the left atrial appendage and interatrial septum in multiple planes. The right atrium and right atrial appendage should also be evaluated in multiple planes. We recommend the routine administration of a small amount of agitated saline contrast intravenously to detect the presence of intracardiac shunting. The use of central venous access, if available, or antecubital venous access provides the best routes for the administration of agitated saline contrast. The contrast is prepared by mixing 5 to 10 cc of saline through a three-way stopcock with two 10-cc syringes. The use of small veins in the hand or wrist often results in delayed and diminished visualization of the contrast. To ensure a thorough examination for a small interatrial communication, we usually perform at least three agitated saline contrast injections. The first injection is performed at rest during normal respiration. If no shunt is visualized, the second injection is performed during the strain and relaxation phases of the Valsalva maneuver, and a third injection is performed during a cough.

CARDIAC ABNORMALITIES OFTEN DIAGNOSED ONLY BY TEE EXAMINATION

The cardiac structural abnormalities listed in Table 4–1 provide a framework for the clinical evaluation of patients with suspected cardiogenic emboli. Because TEE provides structural and hemodynamic information, the identification of a dilated cardiomyopathy, for example, may be made, but the underlying cause often cannot be determined. Therefore, a slightly modified and shorter list of structural abnormalities should be considered while performing and reviewing TEE studies (Table 4–2). In the sections that follow, many of the abnormalities listed in Table 4–2 will be discussed individually. These sections will review pathologic and TTE findings as well as TEE results to provide a thorough description of the abnormalities and their clinical significance.

Atrial Septal Aneurysm

Incidence

Atrial septal aneurysms are areas of thinning in the fossa ovalis region of the atrial septum that may bulge into the atrial chambers or move excessively during the cardiac cycle. In an autopsy study, atrial septal aneurysms were present in approximately 1% of specimens.[7] The results of four large studies with two-dimensional TTE are summarized in Table 4–3. In these studies, the overall incidence of atrial septal aneurysms was 0.2% among 60,156 patients undergoing routine TTE studies. In our laboratory, among 410 patients referred for TEE, 32 (8%) had atrial septal aneurysm diagnosed by TEE. A similar result was reported by Schneider et al.[8] in which 23 (3%) atrial septal aneurysms were diagnosed from a patient group of 765 undergoing TEE for a variety of indications. From these results, it is clear that TEE is superior to TTE for identifying atrial septal aneurysms. The procedure used for diagnosis must be considered when incidence rates are compared.

Definition

When an atrial septal aneurysm is visualized by TEE, there is usually very little doubt about the presence of this abnormality. Criteria have been proposed, however, to provide a standard for the diagnosis of atrial septal aneurysm. Criteria proposed by Hanley et al.[9] from their evaluation of 80 patients with atrial septal aneurysm detected by TTE are the most widely used. As demonstrated in Figure 4–2, the criteria include either an aneurysm involving at least 1.5 cm of the atrial septum and extending 1.5 cm into either atrial chamber from the plane of the atrial septum or an aneurysm with a 1.5-cm excursion in total during the cardiorespiratory cycle. In our laboratory, we have proposed a slightly modified version of these criteria: a 1.1-cm standard for the excursion of the atrial septal aneurysm. This modification was based on the pathologic study by Silver and Dorsey.[7]

Further classification of the types of atrial septal aneurysms has been described by Hanley et al.[9] This classification was based on the position and motion of the atrial septal aneurysms. The type 1A aneurysm bulges continually to the right atrium with little motion during the cardiorespiratory cycle. The type 1B aneurysm predominantly bulges to the right atrium but has a phasic oscillation into the left atrium during the cardiorespiratory cycle. The type 1C aneurysm, a definition modified by Pearson et al.[5] includes those aneurysms that oscillate between the right and left atrial chambers with each cardiac

TABLE 4–2.
Potential and Definite Cardiac Sources of Emboli Often Diagnosed by TEE

Possible
Valvular disease
Wall motion abnormality
Probable
Patent foramen ovale
Atrial septal defect
Spontaneous contrast
Atrial septal aneurysm
Definite
Left atrial thrombus
Left ventricular thrombus
Tumor (myxoma)
Vegetation
Aortic protruding plaque

TABLE 4–3.
Incidence of Atrial Septal Aneurysms in Routine Transthoracic Studies

First Author	No. of Patients	Atrial Septal Aneurysm Present (%)
Hanley[9]	36,200	80 (0.2)
Schneider[8]	12,137	23 (0.2)
Belkin[10]	6,979	36 (0.5)
Gallet[11]	4,840	10 (0.2)
Total	60,156	149 (0.2)

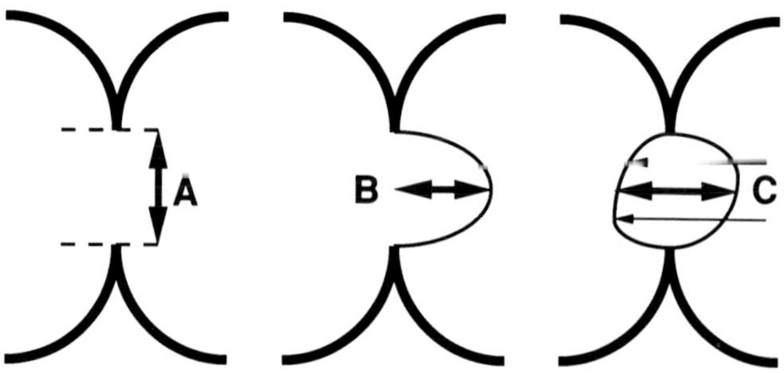

FIG 4–2.
The dimensions defining atrial septal aneurysms must involve 1.5 cm of the septum *(A)* and protrude 1.1 cm into either atrial chamber *(B)* or have a total excursion of 1.1 cm *(C)* during the cardiorespiratory cycle.

TABLE 4–4.
Incidence and Characteristics of Atrial Septal Aneurysms in Patients With Suspected Cardiogenic Emboli

			Other Findings in Patients With ASA Present			
First Author	No. of Patients	ASA* Present(%)	MVP*	Chiari Network	Shunt	Thrombus
Pearson[5]	133	20 (15)	2	4	4	1
Schneider[8]	113	12 (11)	1	0	8	2

*ASA = atrial septal aneurysm; MVP = mitral valve prolapse.

cycle. Type 2 atrial septal aneurysms protrude exclusively into the left atrium.

Association With Cardiogenic Emboli

The clinical histories of patients found to have atrial septal aneurysms by either TEE, TTE, or autopsy include a high percentage of patients with possible cardiogenic emboli. Among the 149 patients with atrial septal aneurysms diagnosed by TTE and listed in Table 4–3, 40 (27%) had a history of cerebral ischemic events (either cerebrovascular accidents or transient ischemic attacks [TIA]) or cardiogenic systemic emboli. Using TEE, we[5] studied 132 patients admitted with unexplained cerebral ischemic events to the stroke service (Table 4–4). In this selected patient population, atrial septal aneurysms were diagnosed in 20 (15%) patients. Based on these studies, there appears to be an association between atrial septal aneurysms and cardiogenic emboli (Fig 4–3). The mechanism by which atrial septal aneurysms may cause cardiogenic emboli remains unclear. One possible explanation is the association of atrial septal aneurysms with other cardiac structural abnormalities that may be potential sources of cardiogenic emboli, including patent foramen ovale, mitral valve prolapse, or thrombus.

In the series reported by Pearson et al.,[5] an associated patent foramen ovale detected by contrast injection was present in 77% of patients who received intravenous contrast. Similar results have been reported by other authors that ranged from 49% to 90%[8–11] of patients with atrial septal aneurysms studied for the presence of atrial communication by TTE and TEE. In view of the large percentage of atrial septal aneurysms with patent foramen ovale present, paradoxical embolization from the venous

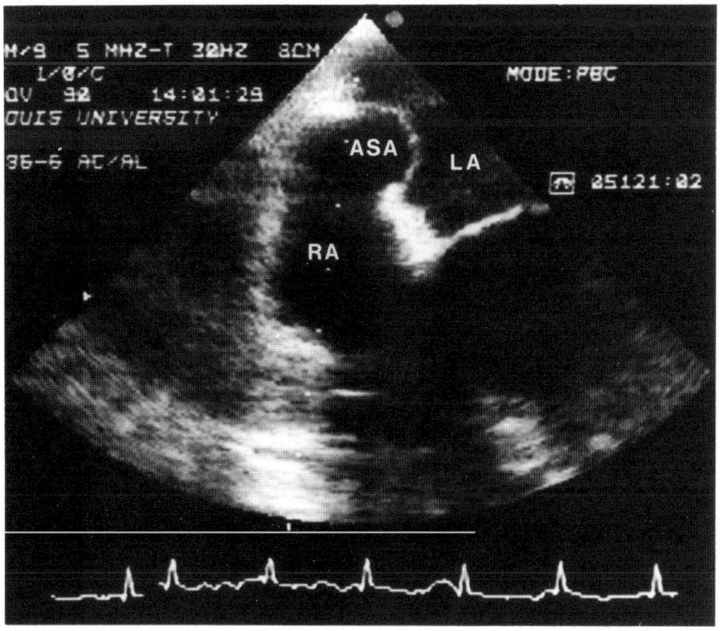

FIG 4–3.
Atrial septal aneurysm *(ASA)* that was detected in a 26-year-old woman with a history of transient ischemic attack. No intracardiac shunt was detected with agitated saline contrast. *LA* = left atrium; *RA* = right atrium.

to the arterial circulation must be considered a possible cause for cardiogenic embolization in patients with atrial septal aneurysms.

Mitral valve prolapse has been associated with stroke in several reports. It has also been shown to have a potential association with the presence of atrial septal aneurysms. In a report by Abinader and associates,[12] 24 (3.8%) patients out of a study group of 630 with mitral valve prolapse detected by TTE had atrial septal aneurysms. Although the reports of mitral valve prolapse in patients with atrial septal aneurysms are slightly lower, about 15%,[5, 8, 9] there may be more than a chance association. The clinical significance of this possible association is not clear.

The presence of a thrombus in the area of the atrial septal aneurysm is another possible cause for cardiogenic emboli. Thrombi have been visualized by TEE adjacent to atrial septal aneurysms in several

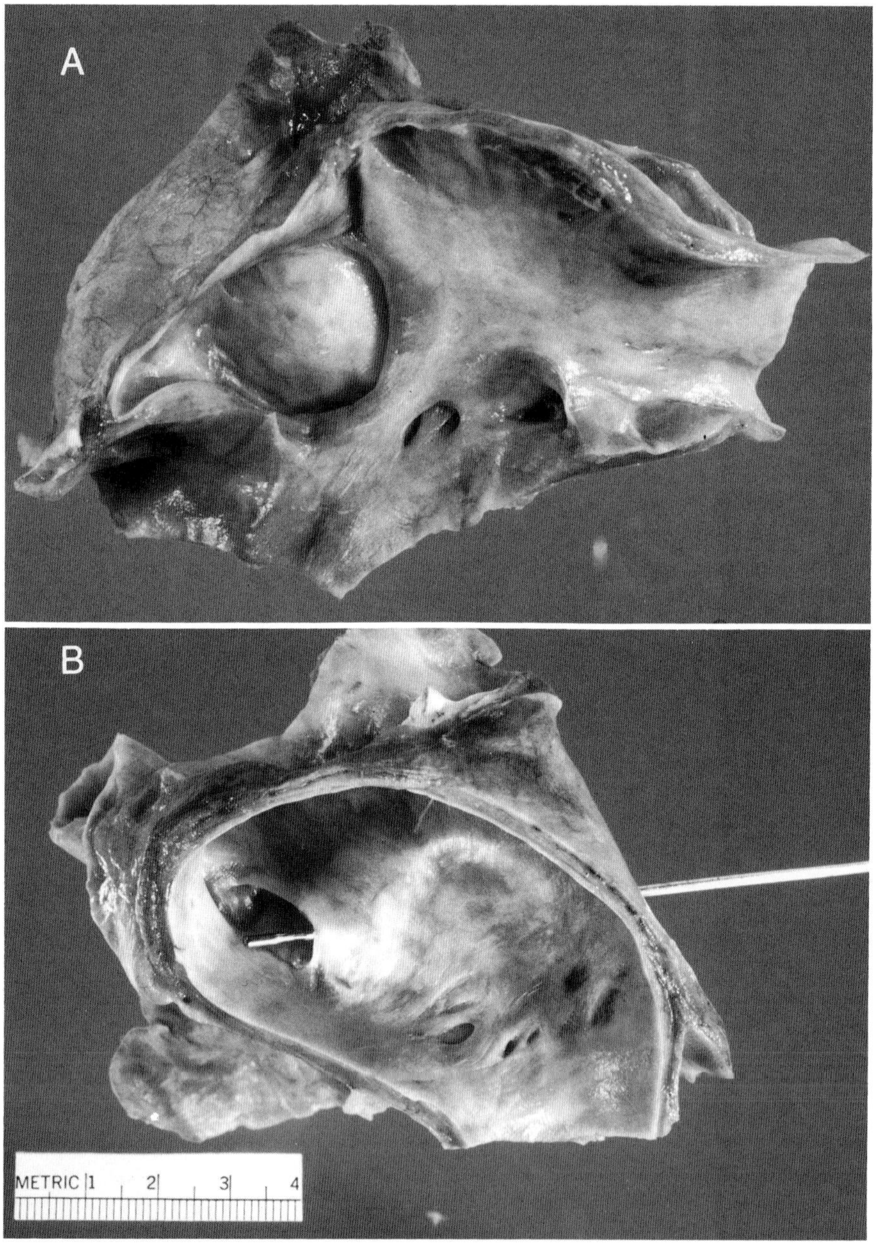

FIG 4–4.
Atrial septal aneurysm and patent foramen ovale present in a 65-year-old man who died following a massive myocardial infarction. **A,** the atrial septal aneurysm can be seen as it protrudes into the right atrium in an isolated atrial preparation. **B,** a probe is passed into the left atrium via a patent foramen ovale in the same specimen. (Courtesy of Frederick A. Dressler, M.D.).

reports. Among 20 patients with suspected cardiogenic emboli and atrial septal aneurysms present on TEE who were reported by Pearson et al.,[5] 1 left atrial thrombus was identified. In a similar study by Schneider et al., 2 of 12 patients with cerebral ischemia had left atrial thrombi seen by TEE.[8] Although the published reports of thrombus associated with atrial septal aneurysms are limited, an association may be present. The TEE evaluation of patients with suspected cardiogenic emboli should include careful evaluation for a thrombus in the area of an atrial septal aneurysm, if identified.

Patent Foramen Ovale

Paradoxical embolization through either a patent foramen ovale or atrial septal defect has been reported as a rare cause of cardiogenic embolization for many years.[13, 14] Recently, observations have been made that suggest that paradoxical embolization through a patent foramen ovale may be a much more common cause of cardiogenic emboli than previously suspected.[15–20] The use of TEE has improved the diagnosis and characterization of patent foramen ovale and atrial septal defects.[21–24]

Pathologic Observations

Patent foramen ovale is the most common component of the fetal circulation that persists into adult life (Fig 4–4). In an autopsy study of 965 normal hearts, a probe-patent foramen ovale was present in 27%.[19] The authors observed a decline in the incidence of patent foramen ovale from 34% in the first decade of life to 22% in the tenth decade. The size of the patent foramen ovale was noted to increase with advancing age from an average size of 3.4 mm during the first decade of life to 5.8 mm during the tenth decade. In this report, no clinical history of cerebrovascular events or pathologic evaluation for emboli was reported.

Transthoracic Contrast Echocardiography Results

Populations of normal[17] and abnormal patients[15, 16, 18] have been studied by using agitated saline contrast and TTE. As demonstrated in Figure 4–5, the presence of a patent foramen ovale was detected in about 15% of the normal or control subjects. In the two large[15, 16] and one small[18] series of young stroke patients, a higher prevalence of patent foramen ovale was noted that ranged from 40% to 73%. Clearly, there appears to be an association between the occurrence of stroke and the presence of a patent foramen ovale.

The observations that right-to-left shunting can occur across a patent foramen ovale in patients with normal left and right heart pressures[20] and that up to 50% of patients with pulmonary emboli have no detectable deep-vein thrombosis strengthen the case for patent foramen ovale as a mechanism for paradoxical embolization. It seems reasonable to postulate that small thrombi could form peripherally in some patients and, in the presence of a patent foramen ovale, paradoxical embolization could occur that could cause cerebral ischemia. The fact that pulmonary emboli and patent foramen ovale are both fairly common entities suggests that paradoxical embolization may be a cause of cerebral ischemia in pa-

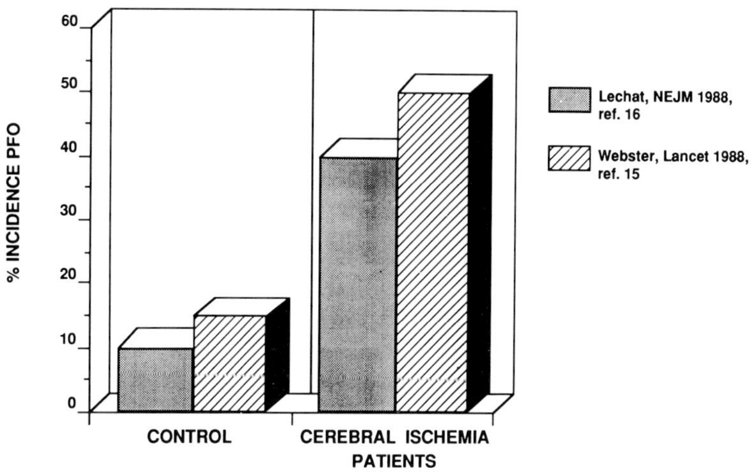

FIG 4–5.
Incidence of patent foramen ovale *(PFO)* reported in two studies utilizing TTE and agitated saline contrast. Multiple contrast injections and provocative maneuvers were used in both studies.

tients with patent foramen ovale and no other demonstrable cause.

The Role of TEE in Evaluating Patients With Patent Foramen Ovale

With the use of agitated saline contrast, TTE can identify patients with patent foramen ovale present. Unfortunately, two factors limit the usefulness of TTE. First, poor-quality images are often obtained that do not allow for reliable detection of patent foramen ovale. For example, in 15% of patients reported by Webster et al.[15] and 14% of the patients reported by Lechat et al.,[16] poor quality images were obtained that could not be analyzed. Second, the use of coughing and the Valsalva maneuver to transiently elevate the right atrial pressure can cause increased lung impedance to the ultrasound beam and alter the orientation of the chest wall and heart so as to cause loss of image. With TEE, high-quality images are obtained in almost all patients, and maneuvers can be performed by the patient without reducing image quality (Fig 4–6).

In studies comparing TTE and TEE for the identification of patent foramen ovale, TEE has been proved to be more sensitive. In a report from our laboratory,[4] nine patients had patent foramen ovale and atrial septal aneurysms identified by TEE. In only one of the nine patients was the diagnosis made by TTE. In a report by Zenker et al., atrial septal defects were diagnosed by TEE in 2 of 40 young patients with a history of cerebral ischemic events.[25] Evaluation of the same group of 40 patients with TTE did not allow a diagnosis of either atrial septal defect. TEE has also been shown to be superior to TTE for characterization of atrial septal defects. Using TEE color flow mapping, Mehta et al.[22] demonstrated that TEE was useful for detection of the classification of atrial septal defects and the evaluation of shunt volumes. Mügge et al.[21] demonstrated the presence of a patent foramen ovale in three patients with the use of color Doppler. TEE was evaluated in comparison to TTE for the diagnosis of a sinus venosus atrial septal defect by Kronzon et al.[24] In this study, 41 patients with the clinical diagnosis of atrial septal defect were studied with both TEE and TTE. Correct identification of the atrial septal defect was possible in 33 patients with TTE and in all patients with TEE. Overall, TEE appears to be superior to TTE for identification and characterization of patent foramen ovale and atrial septal defects.

Clinical Implications

The observed association between patent foramen ovale and the occurrence of cardiogenic emboli described in this section raises several questions about the clinical significance of this association. In particular, the prognostic importance of patent foramen ovale and the role of treatment to prevent neurologic events remain to be proved.[26] In our experience, one recurrent event (TIA) occurred among 11

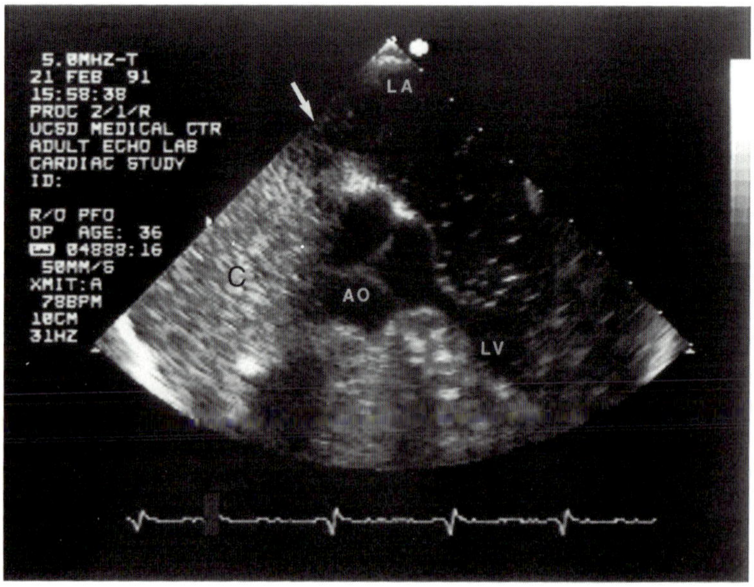

FIG 4–6.
Intravenous injection of agitated saline contrast (*C*), with passage *(arrow)* of the echogenic contrast material from the right atrium to the left atrium *(LA)* consistent with a patent foramen ovale. Note the bubbles passing through the mitral valve orifice. *AO* = aorta; *LV* = left ventricle.

patients with previous TIA or stroke and patent foramen ovale diagnosed by TEE during an 8-month follow-up interval.[27] No large follow-up series of patients with patent foramen ovale has been reported to date. Information on treatment is also limited. In a report by Harvey et al.,[18] four patients with 5- to 10-mm patent foramen ovale had surgical closure and no recurrent neurologic events during a 7- to 21-month follow-up period. In general, it has been our practice to treat patients with suspected cardiac embolic events and patent foramen ovale with antithrombotic or anticoagulant therapy. Patients with recurrent cardiac embolic events are more often treated with anticoagulant therapy. Surgical closure of patent foramen ovale for patients with recurrent embolic events has not been routinely employed in our center; however, randomized trials examining the role of surgical or percutaneous balloon closure as well as antithrombotic therapy may alter the management of these patients.

Left Atrial Thrombus

With TEE, the proximity of the imaging probe to the left atrium and the high-frequency transducer enhance visualization of thrombi in the left atrium and left atrial appendage. Several studies have compared TTE and TEE for the detection of thrombi in the left atrium in patients with mitral stenosis and demonstrated the superiority of TEE.[28–32] Because many of the patients later had surgical procedures, the presence of a thrombus could be confirmed directly.[28–31] Based on the knowledge that TEE is useful for identifying an atrial thrombus, some authors have studied patients with suspected cardiogenic emboli to determine whether atrial thrombi were present.[4, 33] Other studies have reviewed the clinical characteristics of patients found to have atrial thrombi to discern the possible underlying mechanisms for thrombus formation and to determine whether clinical events may have occurred that could have been caused by cardiogenic emboli.[31]

Left Atrial Thrombi in Patients With Cerebral Ischemia

The results of studies employing routine TEE evaluation for left atrial thrombi in patients with cerebral ischemia are summarized in Table 4–5[4, 33] (Figs 4–7 and 4–8). In both series, about 5% of patients had thrombi identified. Of those, thrombi in the left atrial appendage were most common (six of eight, or 75%) (Fig 4–9). None of the thrombi detected were visualized by TTE. In the study by Pearson et al.[4] left atrial thrombi were identified only in patients with clinical cardiac disease. In the series reported by Pop et al.,[33] one thrombus was found in a patient in sinus rhythm with normal left atrial size. In a study of patients with mitral stenosis by

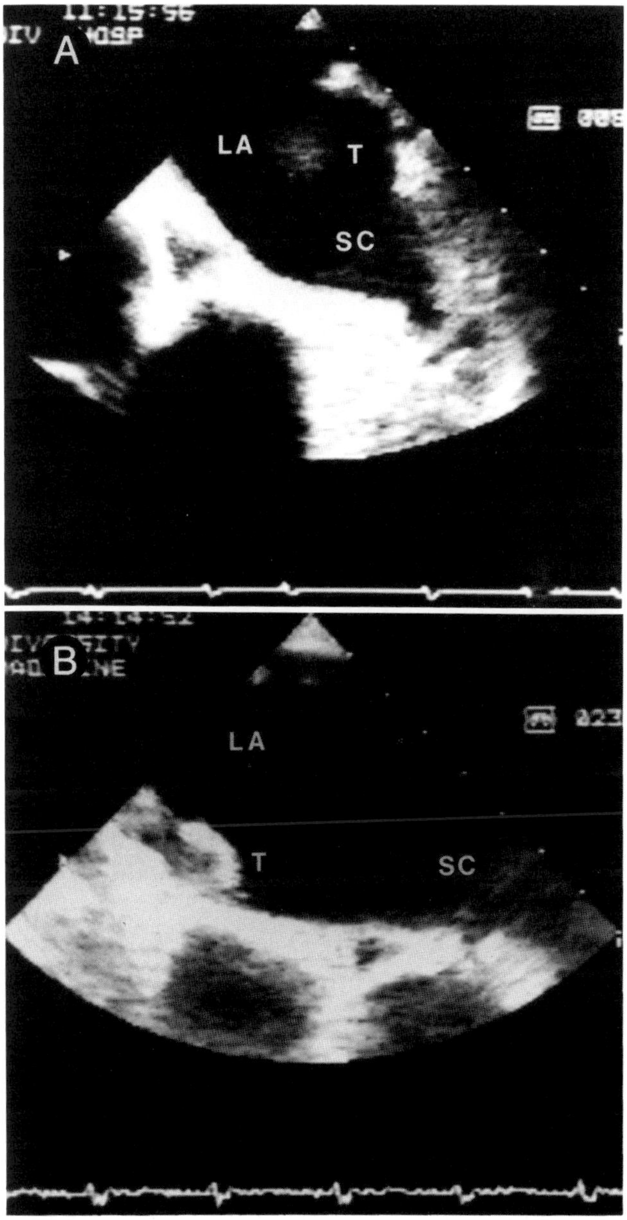

FIG 4–7.
Examples of thrombus *(T)* and spontaneous contrast *(SC)* in the left atrium *(LA)*. **A,** a thrombus is seen in the left atrium of a 78-year-old patient with a history of multiple strokes. The characteristic low-intensity spiral shapes of spontaneous contrast are present in the area near the left atrial appendage. **B,** a thrombus is seen adjacent to the left atrial wall, and spontaneous contrast is seen near the left atrial appendage. The example shown in **B** is from a 66-year-old woman with a history of TIA and atrial fibrillation.

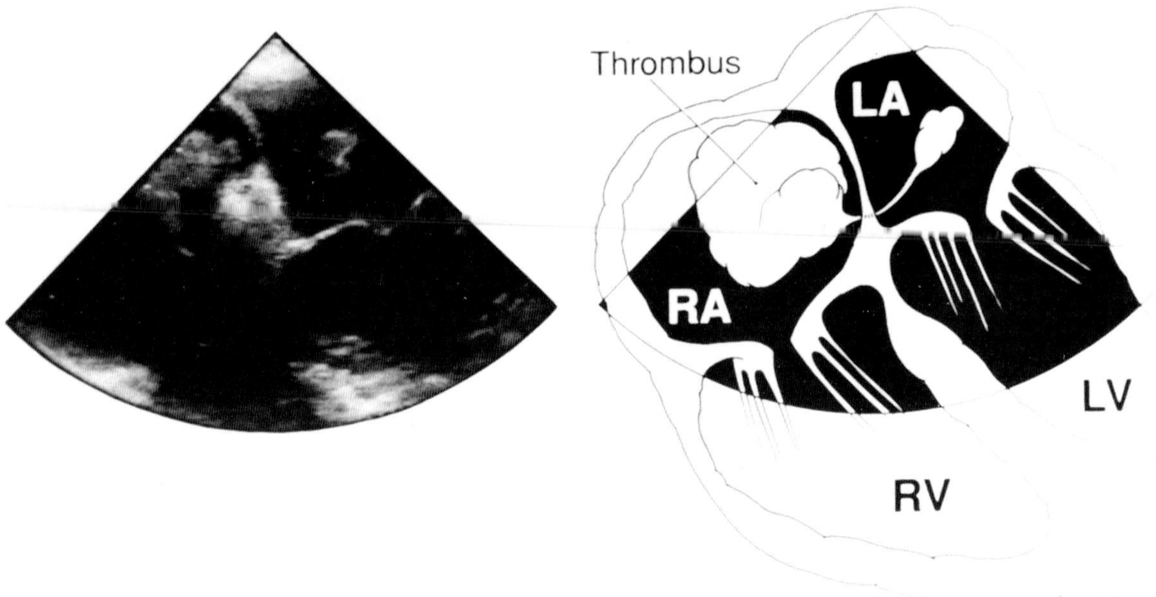

FIG 4–8.
Large, mobile thrombus present in the right atrium *(RA)* and left atrium *(LA)*. The same thrombus extended from the right atrium to the atrial septum and then via a patent foramen ovale into the left atrium as shown in the schematic diagram on the right. The patient had a history of pulmonary embolus and embolus to the left leg that required surgical removal. *RV* = right ventricle; *LV* = left ventricle.

Shrestha et al.,[34] none of the 11 left atrial appendage thrombi documented at the time of surgery were detected by TTE. Overall, left atrial and left atrial appendage thrombi are identified by TEE in about 5% of patients with cerebral ischemia of unknown etiology. Thrombi may rarely occur in patients without underlying heart disease. Improved detection of left atrial and left atrial appendage thrombi is possible with TEE.

Clinical Implications

In patients with suspected cardiogenic emboli, the presence of left atrial or left atrial appendage thrombi on TEE examination would seem to predict a high likelihood for recurrent events. In a series of 23 patients reported by Mügge et al.[31] who had sequential TEE examinations, none of the patients had embolic events during a 7-month interval before a follow-up study. Of the 23 patients, 19 were taking phenprocoumon, and 2 were taking heparin during the interval. Repeat examinations, however, showed that complete or partial clot dissolution occurred in 16 of the 19 patients taking phenprocoumon and 1 of the 2 taking heparin. No change in thrombus size was detected in the 2 patients not treated with anticoagulant therapy. In our experience, 3 of 11 patients with left atrial thrombi identified by TEE and a history of a recent cerebral ischemic event had a recurrent event during an 8-month follow-up interval despite treatment with warfarin in all 3 patients.[27] We did not perform repeat TEE examinations in these patients. In addition, there has been a report of right atrial thrombus that disappeared after 3 days of intravenous urokinase therapy.[35] In summary, al-

TABLE 4–5.
Incidence of Left Atrial Thrombi in Patients With Cerebral Ischemia

First Author	No. of Patients	Left Atrial Thrombus Present		Thrombus Present Only in Left Atrial Appendage	
		TTE	TEE	TTE	TEE
Pearson[4]	79	0	5 (6%)	0	4 (5%)
Pop[33]	72	0	3 (4%)	0	2 (3%)

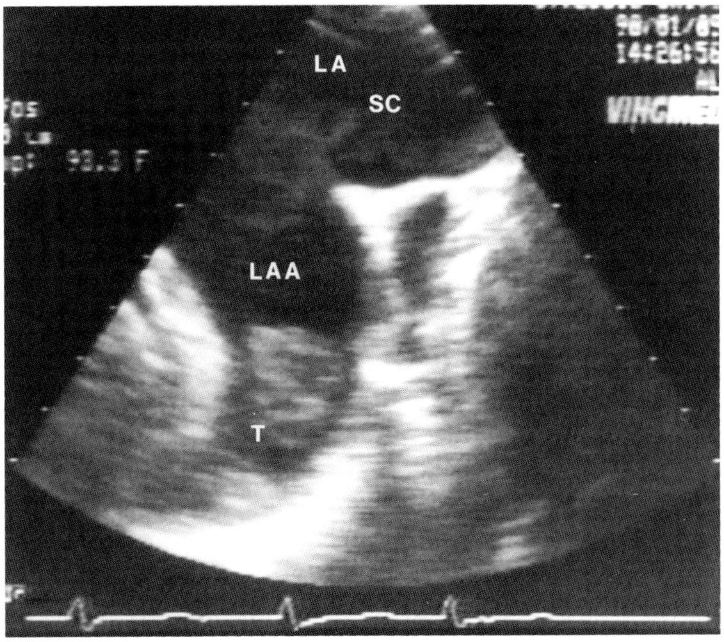

FIG 4–9.
A thrombus *(T)* is seen in the left atrial appendage *(LAA)* in an 81-year-old woman with a history of stroke and atrial fibrillation. Spontaneous contrast *(SC)* is also seen in the left atrial appendage and the left atrial chamber *(LA)*.

though limited data are available, patients with left atrial thrombi appear to be at increased risk for recurrent cardioembolic events. Dissolution of left atrial thrombi has been reported in patients treated with anticoagulant therapy, although the small number of observations made in untreated patients cannot serve as a control group to verify the effects of treatment. Further investigation will be required to definitively determine the prognostic significance of left atrial thrombi for recurrent embolic events and to demonstrate the benefits of treatment.

Spontaneous Contrast

Definition

Spontaneous echo contrast is often described as a swirling smokelike ultrasound reflection most often seen in the left atrium in patients with low flow states, including mitral valve disease. In an early description of this abnormality in humans by Iliceto et al.,[36] spontaneous contrast was seen in the left atrium of ten patients with mitral stenosis when TTE with a 3.5-mHz transducer was used. Described as dynamic intracavitary echoes, spontaneous contrast was seen as low-intensity echoes slowly moving in a circular or spiral shape within the left atrial cavity. In our laboratory, we define spontaneous contrast as the presence of dynamic echoes curling in a circular pattern within the cardiac chambers (see Figs 4–7 and 4–9). Gain settings must be routinely adjusted to exclude the possibility of noise artifact,[37] which can mimic spontaneous contrast.

Incidence

The reported incidence of spontaneous contrast varies depending on the type of patients studied. With TTE, Beppu et al.[38] demonstrated spontaneous contrast in 37 of 116 (32%) patients with rheumatic mitral valve disease. Using TEE, Daniel and associates[39] found spontaneous contrast in 61 of 122 (50%) patients with mitral stenosis. In a random series of 314 patients, Erbel et al.[40] demonstrated spontaneous contrast by TEE in 10 patients (3%), all of whom had mitral stenosis or mitral valve prostheses. In 150 consecutive patients studied by TEE for a variety of indications in our laboratory, Castello et al. reported a 19% incidence of spontaneous contrast. The majority of the patients were studied to evaluate either cardiac sources of emboli (34%), prosthetic or native valve disease (30%), or left ventricular function (10%).

Association of Spontaneous Contrast With Other Abnormalities

The presence of spontaneous contrast is usually associated with other cardiac abnormalities. Multivariate analysis of the clinical characteristics of 29 patients with spontaneous contrast among 150 consecutive TEE patients by Castello et al.[37] showed that left atrial enlargement, atrial fibrillation, mitral regurgitation, and mitral valve prostheses were associated with the presence of spontaneous contrast. Other authors have also reported high percentages of patients with spontaneous contrast who had associated atrial fibrillation.[38-40] Spontaneous contrast, however, can be detected in patients with normal left atrial size and sinus rhythm.[37, 39]

Risk for Cardiogenic Emboli

The observation that left atrial thrombi were present in many patients with left atrial spontaneous contrast has led some authors to conclude that patients with spontaneous contrast are at increased risk for cardiogenic emboli.[39, 40] With TEE, left atrial thrombus has been detected in 18% to 36% of patients with spontaneous contrast.[37, 39, 40] Daniel et al. reported a history of cardiogenic emboli in 21 of 61 patients with spontaneous contrast in the left atrium.[39] Castello et al., however, have shown that thrombus in the left atrium is almost as likely to occur in patients without spontaneous contrast (four of nine patients) as those with spontaneous contrast (five of nine patients).[37] Although there appears to be an association between spontaneous contrast and cardiogenic emboli, further information about the incidence and prognostic value of spontaneous contrast in patients with various cardiac disease states is needed to assist clinical decision making. Currently the prognostic implications of spontaneous contrast in patients without other identifiable causes of cardiogenic emboli are unknown. Furthermore, the prognostic implication of spontaneous contrast seen in patients having TEE examinations for reasons other than a suspected embolic source is unknown.

Effects of Treatment

Limited information is available about the effects of treatment on spontaneous contrast. Resolution of spontaneous contrast has been reported with trifluoperazine in one patient in whom heparin infusion was not successful.[41] Castello et al. reported resolution of a left atrial thrombus in a patient receiving warfarin therapy with persistent spontaneous contrast.[37] Follow-up information on nine patients with spontaneous contrast in our laboratory revealed one recurrent cerebral ischemic event during a mean follow-up of 8 months despite warfarin therapy.[27] Further information about the effects of various treatment modalities on spontaneous contrast and the prognostic implications of the presence of spontaneous contrast is needed before specific recommendations for therapy can be made.

Aortic Debris

Several recent studies have described protruding aortic atherosclerotic plaque as a potential embolic source.[42-44] Slight modification of the standard TEE examination of cardiac structures allows visualization of the ascending aorta and aortic arch. The de-

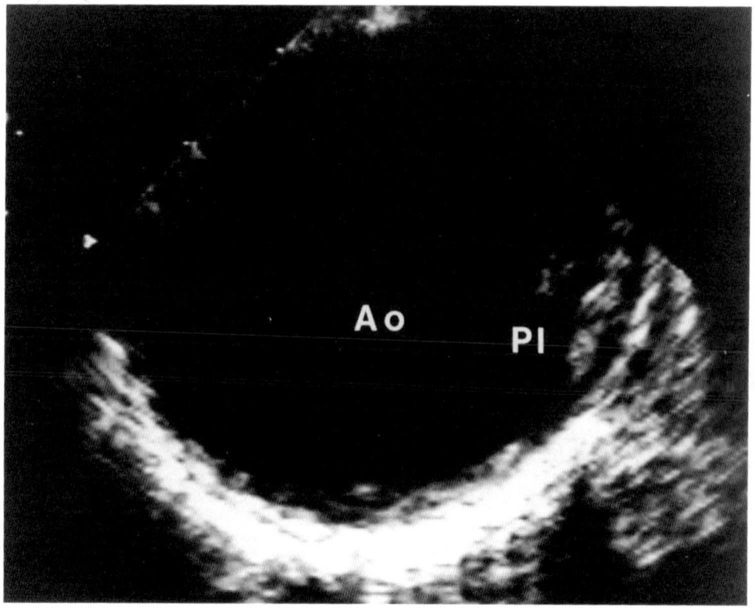

FIG 4–10.
Atherosclerotic plaque and mobile intraluminal plaque *(Pl)* present in the descending aorta *(Ao)* of a 74-year-old man with a history of stroke.

scending aorta can also be visualized in patients with suspected abdominal, pelvic, or lower extremity emboli. With the high-frequency TEE probe positioned in close proximity to the aorta, the lumen of the aorta can be evaluated in detail (Fig 4–10).

In the first reported cases involving TEE by Tunick and Kronzon,[44] three patients with large protruding and freely mobile aortic plaques were described. All three patients had histories of possible embolic events. Routine TEE examination for a cardiac source of emboli showed the mobile plaques. A patient with a history of multiple embolic events and multiple mobile plaques seen in the aorta by TEE was also described by Tunick and colleagues.[43] This patient had endarterectomy with good results and no subsequent embolic events. In a study by Karalis et al., 36 patients with aortic atherosclerotic debris were described.[42] A history of an embolic event was present in 8 of the 11 patients with pedunculated and mobile thrombi and 3 of the 25 patients with immobile plaques. Invasive procedures involving the thoracic aorta were performed in 15 patients within 1 week of the TEE examination. Embolic events occurred in 4 patients, all of whom had mobile plaques seen by TEE. In 2 other patients with mobile plaques, the procedures were successfully altered to minimize the chance for embolization.

In summary, TEE allows the recognition and characterization of atherosclerotic plaques in the aorta. Patients with mobile pedunculated plaques are at increased risk for embolic events. A high risk of embolization is present in patients with mobile plaques if they have invasive procedures involving the abnormal aortic region.

OTHER CARDIAC CONDITIONS ASSOCIATED WITH A RISK FOR CARDIOGENIC EMBOLI

Atrial Fibrillation

Nonvalvular atrial fibrillation is associated with approximately 45% of embolic strokes.[45] The risk of stroke in patients with atrial fibrillation is about 5% annually and increases with age. Overall, 35% of patients with nonvalvular atrial fibrillation may eventually develop cerebral infarction.[46, 47] Recently, three studies[48–50] have demonstrated the benefit of preventive therapy in patients with nonvalvular atrial fibrillation. All three studies showed a reduction in stroke rates with warfarin. Aspirin was beneficial in selected patient groups in the Stroke Prevention in Atrial Fibrillation trial.[49] In this section, the role of TEE evaluation of patients with atrial fibrillation is reviewed.

Nonvalvular atrial fibrillation probably enhances the risk of stroke by causing stasis of blood in the left atrium and increasing the chances for thrombus formation. It may also be that pre-existing structural abnormalities such as atrial septal aneurysms, mitral valve prolapse, or segmental left ventricular wall abnormalities are more thrombogenic in the presence of atrial fibrillation. Left atrial thrombus and spontaneous contrast are more commonly visualized by TEE in patients with atrial fibrillation.[37] Both abnormalities are consistent with a low flow state within the left atrium. One possible role for TEE is that evaluation of patients with nonvalvular atrial fibrillation may help to identify subgroups of patients at increased risk for cardiogenic emboli. The presence or absence of cardiac abnormalities as demonstrated by TEE may allow stratification of patients for whom the antiplatelet effects of aspirin or the antithrombotic effects of warfarin may be more effective preventive therapy. Further study is needed to define the role of TEE in the evaluation and risk stratification of patients with nonvalvular atrial fibrillation.

In patients with atrial fibrillation who are undergoing electrical cardioversion, anticoagulation with warfarin prior to the procedure is common clinical practice. Some physicians have advocated TEE evaluation for a thrombus or spontaneous contrast in patients scheduled for cardioversion. In those patients with left and right atrial chambers that appear normal on TEE, routine preprocedure anticoagulation may not be considered necessary. It may be difficult to validate this approach with clinical studies, however, because the incidence of cardiogenic emboli following cardioversion is very low. Therefore, a large number of patients would need to be studied in a randomized trial to establish the safety of not using warfarin therapy in patients with normal TEE evaluation prior to cardioversion. One additional note of caution is that mechanical activity of the left atrium may not recover for weeks following the restoration of electrical activity. This may mean that the risk of thrombus formation would continue following the cardioversion procedure and a new thrombus, not seen by the initial TEE evaluation, could develop and then embolize even in patients with normal TEE findings prior to cardioversion.

Endocarditis

Endocarditis is discussed separately in Chapters 5 and 6. It is well known that endocarditis is frequently associated with embolic events. TEE permits excellent visualization of the mitral, aortic, and tricuspid valves for vegetations. Some authors have described an increased risk of embolization in the presence of large vegetations.[51] In addition, vegetations may be detected in patients with cardiogenic emboli in whom the diagnosis of endocarditis was only suspected. Therefore, the possibility of bacterial, fungal, or marantic endocarditis must always be kept in mind when evaluating patients for sources of cardiogenic emboli.

Left Ventricular Thrombi

Left ventricular thrombi are known to have potential for embolization. Thrombi most commonly form in the presence of left ventricular wall motion abnormalities such as acute myocardial infarction, aneurysm, or dilated cardiomyopathy.[52] There have been case reports of left ventricular thrombi occurring in patients with normal left ventricular function.[53] The use of TEE for the identification of left ventricular thrombi has some limitations. In the transverse four-chamber view the left ventricular apex is the region of the heart most distant from the imaging probe. In the transverse short-axis views obtained from the transgastric location of the TEE probe, the left ventricular apex is often difficult to visualize. Imaging of the apex is improved with the longitudinal long-axis or two-chamber views, although the apex may still defy visualization. The presence of regional wall motion abnormalities can be a marker for the possible presence of a left ventricular thrombus. In patients in whom thrombi are clearly identified, the information is a useful guide to treatment. In patients with no thrombi visualized by TEE, however, the possibility of a thrombus cannot be completely excluded. Other techniques such as TTE, cardiac catheterization, magnetic resonance imaging (MRI), or ultrafast computed tomographic (CT) scanning may provide additional diagnostic information.[54]

Intracardiac Tumors

Numerous authors have described enhanced visualization of intracardiac tumors with TEE. Intracardiac tumors may be a potential source of cardiogenic emboli either by direct embolization or embolization of a thrombus that is formed adjacent to the tumor. In addition, TEE provides important information about the mobility of intracardiac tumors such as left atrial myxoma and sites of attachment to the endocardial surface that may not be well visualized by TTE (see Chapter 6). Therefore, TEE evaluation for cardiogenic emboli should always include an evaluation for intracardiac tumors. In patients with suspected intracardiac tumors visualized by TTE, additional diagnostic information can often be derived from TEE evaluation.[55, 56]

Intracardiac Devices

Prosthetic Cardiac Valves

Prosthetic cardiac valves are associated with an increased risk for cardiogenic emboli. Frequently, TTE evaluation of patients with prosthetic valves for sources of emboli are complicated by the presence of the echogenic prosthetic valve, which impairs visualization of the left atrium. With TEE, the prosthetic valve and the left atrial chamber can be imaged without interference. In a recent study comparing TTE and TEE for the evaluation of valve prostheses, 89 patients with mitral valve prostheses were studied.[57] Of those 89 patients, 37 patients were observed to have left atrial spontaneous contrast; 6 were observed to have thrombi in the left atrium, in the left atrial appendage, or adherent to the sewing ring; and 2 had vegetations seen. In comparison, only 1 abnormality, a left atrial thrombus, was noted by TTE.

In our experience, vegetations and thrombi have been visualized in patients with valve prostheses and a history of cardiogenic emboli. One additional abnormality has recently been noted that may be associated with a risk of embolism. We have observed very small filamentous projections from the atrial surface of mitral valve prostheses. These projections may represent thrombotic material with a potential for embolization (see Fig 5–14). Further study will be required to determine the association between these projections and the risk of cardiogenic emboli.

Permanent Pacemakers

We have observed thrombi adherent to the intracardiac leads of permanent transvenous pacemakers in several patients. Thrombi have been seen adhering to the leads in the right atrial and right ventricular chambers. In one case in which a pacemaker lead was inadvertently placed through a patent foramen ovale into the left atrium, multiple thrombi adhering to the lead were noted in the left atrial chamber (Fig 4–11). In patients with permanent pacemakers and suspected cardiogenic emboli, transesophageal evaluation for the presence of thrombi adherent to the pacemaker leads should be considered.

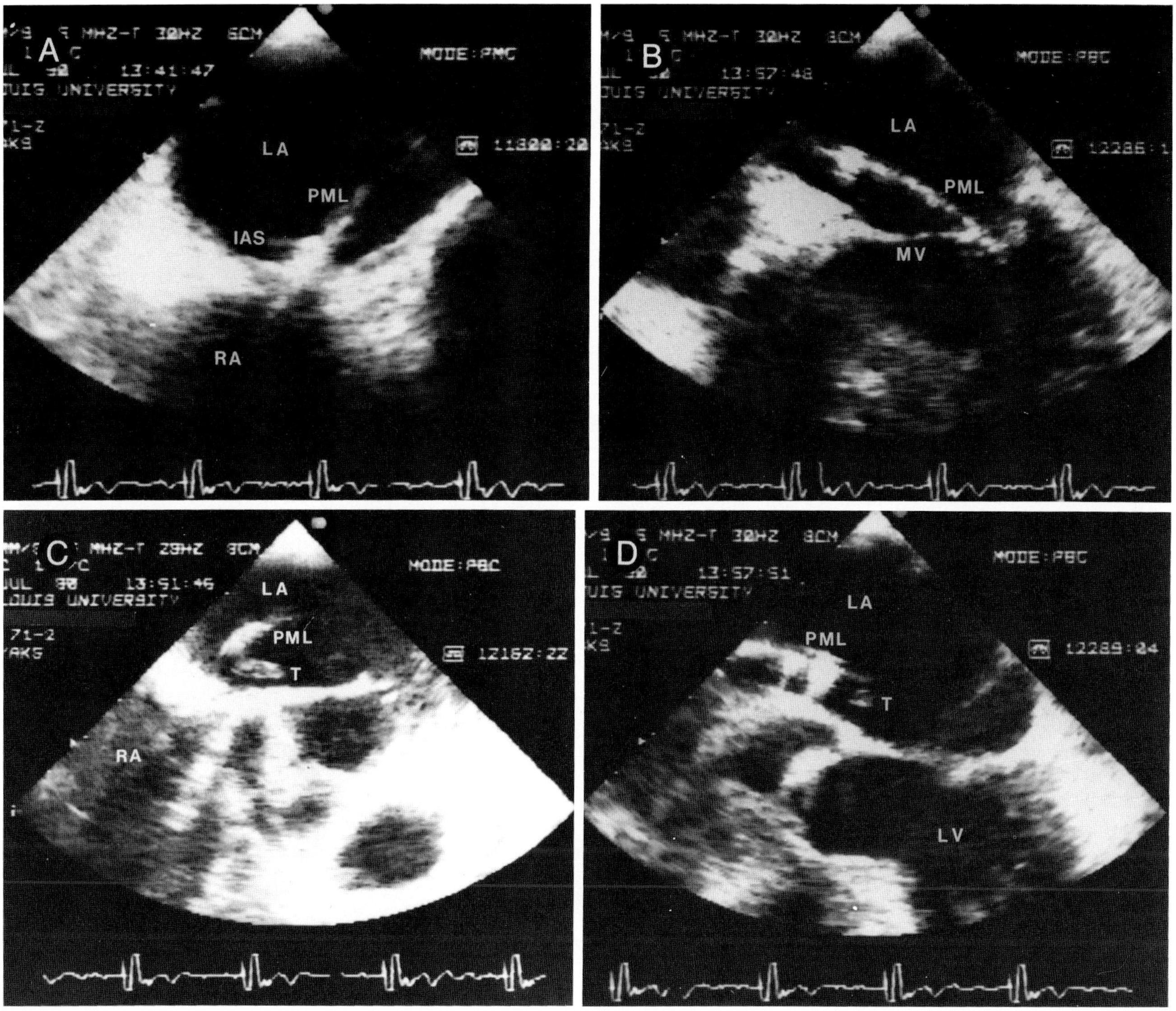

FIG 4–11.
A permanent pacemaker lead *(PML)* placed through a patent foramen ovale is shown in **A. B,** the pacemaker lead is seen to extend into the left atrium *(LA)* to the area of the mitral valve *(MV)*. **C** and **D,** at least two mobile thrombi *(T)* are seen adherent to the pacemaker lead. The patient is a 72-year-old woman with a history of recent TIA. The permanent pacemaker lead had been in place in this position for 11 years. *IAS* = interatrial septum; *LV* = left ventricle; *RA* = right atrium.

SUMMARY AND CONCLUSIONS

For the evaluation of patients with unexplained cerebral ischemia or suspected systemic emboli of cardiac origin, TEE is a valuable clinical tool. This technique appears to be much more sensitive than conventional TTE in that it identifies potential abnormalities in up to 50% of patients with suspected cardiac sources of emboli. Accordingly, evaluation of patients for cardiac sources of emboli has become the leading indication for TEE and accounts for approximately a third of the procedures performed.

The apparent association of embolic events with new or previously unsuspected abnormalities such as atrial septal aneurysms has also raised many questions regarding patient management based on the information obtained by TEE examination. Further investigation of the natural history of patients with cardiogenic emboli and abnormalities visualized by TEE examination is needed. The natural history of asymptomatic patients with potential causes for emboli found during TEE examinations for other indications also remains uncertain. Finally, the effects of treatment guided by TEE findings on primary and recurrent events warrant further investigation. Plans are underway for multicenter randomized trials comparing treatment protocols.

REFERENCES

1. Centers for Disease Control: Progress in chronic disease prevention: Chronic disease reports: Mortality trends—United States, 1979–1986. *MMWR* 1989; 38:189–201.
2. Foulkes MA, Wolf PA, Price TR, et al: The Stroke Data Bank: Design, methods, and baseline characteristics. *Stroke* 1988; 19:547–554.
3. Cerebral Embolism Task Force: Cardiogenic brain embolism. *Arch Neurol* 1989; 46:727–743.
4. Pearson AC, Labovitz AJ, Tatineni S, et al: Superiority of transesophageal echocardiography in detecting cardiac source of embolism in patients with cerebral ischemia of uncertain etiology. *J Am Coll Cardiol* 1991; 17:66–72.
5. Pearson AC, Nagelhout D, Camp A, et al: Atrial septal aneurysm and stroke: A transesophageal echocardiographic study. *J Am Coll Cardiol* 1991; 18:1223–1229.
6. Fagan LF, Weiss R, Schwartz M, et al: Transtracheal placement and imaging with a transesophageal echocardiographic probe. *Am J Cardiol* 1991; 67:909–910.
7. Silver MD, Dorsey JS: Aneurysms of the septum primum in adults. *Arch Pathol Lab Med* 1978; 102:62–65.
8. Schneider B, Hanrath P, Vogel P, et al: Improved morphologic characterization of atrial septal aneurysm by transesophageal echocardiography: Relation to cerebrovascular events. *J Am Coll Cardiol* 1990; 16:1000–1009.
9. Hanley PC, Tajik AJ, Hynes JK, et al: Diagnosis and classification of atrial septal aneurysm by two-dimensional echocardiography: Report of 80 consecutive cases. *J Am Coll Cardiol* 1985; 6:1370–1382.
10. Belkin RN, Hurwitz BJ, Kisslo J: Atrial septal aneurysm: Association with cerebrovascular and peripheral embolic events. *Stroke* 1987; 18:856–862.
11. Gallet B, Malergue MC, Adams C, et al: Atrial septal aneurysm—a potential cause of systemic embolism. *Br Heart J* 1985; 53:292–297.
12. Abinader EG, Rokey R, Goldhammer E, et al: Prevalence of atrial septal aneurysm in patients with mitral valve prolapse. *Am J Cardiol* 1988; 62:1139–1140.
13. Belkin RN, Kisslo J: Atrial septal aneurysm: Recognition and clinical relevance. *Am Heart J* 1990; 120:948–957.
14. Sweeney LJ, Rosenquist GC: The normal anatomy of the atrial septum in the human heart. *Am Heart J* 1979; 98:194–199.
15. Webster AWI, Smith HJ, Sharpe DN, et al: Patent foramen ovale in young stroke patients. *Lancet* 1988; 2:11–12.
16. Lechat P, Mass LJ, Laschault G, et al: Prevalence of patent foramen ovale in patients with stroke. *N Engl J Med* 1988; 318:1148–1152.
17. Lynch JJ, Schuchard GH, Gross CM, et al: Prevalence of right-to-left atrial shunting in a healthy population: Detection by Valsalva maneuver contrast echocardiography. *Am J Cardiol* 1984; 53:1478–1480.
18. Harvey JR, Teague SM, Anderson JL, et al: Clinically silent atrial septal defects with evidence for cerebral embolization. *Ann Intern Med* 1986; 105:695–697.
19. Hagen PT, Scholz DG, Edwards WD: Incidence and size of patent foramen ovale during the first 10 decades of life: An autopsy study of 965 normal hearts. *Mayo Clin Proc* 1984; 59:17–20.
20. Strunk BL, Cheitlin MD, Stulbarg MS, et al: Right-to-left interatrial shunting through a patent foramen ovale despite normal intracardiac pressures. *Am J Cardiol* 1987; 60:413–415.
21. Mügge A, Daniel WG, Klopper JW, et al: Visualization of patent foramen ovale by transesophageal color-coded Doppler echocardiography. *Am J Cardiol* 1988; 62:837–838.
22. Mehta RH, Helmcke F, Nanda NC, et al: Transesophageal Doppler color flow mapping assessment of atrial septal defect. *J Am Coll Cardiol* 1990; 16:1010–1016.
23. Hanrath P, Schlüter M, Langenstein BA, et al: Detection of ostium secundum atrial septal defects by transesophageal cross-sectional echocardiography. *Br Heart J* 1983; 49:350–358.
24. Kronzon I, Tunick PA, Freedberg RS, et al: Transesophageal echocardiography is superior to transthoracic echocardiography in the diagnosis of sinus venosus atrial septal defect. *J Am Coll Cardiol* 1991; 17:537–542.
25. Zenker G, Erbel R, Kramer G, et al: Transesophageal two-dimensional echocardiography in young patients with cerebral ischemic events. *Stroke* 1988; 19:345–348.
26. Falk RH: PFO or UFO? The role of a patent foramen ovale in cryptogenic stroke. *Am Heart J* 1991; 121:1264–1266.
27. Camp AD, Pearson AC, Sullivan NA, et al: Evaluation of patients with transesophageal echocardiography following cerebral ischemia: Followup experience (abstract) *J Am Coll Cardiol* 1991; 17:315.
28. Aschenberg W, Schlüter M, Kremer P, et al: Transesophageal two-dimensional echocardiography for the detection of left atrial appendage thrombus. *J Am Coll Cardiol* 1986; 7:163–166.
29. Chen YT, Kan MN, Chen JS, et al: Transesophageal two-dimensional echocardiography for detection of left atrial masses. *Am J Noninvas Cardiol* 1989; 3:337–341.
30. Taams MA, Gussenhoven EJ, Lancee CT: Left atrial vascularised thrombus diagnosed by transesophageal

cross sectional echocardiography. *Br Heart J* 1987; 58:669–671.

31. Mügge A, Daniel WG, Hausmann D, et al: Diagnosis of left atrial appendage thrombi by transesophageal echocardiography: Clinical implications and follow-up. *Am J Card Imaging* 1990; 4:173–179.
32. Kronzon I, Tunick PA, Glassman E, et al: Transesophageal echocardiography to detect atrial clots in candidates for percutaneous transseptal mitral balloon valvuloplasty. *J Am Coll Cardiol* 1990; 16:1320–1322.
33. Pop G, Sutherland GR, Koudstaal PJ, et al: Transesophageal echocardiography in the detection of intracardiac embolic sources in patients with transient ischemic attacks. *Stroke* 1990; 21:560–565.
34. Shrestha NK, Moreno FL, Narciso FV, et al: Two-dimensional echocardiographic diagnosis of left atrial thrombus in rheumatic heart disease. *Circulation* 1983; 67:341–347.
35. Dall'Aglio V, Nicolosi GL, Zanuttini D: Transthoracic and transesophageal echocardiographic documentation of disappearance of massive right atrial and pulmonary artery thromboemboli after fibrinolytic therapy and normalization of left ventricular dimensions and function. *Eur Heart J* 1990; 11:863–865.
36. Iliceto S, Antonelli G, Sorino M, et al: Dynamic intracavitary left atrial echoes in mitral stenosis. *Am J Cardiol* 1985; 55:603–606.
37. Castello R, Pearson AC, Labovitz AJ: Prevalence and clinical implications of atrial spontaneous contrast in patients undergoing transesophageal echocardiography. *Am J Cardiol* 1990; 65:1149–1153.
38. Beppu S, Nimura Y, Sakakibara H, et al: Smoke-like echo in the left atrial cavity in mitral valve disease: Its features and significance. *J Am Coll Cardiol* 1985; 6:744–749.
39. Daniel WG, Nellessen U, Schroder E, et al: Left atrial spontaneous echo contrast in mitral valve disease: An indicator for an increased thromboembolic risk. *J Am Coll Cardiol* 1988; 11:1204–1211.
40. Erbel R, Stern H, Ehrenthal W, et al: Detection of spontaneous echocardiographic contrast within the left atrium by transesophageal echocardiography: Spontaneous echocardiographic contrast. *Clin Cardiol* 1986; 9:245–252.
41. Mahony C, Sublett KL, Harrison MR: Resolution of spontaneous contrast with platelet disaggregatory therapy (trifluoperazine). *Am J Cardiol* 1989; 63:1009–1010.
42. Karalis DG, Chandrasekaran K, Victor MF, et al: Recognition and embolic potential of intraaortic atherosclerotic debris. *J Am Coll Cardiol* 1991; 17:73–78.
43. Tunick PA, Culliford AT, Lamparello PJ, et al: Atheromatosis of the aortic arch as an occult source of multiple systemic emboli. *Ann Intern Med* 1991; 114:391–392.
44. Tunick PA, Kronzon I: Protruding atherosclerotic plaque in the aortic arch of patients with systemic embolization: A new finding seen by transesophageal echocardiography. *Am Heart J* 1990; 120:658–660.
45. Cerebral Embolism Task Force: Cardiogenic brain embolism. *Arch Neurol* 1986; 43:71–84.
46. Kannel WB, Abbott RD, Savage DD, et al: Epidemiologic features of chronic atrial fibrillation. *N Engl J Med* 1982; 306:1018–1022.
47. Wolf PA, Abbott RD, Kannel WB: Atrial fibrillation: A major contributor to stroke in the elderly. *Arch Intern Med* 1987; 147:1561–1564.
48. Petersen P, Boysen G, Godtfredsen J, et al: Placebo-controlled, randomised trial of warfarin and aspirin for prevention of thromboembolic complications in chronic atrial fibrillation. *Lancet* 1989; 1:175–179.
49. The SPAF investigators: Preliminary report of the Stroke Prevention in Atrial Fibrillation study. *N Engl J Med* 1990; 322:863–868.
50. The Boston Area Anticoagulation Trial for Atrial Fibrillation Investigators: The effect of low-dose warfarin on the risk of stroke in patients with nonrheumatic atrial fibrillation. *N Engl J Med* 1990; 323:1505–1511.
51. Mügge A, Daniel WG, Frank G, et al: Echocardiography in the infective endocarditis: Reassessment of prognostic implications of vegetation size determined by the transthoracic and the transesophageal approach. *J Am Coll Cardiol* 1989; 14:631–638.
52. Meltzer RS, Visser CA, Fuster V: Intracardiac thrombi and systemic embolization. *Ann Intern Med* 1986; 105:689–698.
53. Stoddard MF, Pearson AC, Kanter KR, et al: Left ventricular thrombus with normal left ventricular wall motion in a patient with myelofibrosis. *Am Heart J* 1989; 117:966–968.
54. Love BB, Struck LK, Stanford W, et al: Comparison of two-dimensional echocardiography and ultrafast cardiac computed tomography for evaluating intracardiac thrombi in cerebral ischemia. *Stroke* 1990; 21:1033–1038.
55. Fagan LF, Castello R, Barner H, et al: Transesophageal echocardiographic diagnosis of recurrent right ventricular myxoma two years after excision of right atrial myxoma. *Am Heart J* 1990; 120:1456–1458.
56. Kuecherer HF, Lee E, Schiller NB: Enhanced detection of intracardiac masses by transesophageal echocardiography. *Am J Card Imaging* 1990; 4:180–186.
57. Daniel LB, Grigg LE, Weisel RD, et al: Comparison of transthoracic and transesophageal assessment of prosthetic valve dysfunction. *Echocardiography* 1990; 7:83–95.

Chapter 5

Assessment of Native and Prosthetic Valves

Hugh A. McCann, M.D.

Howard C. Dittrich, M.D.

As medical therapies and surgical techniques become increasingly more sophisticated, the demands for diagnostic accuracy expand accordingly. The refinement in transducer technology and improvement in ultrasonic imaging systems have resulted in the relatively widespread application of transesophageal echocardiography (TEE) in medical practice.[1] The precise role of TEE in the clinical evaluation of some pathologic entities is still being assessed, while in some other conditions, such as acute aortic dissection, the procedure has already become the diagnostic "gold standard."[2] The inherent safety of the procedure has encouraged its wide clinical application.[3, 4] With the development of the biplane transesophageal probe[5] and, more recently, the omniplane probe,[6] it is difficult to predict with confidence the eventual extent of the procedure's clinical application. It is already clear, however, that TEE is a major advance in the diagnosis and characterization of valvular heart disease.

Indeed, few other clinical entities, if any, have enjoyed the benefit of TEE's improved spatial resolution and clearer anatomic depiction more than the assessment of native and prosthetic cardiac valves. The reasons for this are essentially fourfold. First, the proximity of the transducer to the region of interest (namely, the cardiac valves) allows for the utilization of a high-frequency, near-focused transducer, which greatly improves spatial resolution and image clarity. Second, the unique spatial relationship of the probe in the lower portion of the esophagus to the valves facilitates the assessment of clinical issues that were heretofore not satisfactorily described (such as regurgitant jets associated with dysfunctional prosthetic valves in the mitral position). Third, the transesophageal window obviates the comparatively long pathway traveled by the ultrasonic impulse from the precordial window to the structure of interest and back to the transducer, which is associated with signal attenuation, shadowing, and complex interactions between ultrasound and biologic tissues. All of these phenomena may conspire to mislead the diagnostician because of artifact, missing data, or poor spatial resolution in the distal field. This can be particularly frustrating in the assessment of valvular anatomy and function. Finally, TEE has the advantage of virtually ensuring adequate visualization of cardiac structures, which may simply not be feasible from the precordial windows in a substantial proportion of patients because of poor acoustic access.

ASSESSMENT OF NATIVE VALVES

Vegetations

Echocardiography is now recognized as the procedure of choice for the noninvasive assessment of valvular morphology, most notably for valvular vegetations. The superiority of TEE over transthoracic echocardiography (TTE) has been unequivocally established by the study of Erbel et al.,[7] which prospectively evaluated 96 patients with suspected endocarditis and 70 controls. These investigators showed a measured sensitivity of 63% and 100% in identifying vegetations for TTE and TEE, respectively. The specificity was 98% and 98%, the positive predictive value was 92% and 95%, and the negative predictive value was 91% and 100%, respectively. The main advantage of TEE over TTE was seen in vegetations of less than 11 mm in diameter. In those patients with lesions of 6 to 10 mm in diameter, TTE had a sensitivity of 69% (9 of 13 lesions), while that of TEE was 100%. In lesions less than 6 mm, the sensitivity of TTE fell to 25% (6 of 24 lesions) as compared with 100% for TEE. Despite a bias in patient selection toward those patients proceeding to surgery, this study clearly established the superior sensitivity of TEE for small vegetations.

Mügge et al.[8] also found TEE to be more sensitive than TTE in identifying vegetations (90% vs. 58% in patients subsequently undergoing surgery or necropsy) but also showed that the superior resolution of TEE in accurately describing the vegetations' size, site, and shape was important because those patients with a vegetation diameter of greater than 10 mm had a significantly higher incidence of embolic events than did those with a vegetation diameter of 10 mm or less (47% vs. 19%). Vegetation size did not vary significantly in patients with or without heart failure or in patients dying or surviving during acute endocarditis.

More recently, Schively and coworkers[9] reported a prospective study in which they compared TEE with TTE in 66 episodes of suspected endocarditis in 62 patients. The echocardiographic results were compared with the presence or absence of endocarditis determined by pathologic or nonechocardiographic data from the subsequent clinical course. Ultimately, the diagnosis of endocarditis was made in 16 of the 66 episodes. In 7 of 16 TTE and 15 of 16 TEE examinations endocarditis was diagnosed. This resulted in a sensitivity rate for TTE of 44% and TEE of 94% ($P < .01$). The overall specificity of TTE was found to be 98%, while that of TEE was 100%. With regard to specific valves, their data suggested that TEE provided superior imaging of mitral and aortic leaflets when compared with TTE. On the other hand, no important difference was shown for imaging of the tricuspid valve by the two techniques. This study was done by using single-plane technology, and as a consequence, no information concerning the pulmonic valve was obtained. With the addition of biplane imaging, the overall sensitivities of TEE for all valves may ultimately improve further.

The authors concluded that the high diagnostic sensitivity of TEE helps define patients with a low probability of the disease when the study yields negative results, especially in those patients with only an intermediate likelihood of endocarditis by clinical criteria.

Pulmonic Valve

The pulmonic valve is seldom adequately seen from the transverse plane, but it is more readily seen when viewed from the longitudinal (see Fig 2–13) plane, where vegetations are best identified (Fig 5–1) and are often accompanied by some degree of color flow insufficiency.

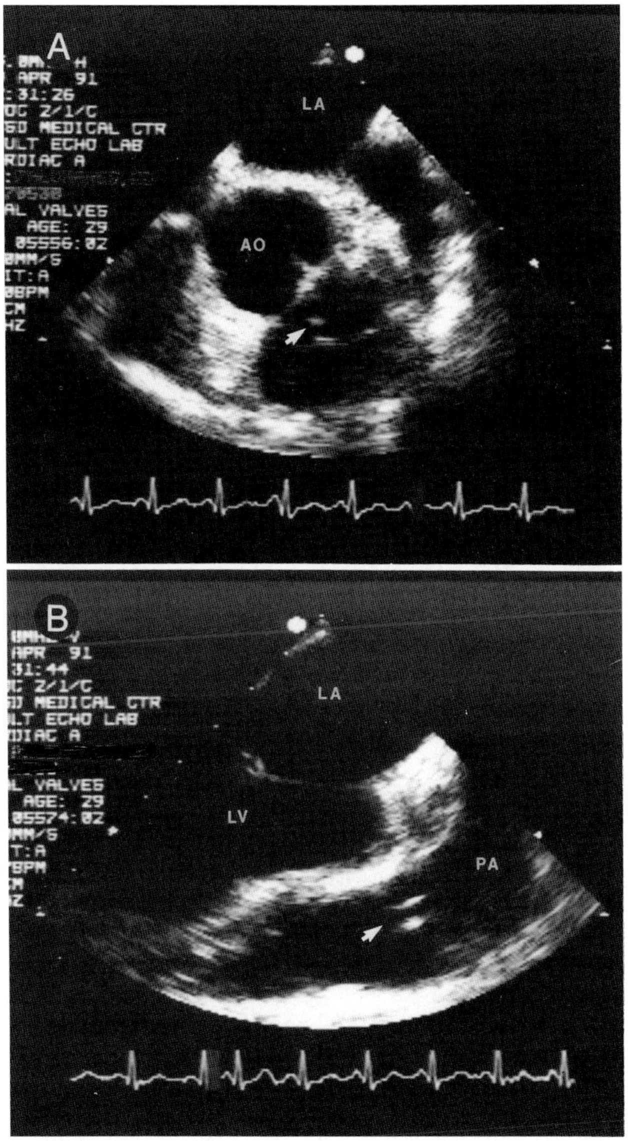

FIG 5–1.
The transverse plane **(A)** demonstrates an echo density on the pulmonic valve *(arrow)* in a patient with prior pulmonic valve endocarditis. The longitudinal plane **(B)** more clearly demonstrates the vegetation *(arrow)*. *AO* = aorta; *LA* = left atrium; *LV* = left ventricle; *PA* = pulmonary artery.

Tricuspid Valve

Vegetations of the tricuspid valve can be well seen, especially when arising from the posterior or septal leaflets (Fig 5–2). Anterior leaflet vegetations often require evaluation from the transgastric transverse short-axis view or the longitudinal plane obtained at the base (see Fig 2–17). Evaluation of tricuspid valve vegetations from the four-chamber transverse view can be made extremely difficult by a dilated aortic root, aortic valve calcification, or the presence of a prosthesis in the aortic position. All of these can obscure visualization of the tricuspid leaflets because of anatomic distortion (in the former case) or attenuation of the signal (in the latter two situations).

Mitral Valve

Vegetations on the mitral valve are in general easily seen, especially from the transverse four-chamber and longitudinal two-chamber views (Fig 5–3). The latter view in particular allows for careful evaluation of the subvalvular apparatus where smaller vegetations may exist. A potentially difficult area to assess for vegetations is the ventricular aspect of the posterior leaflet base, a region sometimes shielded by the leaflet, particularly if calcified. The longitudinal two-chamber view corresponds well to the parasternal long-axis view, the best view for assessing leaflet redundancy and mitral valve prolapse.[10] This view can be utilized to assess mitral

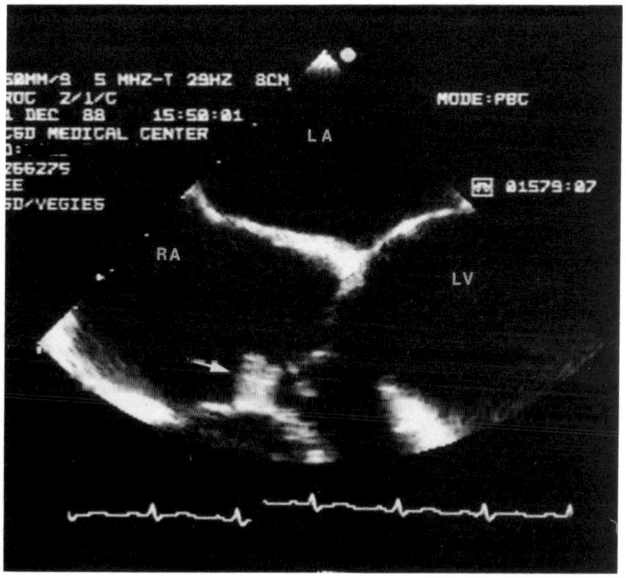

FIG 5–2.
Tricuspid valve vegetation. A large growth *(arrow)* is seen principally on the right atrial *(RA)* aspect of the tricuspid valve. Although the vegetation was seen from the surface echo, this transverse four-chamber view provides vastly superior images of the vegetation. *LA* = left atrium; *LV* = left ventricle.

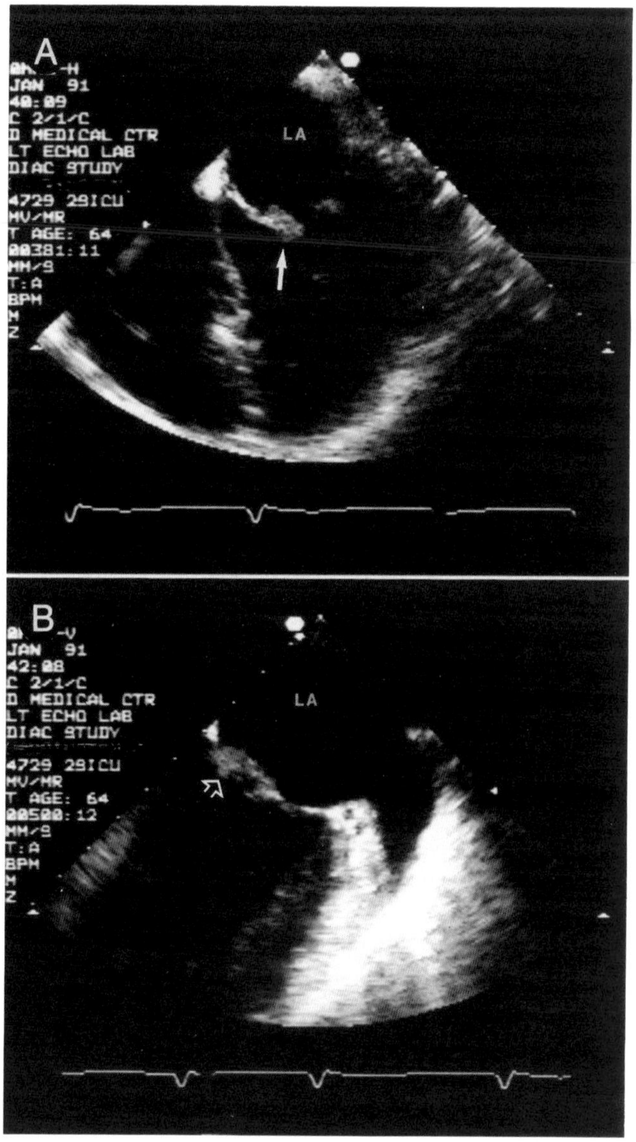

FIG 5–3.
Shown are mitral valve vegetations on both the anterior *(closed arrow)* and the posterior *(open arrow)* mitral valve leaflets. The transverse plane **(A)** demonstrates the anterior vegetation better, while the horizontal plane **(B)** is preferred for posterior leaflet vegetations. *LA* = left atrium.

anatomy with regard to redundancy and prolapse. However, our experience has been that the transesophageal window offers little advantage over the precordial window in this situation, and we do not consider assessment for the presence of mitral valve prolapse to be an indication for TEE.

Aortic Valve

Vegetations of the aortic valve are well seen, although the left coronary cusp sometimes evades thorough examination. More importantly, a tangential course through the left coronary cusp can sometimes give the appearance of a vegetation or "pseudomass" effect (see Fig 3–4). These normal findings, not previously well visualized with TTE, point out the need to adjust one's threshold for reading vegetations, etc. In addition, Lambdl's excrescence, a normal thickening of the raphe of the aortic cusp in the elderly, can appear quite dramatic. In addition to the improved sensitivity of TEE in detecting vegetations when present, the higher resolution can offer other advantages in a qualitative sense. In one patient in whom a mass suggestive of a vegetation was seen on precordial echo, TEE confirmed its presence but showed that the homogeneous appearance was atypical for vegetation (Fig 5–4). The patient subsequently underwent surgery for recurrent pulmonary emboli, and a thrombus was removed from the valve. All cultures were negative, and the patient was ultimately found to have an antithrombin III deficiency, the obvious substrate for her recurrent thromboembolism and valve thrombosis.

Paravalvular Disease

In addition to abnormal mass echoes, TEE can also demonstrate abnormalities in anatomy such as ring abscesses, mycotic lesions, sinus of Valsalva aneurysms, or even valve destruction,[11] and the detailed anatomic description of endocarditis and its complications (e.g., flail leaflet) has been well described.[12, 13] Our experience[14] has been that TEE often yields valuable anatomic information regarding the presence of paravalvular pathology such as an abscess, fistula, aneurysm, or membrane. These abnormalities were frequently not appreciated on the precordial study and had a major impact on clinical decision making and patient management.

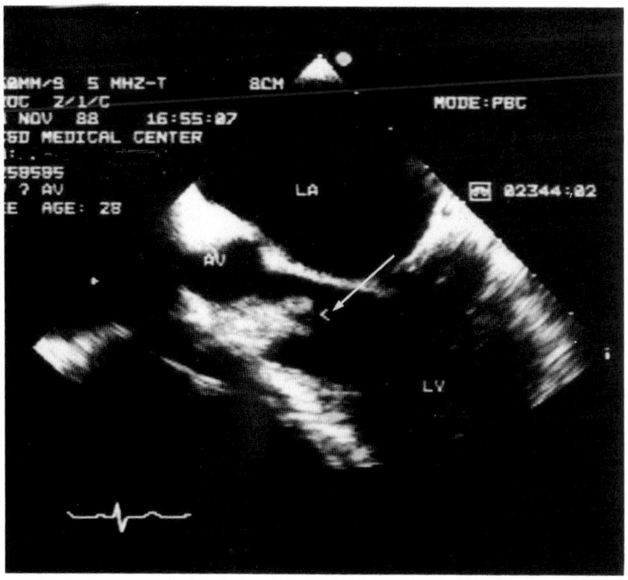

FIG 5–4.
This large, homogeneous vegetation of the aortic valve *(arrow)* was seen on a routine preoperative precordial study. The study was not of sufficient quality to assess the atypical appearance of the vegetation, which was subsequently found to be a thrombus secondary to a hypercoagulable state. (See the text for details.) *AV* = aortic valve; *LA* = left atrium; *LV* = left ventricle.

These findings were recently confirmed by Daniel et al.,[15] who found TEE's sensitivity in the detection of abscess far superior to TTE (87% vs. 28%). Paravalvular abscesses were more commonly associated with aortic endocarditis. The clinical importance of making the diagnosis of paravalvular abscess when present was emphasized by the higher mortality in patients with abscess formation (23% vs. 14% in-hospital mortality). The para-aortic abscess is very frequently located between the noncoronary cusp and intervalvular fibrosa (Fig 5–5). This may be due to the relative absence of coronary blood flow to "drain" the sinus of infected material in this location.[16] This area is difficult to thoroughly evaluate from the precordium. The TEE probe is ideally located to evaluate this area of the aortic root. Even in the presence of a heavily calcified native valve or prosthetic valve, the region of interest is proximal to the attenuating structures and can therefore still be effectively interrogated in these situations.

Sometimes infection in this area has caused the development of a sinus of Valsalva aneurysm, which can also be well seen and interrogated for the presence of any fistulas or connections to other cardiac structures. Although the presence of a fistula created by erosion through to the left atrium (Fig 5–6) or, more frequently, the right atrium can also be seen by color flow Doppler imaging from TTE,[17] the transesophageal images are superior for precise definition of the pathology involved.

Finally, subvalvular structures such as membranes or fibrous ridges can be seen by precordial echo but are much better evaluated from the transesophageal window. Specific data regarding the attachment of the membrane to the aortic leaflets and other anatomic details that are important in the surgical planning as corrective procedures are clearly visible from the transesophageal window but cannot be adequately assessed from precordial studies or angiographic images (Fig 5–7).

Regurgitation

Combined echocardiography and Doppler color flow mapping from transthoracic imaging windows

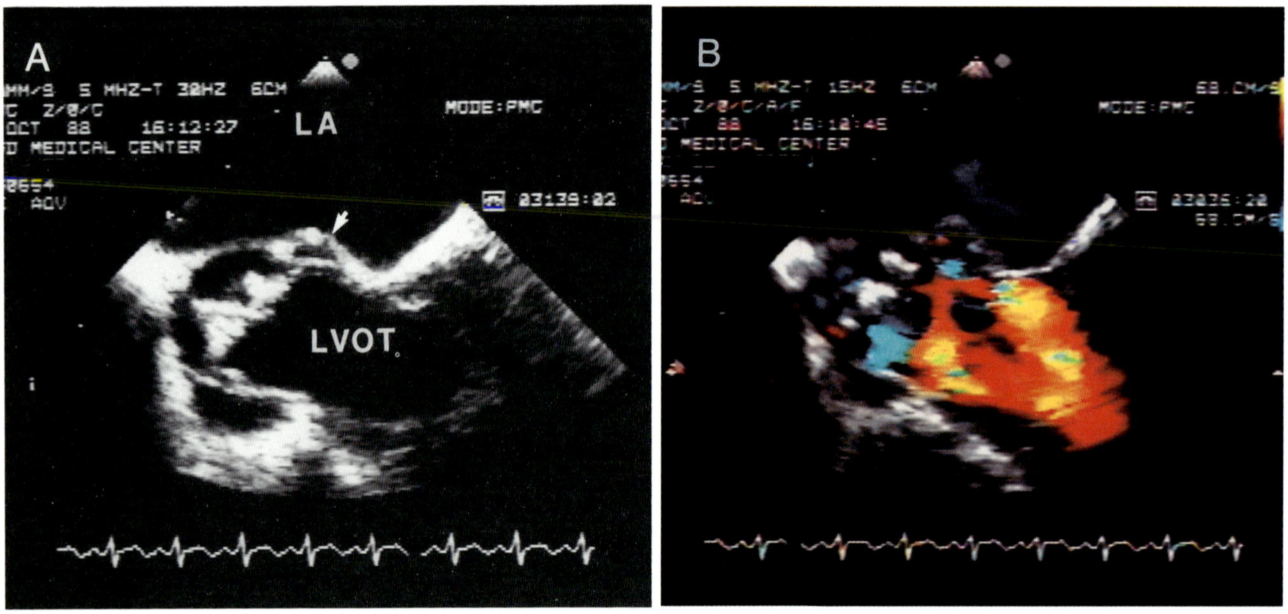

FIG 5–5.
A, an aortic valve shows large vegetations and a paravalvular abscess *(arrow)* in the fibrous region between the aortic and mitral valves. **B,** color flow Doppler in systole demonstrates some flow into the abscess cavity. The individual in this case had persistent fevers despite adequate antibiotics for a sensitive organism. *LA* = left atrium; *LVOT* = left ventricular outflow tract. (From Dittrich HC, et al: *Am J Cardiol* 1990; 66:758–761. Used by permission.)

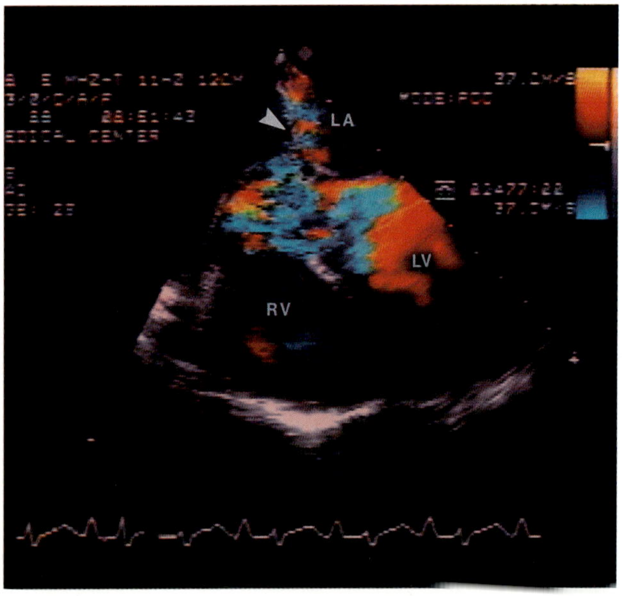

FIG 5–6.
A systolic frame from the transverse plane demonstrates a fistulous communication between the left ventricular outflow tract immediately below the aortic valve and the left atrium *(LA)*. The systolic color flow jet *(arrowhead)* was mistakenly thought to represent an eccentric mitral regurgitant jet on transthoracic echo. *LV* = left ventricle; *RV* = right ventricle. (From Dittrich HC, et al: *Am J Cardiol* 1990; 66:758–761. Used by permission.)

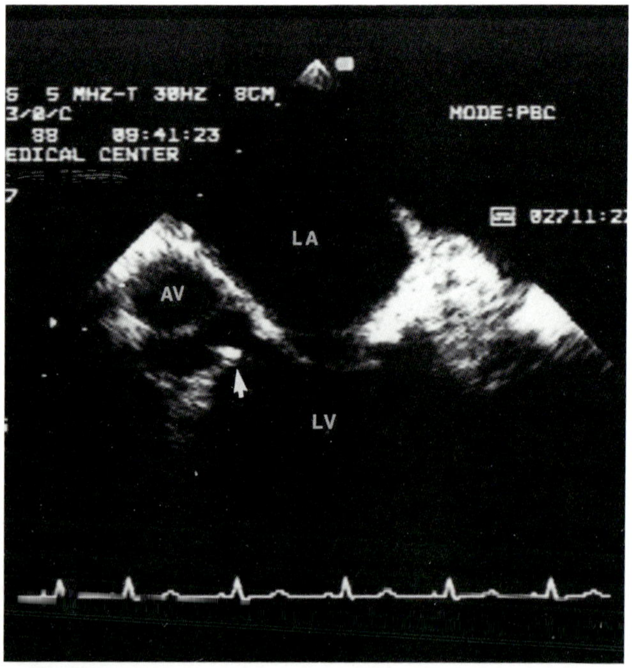

FIG 5–7.
A transverse plane through the left ventricular outflow tract demonstrates a subvalvular membrane *(arrow)* with a faint filamentous communication to the aortic valve *(AV)*. In real time, several filamentous communications were noted between the subvalvular membrane and the aortic valve. This information was valuable at the time of surgery for this congenital defect. *LA* = left atrium; *LV* = left ventricle.

is the standard method for noninvasive assessment of valvular regurgitation. A comparison of regurgitant jet size by TEE and TTE shows that more regurgitant lesions are seen from the transesophageal window for mitral, aortic, and tricuspid valves.[18] Although the overall correlation between maximal jet areas determined by TEE and TTE was good (r = 0.85; SEE = 2.8 cm^2), there was a systematic overestimation by the transesophageal technique. The same caveats that apply to the quantification of regurgitant lesions by color flow Doppler as seen from the precordial window pertain equally to the transesophageal window, namely, variations in loading conditions, the inherent error involved in tomographic sampling of a complex three-dimensional entity, and alterations in compliance of the receiving chamber. Although these obvious potential pitfalls persist for transesophageal imaging as they do for transthoracic echo, underestimation because of image attenuation, incomplete sampling of eccentric jets due to poor visualization, or poor signals because of poor image quality are for the large part overcome by TEE. The tendency, however, is to overestimate the severity of the regurgitation for the reasons described above. One must therefore be careful in labeling a regurgitant jet seen by color flow from the transesophageal window as pathologic, particularly if the jet is small in area, of low velocity, centrally located, and associated with a morphologically normal appearing valve.

Mitral Regurgitation

Evaluation of the severity of mitral regurgitation is most effectively accomplished by assessing a combination of several factors. Although some individuals have emphasized the importance of the mitral regurgitant color Doppler jet area from either single or biplane technique,[19] others have found this to be the least helpful in terms of quantitation of mitral regurgitation. The transesophageal window, however, does allow detailed interrogation of the left atrium to map the full extent of the regurgitant jet. This can be particularly important in patients with deflected jets along the left atrial wall, in whom the jet size and hence the severity of regurgitation can be seriously underestimated. A wall-hugging mitral regurgitant jet that wraps around the posterior left atrium can often represent a significant amount of mitral regurgitation and yet appear rather small in area from any single plane or virtually missed if the left atrium is not carefully interrogated (Fig 5–8). These jets may represent a much larger volume of mitral regurgitation than a central jet with a narrow base and broad distal component. Seeing a large systolic color jet entering the left atrial appendage often suggests a significant degree of mitral regurgitation (Fig 5–9,A and B). In individuals with relatively normal left ventricular function and no mitral stenosis, the appearance of an area of color flow convergence on the ventricular aspect of the mitral valve suggests a high flow state (Fig 5–9,C). The absence of this flow con-

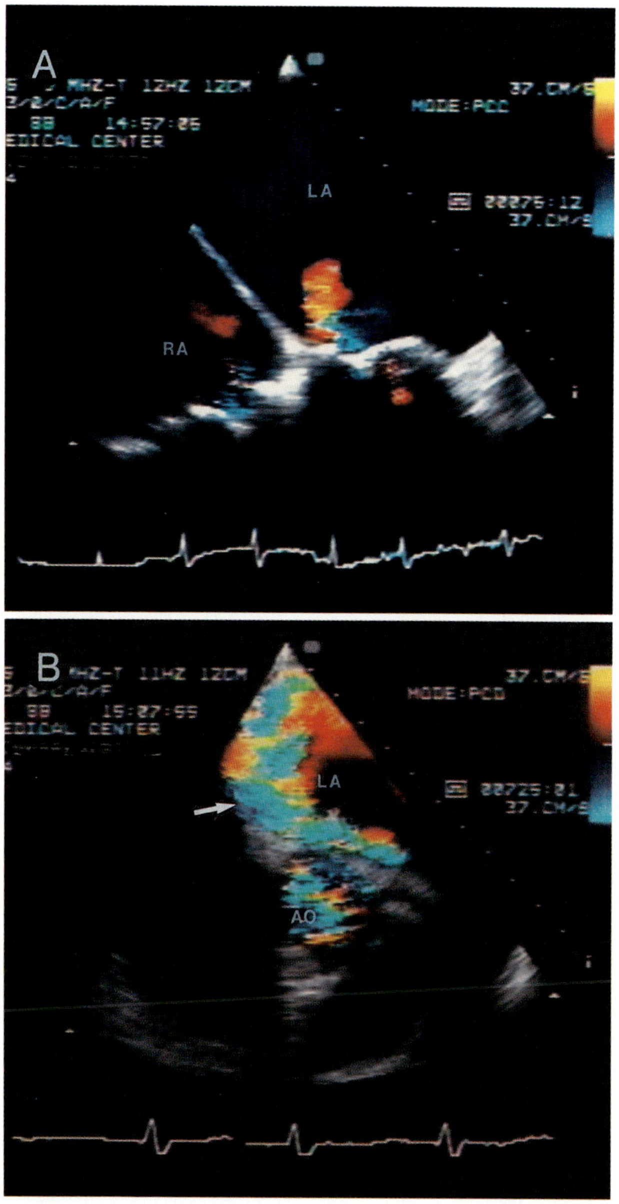

FIG 5–8.
A, a small regurgitant jet was noted when imaging with the transverse plane in the central portion of the valve. **B,** When the probe was withdrawn to the level of the aortic root *(AO)* at the left main coronary artery, a large mitral regurgitant color flow jet *(arrow)* was seen to pass medially and along the interatrial septum. *LA* = left atrium; *RA* = right atrium.

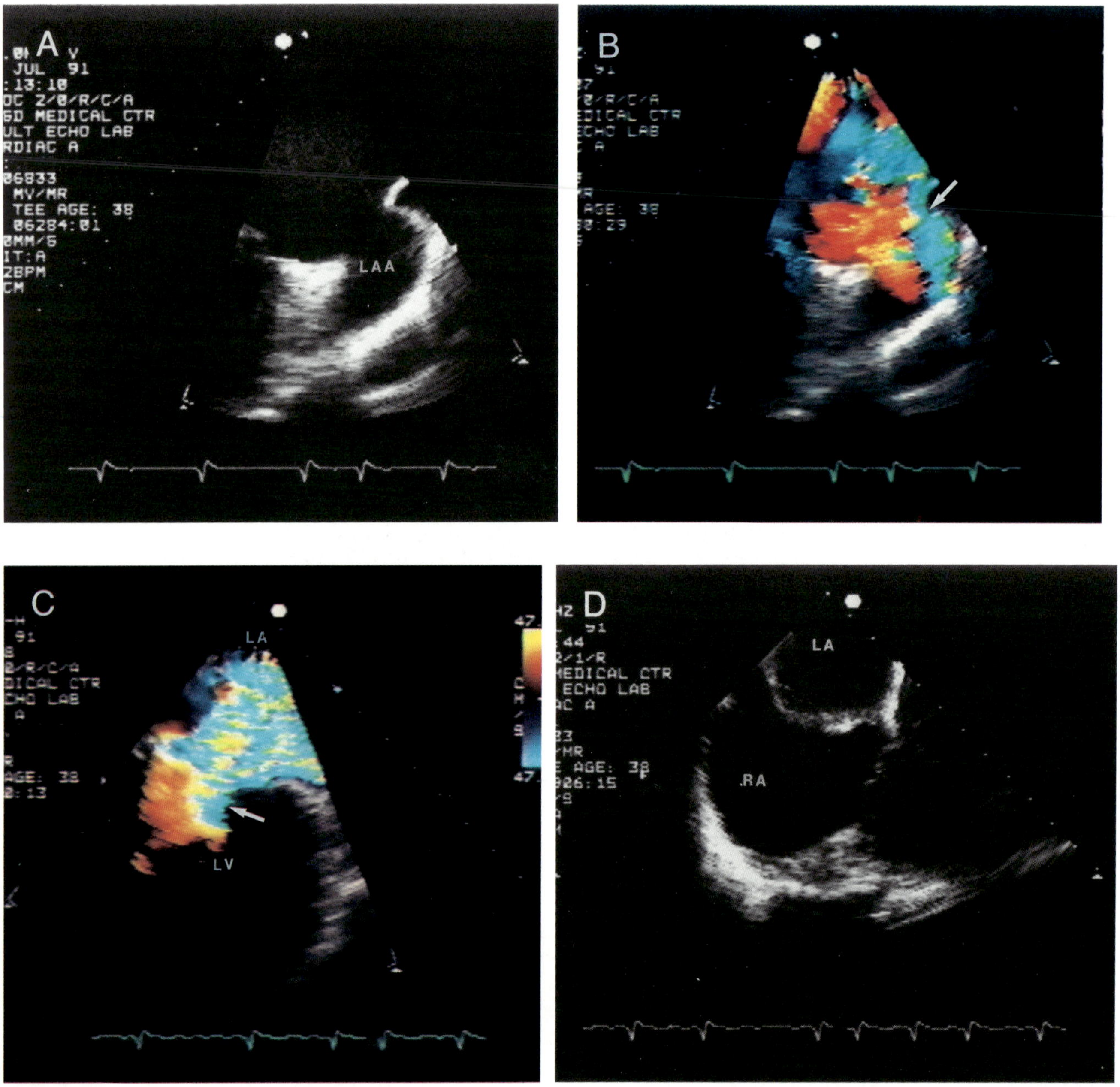

FIG 5–9.
Findings for severe mitral regurgitation: **A,** two-dimensional image of the left atrial appendage *(LAA)* in an individual with severe mitral regurgitation. **B,** systolic flow into the left atrial appendage *(arrow)* is consistent with the finding of severe mitral regurgitation. **C,** the longitudinal two-chamber view demonstrates color flow convergence *(arrow)* on the ventricular aspect of the valve. **D,** pronounced systolic bulging of the interatrial septum into the right atrium *(RA)*. *LA* = left atrium; *LV* = left ventricle.

vergence in the presence of normal left ventricular function almost certainly excludes severe mitral regurgitation.

Other important features in assessing the severity of mitral regurgitation include the presence of systolic expansion of the left atrium, which suggests a significant regurgitant volume. In addition, one will frequently see bulging of the interatrial septum into the right atrium in systole as a consequence of the mitral regurgitant volume causing stretching of the interatrial septum (Fig 5–9,D). Of course, in chronic mitral regurgitation, one would also expect to see a dilated left ventricle with characteristic findings of volume overload.

The pulmonary vein flow characteristics are very helpful in the grading of mitral regurgitation (Fig 5–10). Severe mitral regurgitation can often be excluded if one sees only a low-velocity homogeneous color flow jet within the pulmonary vein. This color Doppler finding coincides with normal pulmonary venous flow velocity from pulsed-wave Doppler (see Fig 2–23,A). Recently, Klein et al. have documented the utility of evaluating the pulmonary venous inflow profile obtained by pulsed-wave Doppler.[20] Systolic reversal of flow and a change in the diastolic portion of the inflow profile has been found to correlate with various grades of mitral regurgitation by angiography (see Fig 9–6). In assessing the pulmonary venous inflow from pulsed-wave Doppler, however, it is important to evaluate more than one pulmonary vein because of the tendency for an eccentric mitral regurgitant jet to disproportionately af-

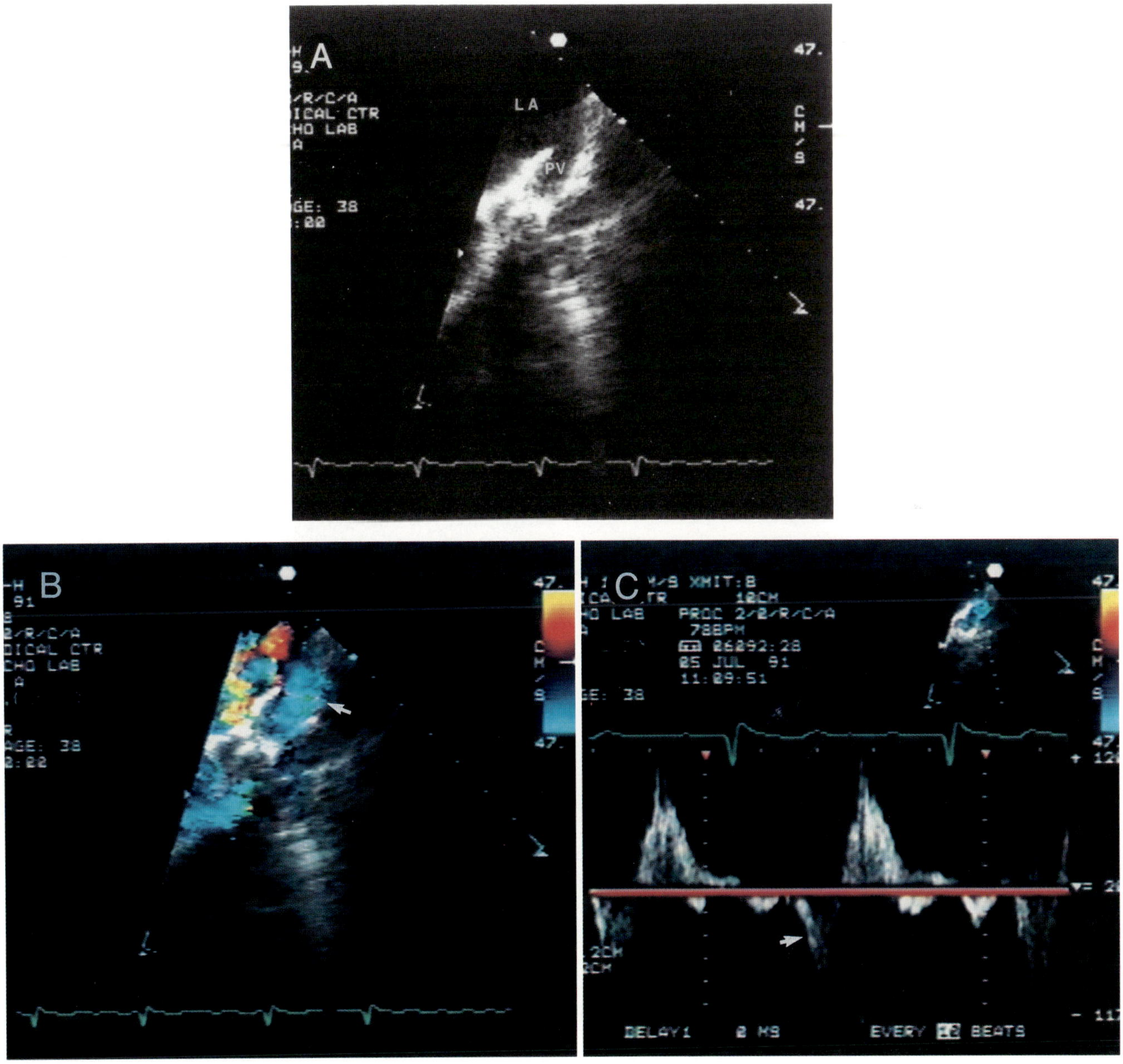

FIG 5–10.
Doppler images of the pulmonary vein in severe mitral regurgitation. **A,** a two-dimensional image of the left upper pulmonary vein *(PV)* emptying into the left atrium *(LA)*. **B,** color Doppler in late systole demonstrates flow reversal *(arrow)* consistent with severe mitral regurgitation. **C,** pulsed-wave Doppler in the left upper pulmonary vein demonstrates the systolic reversal *(arrow)* in this individual with severe mitral regurgitation. (Compare with the normal pulmonary venous Doppler findings in Figure 2–23).

fect the pulmonary vein toward which that jet is directed.

Finally, in evaluating for severe mitral regurgitation, one can assess the mitral inflow velocity profile by pulsed-wave Doppler (see Fig 2–25,A). This mitral inflow profile is influenced by various factors including the transmitral pressure gradient, preload, atrial-ventricular timing, and left ventricular diastolic function. In general, however, one seldom will find a profile with A-wave dominance in the presence of severe mitral regurgitation.

Therefore, although no single criterion exists that is pathognomonic of severe mitral regurgitation, the combination of findings described above will usually allow one to assess the severity of regurgitation with confidence. The utility of TEE for the assessment of mitral valve repair is discussed thoroughly in Chapter 9.

Aortic Insufficiency

The main advantage of TEE over a conventional precordial study in the assessment of insufficiency of the aortic valve is the additional information one can obtain regarding the nature and extent of valvular destruction associated with the regurgitant leak. This includes the determination of whether the jet is valvular or paravalvular in origin and the prognostic significance of the discovery of paravalvular pathology (see above under "Paravalvular Disease"). Indeed, if anything, the guidelines for the quantification of aortic insufficiency from the transesophageal window are less well established than the precordial window where pressure half-time[21] and jet width[22] at the valve have been found useful. One useful maneuver, however, in the assessment of insufficiency of the aortic valve by TEE is to interrogate the aorta by Doppler to look for diastolic reversal of flow suggestive of significant aortic insufficiency (see Fig 9–14).

Stenosis

The hemodynamic significance of valvular abnormalities can be partially assessed by color flow Doppler, which may demonstrate abnormal flow or regurgitation associated with the two-dimensional findings. Because TEE probes did not until recently include continuous-wave Doppler, the Doppler interrogation of cardiac valves heretofore consisted essentially of a detailed color flow description of regurgitant jets (i.e., valvular vs. paravalvular). The inevitable result was that the procedure's value in assessing valvular disease had been founded mainly in the qualitative data obtained from two-dimensional anatomic assessment[23] or the jet's appearance on color flow Doppler.[24] However, it is now reasonable to assume that the addition of continuous-wave Doppler capabilities to new probes will enhance the procedure's clinical value in that quantitative "hemodynamic" data as well as anatomic data and "pseudo-angiographic data" (color flow Doppler) will be acquired. As a consequence, the indications for TEE in valvular heart disease have now expanded to include stenotic lesions (see Fig 9–10).

Mitral Stenosis

TEE is ideally suited for the evaluation of mitral pathology and assessing the degree of its dysfunction (Fig 5–11). A stenotic mitral valve is usually well evaluated from the precordial parasternal window. This is the view routinely used for scoring the degree of pathology in accordance with the Balloon Valvuloplasty Registry criteria. The precordial window, however, has a number of distinct disadvantages. First, the left atrial appendage cannot be examined adequately by TTE. The excellent resolution of the appendage by TEE is well established (see Figs 2–10 through 2–12). Second, the transesophageal window offers an opportunity to examine the interatrial septum prior to attempting a transseptal approach for balloon valvuloplasty. We recently reported the presence of a left atrial myxoma in the fossa ovalis of a patient about to undergo balloon mitral valvuloplasty via the transseptal approach.[25] In this case, the information gained from TEE probably prevented a catastrophic outcome. Third, heavy calcification in the valve can frequently attenuate the ultrasonic signal from the precordial window and cause one to erroneously underestimate the degree of regurgitation. This is obviously an important factor to consider when deciding between balloon valvuloplasty and valve surgery. Finally, the longitudinal plane, which provides a view roughly equivalent to the parasternal long axis (see Fig 2–10,B and C), can add much to the assessment of subvalvular structures. It has therefore been suggested that TEE be performed in all patients being considered for balloon mitral valvuloplasty. The procedure has also met with considerable success in its use as a guide during puncture of the interatrial septum.[26, 27] Finally, TEE has also been used after percutaneous valvuloplasty to assess the echocardiographic and hemodynamic characteristics of atrial septal defects created by the procedure.[28]

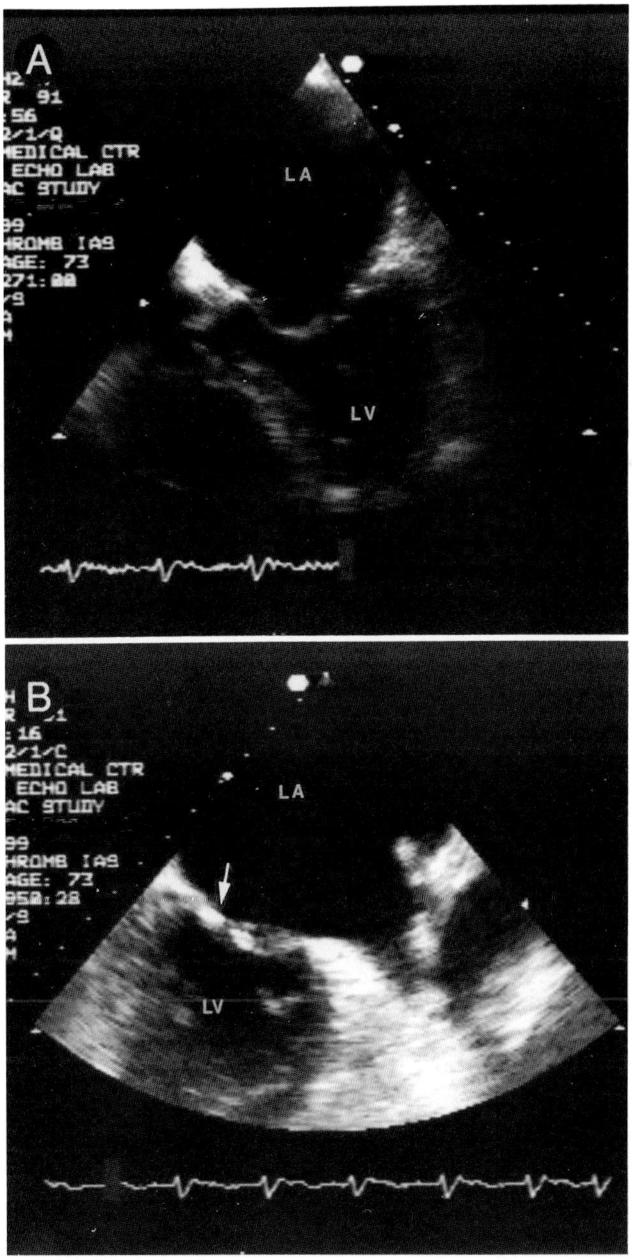

FIG 5–11.
A, the four-chamber transverse plane demonstrates a rheumatic, stenotic mitral valve with doming in late diastole. **B,** the longitudinal plane is superior for defining calcification, particularly in the posterior leaflet *(arrow)*. *LA* = left atrium; *LV* = left ventricle.

Aortic Stenosis

The role of TEE in assessing stenotic aortic valves has been limited because of valve position and orientation[29] and signal attenuation from calcified native or prosthetic structures. Our experience has been that even with prosthetic valves, unique information such as fibrotic deposits or restricted disk motion that was not discernible by TTE can often be appreciated. Obviously, the capabilities provided by continuous-wave Doppler are a major advance in this area, although the angle between the stenotic jet and the Doppler signal may be prohibitive in some cases.

Chandrasekeran et al. have recently described their initial experience with monoplane TEE measurement of the aortic valve area in patients with aortic stenosis.[30] They noted that the required images could be obtained with only moderate transducer manipulation and minimal time. In their population of 95 patients, the authors were able to obtain satisfactory images at the level of the aortic valve, and their correlation coefficients for valve areas measured by the Gorlin equation at cardiac catheterization and the continuity equation by TTE were 0.76 and 0.75 respectively. TEE planimetry consistently overestimated the valve area when compared with catheterization and TTE. This may be due in part to the inability, by monoplane, to obtain the exact minimal valve area. Moreover, the method again would encounter predictable significant limitations in heavily calcified valves where there is signal attenuation or in bicuspid or unicuspid valves where the anatomic distortion would mean that the functional valve orifice could not be represented in one tomographic plane. The procedure would not be feasible in prosthetic valves.

ASSESSMENT OF PROSTHETIC VALVES

The spatial resolution of TEE is most severely tested and can, on occasion, be exceeded when prosthetic valves are evaluated. The procedure's sensitivity in these situations appears to depend to a large degree on the position and orientation of the valve relative to the transducer and its tomographic plane of interrogation. Nellesen et al.[31] and more recently Chan and Walley[32] described shortcomings in the technique to identify cusp tears in bioprosthetic valves. These limitations appear to apply most when the valve prosthesis is situated in the aortic position, in which case attenuation of the ultrasonic signal by the sewing ring causes incomplete leaflet visualization. On the other hand, Nellesen et al.[31] and Taams et al.[24] found TEE to be extremely useful in the evaluation of prosthetic valves in the mitral position. The single most important reason for this is the spatial relationship of the probe to the prosthetic valve, which can attenuate the signal when evaluated from the apical precordial window. This may obviously mask a prosthetic valvular or paravalvular leak or at least cause underestimation of the degree of regurgitation present.

Mitral Prostheses

There is perhaps no other aspect of valvular heart disease where TEE has proved to be such a major diagnostic advance as in the assessment of a dysfunctional prosthesis in the mitral position (Fig 5–12). Valvular or paravalvular leaks are a major complication of prosthetic valves and cannot be adequately assessed from the precordial window.[33] It should be appreciated, however, that all types of normally functioning prosthetic valves have been shown to produce systolic jets in the left atrium by color Doppler from the transesophageal window.[34]

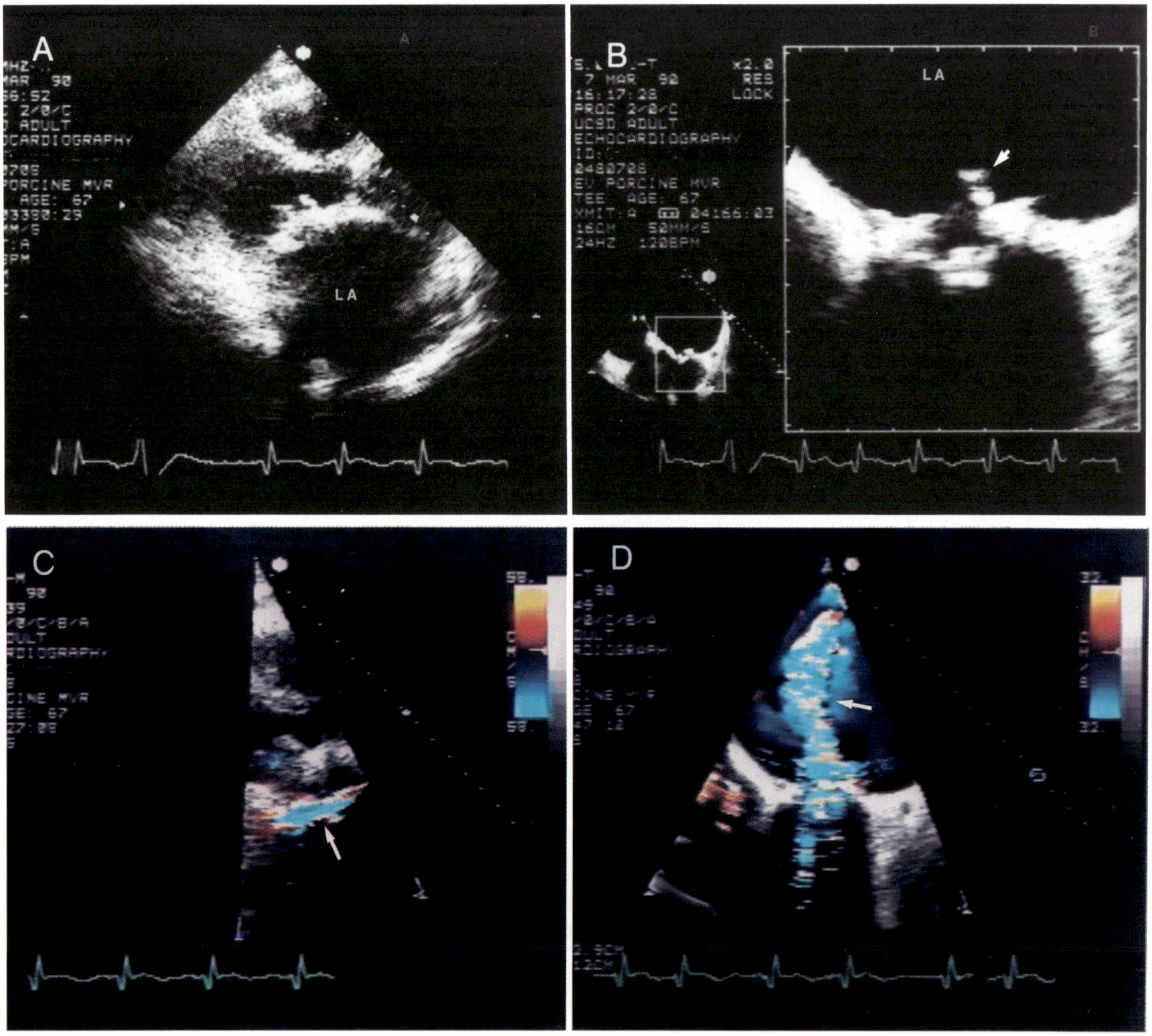

FIG 5–12.
Bioprosthetic mitral valve disease. **A,** a transthoracic image demonstrates a thickened valve with no obvious flail portion. **B,** transverse TEE shows a thickened, flail portion *(arrow)* of a porcine mitral valve. The remainder of the valve is also noted to be thickened. **C,** color Doppler from the transthoracic image demonstrates some color flow in systole, presumably secondary to mitral regurgitation. **D,** a transverse TEE image demonstrates a large color jet of severe mitral regurgitation in this patient with a flail bioprosthesis. *LA* = left atrium.

Each prosthesis type generates its own specific jet pattern. Tilting-disc valves show "closure and leakage backflow" during the entire systolic interval and frequently have more than two jets with an eccentric origin (Fig 5–13). The bileaflet valve (St. Jude) usually has one central jet and two peripheral jets. "Physiologic leaks" are also seen in bioprosthetic valves, although less frequently than with mechanical prostheses, and are usually single and centrally located. Chen et al.[33] found low-velocity, flamelike jets that were small in both length and area in 30% of porcine valves in the mitral position when they were evaluated by TEE. These findings contrast with the experience of Mohr-Kahaly and associates, who saw regurgitant jets of similar size and velocities in 85% of apparently normal porcine prostheses in the mitral position.[35]

Differentiating valvular from perivalvular regur-

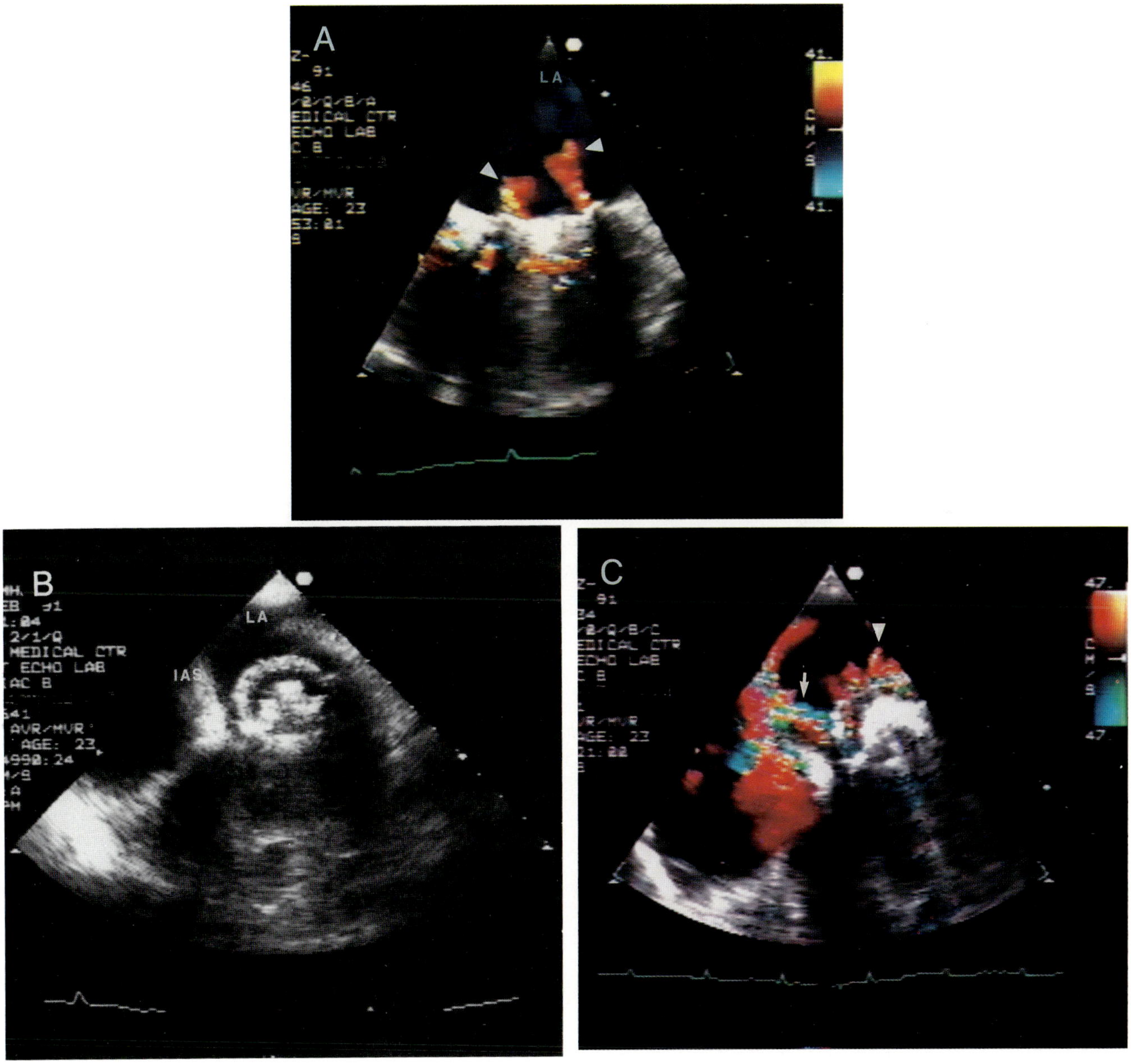

FIG 5–13.
A, transverse-plane image of a Bjørk-Shiley prosthesis seen parallel to the sewing ring. Note the two small color jets *(arrowheads)* normally seen with disc valves. The same prosthesis is imaged obliquely in **B.** Note the round sewing ring and central portion of the prosthesis. **C,** color Doppler demonstrates normal peripheral color jets (*arrowheads*) from a Bjørk-Shiley valve. In addition, a large paravalvular leak *(arrow)* is arising outside the sewing ring and hugging the interatrial septum *(IAS)*. *LA* = left atrium.

gitation is easier with mitral than with aortic prostheses (see Fig 9–16). Both require the combination of color flow and two-dimensional imaging. Freezing a color/two-dimensional image and then electronically removing the color map allows for more precise localization of the color jet relative to the prosthetic ring. In addition, the M/Q-mode, which combines M mode and color flow, helps to localize a paravalvular leak in real time. Khandheria and colleagues studied 50 patients with prosthetic mitral valve disease who underwent confirmatory procedures such as catheterization and surgery.[36] They found that in 48% of these patients TEE demonstrated an abnormality where TTE findings were normal or suboptimal. In 10% of patients, an abscess or vegetation was seen only by TEE. They also found that semiquantitation of the degree of mitral prosthetic regurgitation by TEE is comparable to left ventriculography and superior to TTE. It is important to recognize that semiquantitation of prosthetic regurgitation requires the same careful evaluation of a number of criteria as discussed earlier under native valve regurgitation.

Aortic Prostheses

Our experience has been that although leaflet visualization of prosthetic valves in the aortic position may be incomplete, the procedure is of diagnostic value in the majority of patients.[14] Despite the shadowing produced by the aortic prosthesis, one may see long, filamentous material appear on the aortic side of the valve in systole or in the left ventricular outflow tract side in diastole. In some cases, this material may represent only a small portion of the thrombus in the aortic prosthesis and prove to be the underlying source for the cardiac embolus (Fig 5–14). At other times, the disc(s) of a mechanical valve may be visualized adequately from either the transverse or longitudinal planes, thereby allowing for accurate assessment of clinically important abnormalities (Fig 5–15). In some cases of acute valvular dysfunction secondary to an infectious process, the site of an abnormality may be important and allow for adequate examination by TEE. In these situations, the pathology (abscess, aneurysm, dehiscence, or fistula) often lies in and around the sewing ring, especially near the sinus of Valsalva of the noncoronary cusp or in the mitral-aortic intervalvular fibrosa.[16] All of these pathologies are well seen on TEE. The ability of TEE to differentiate valvular from paravalvular aortic insufficiency in prosthetic valves is certainly an important advantage over surface echo (Fig 5–16), where serious problems have been shown to exist, especially in the case of the Bjørk-Shiley prosthesis.[37] The diagnosis of such periprosthetic pathology has been found by ourselves and others to have a major impact on patient management and prognosis.[14, 15]

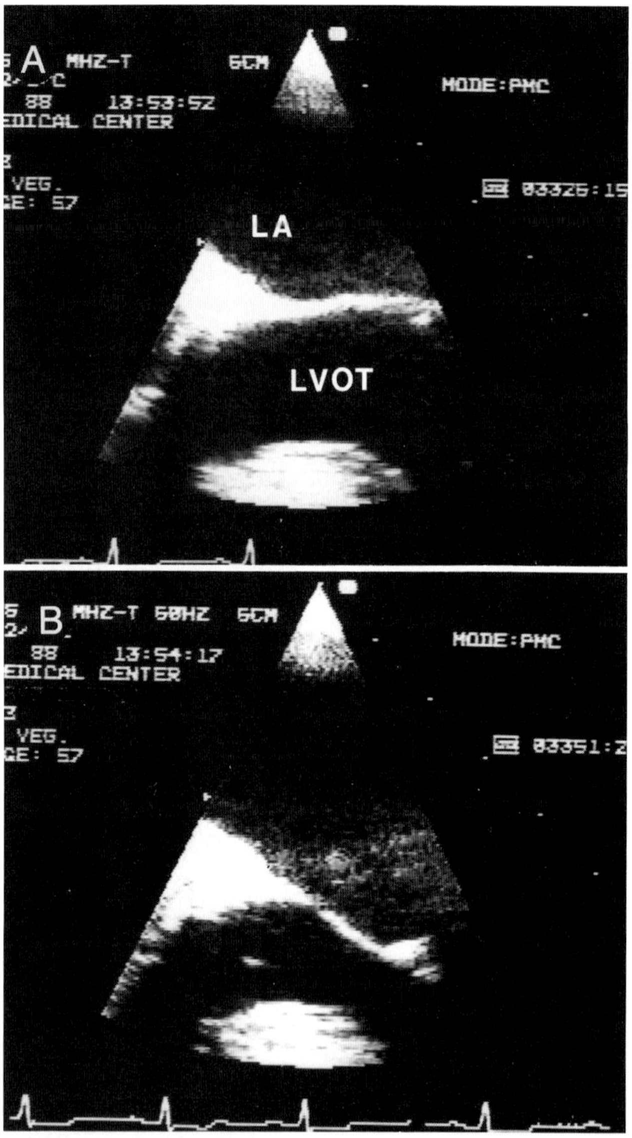

FIG 5–14.
A, a systolic frame demonstrates the left ventricular outflow tract adjacent to a mechanical valve. **B,** during diastole, a serpiginous echodensity appeared in the left ventricular outflow tract, but was found at surgery to represent only a small portion of a large organized thrombus on the mechanical prosthesis. This thrombus had been the source of an embolic event. *LA* = left atrium. (From Dittrich HC, et al: *Am J Cardiol* 1990; 66:758–761. Used by permission.)

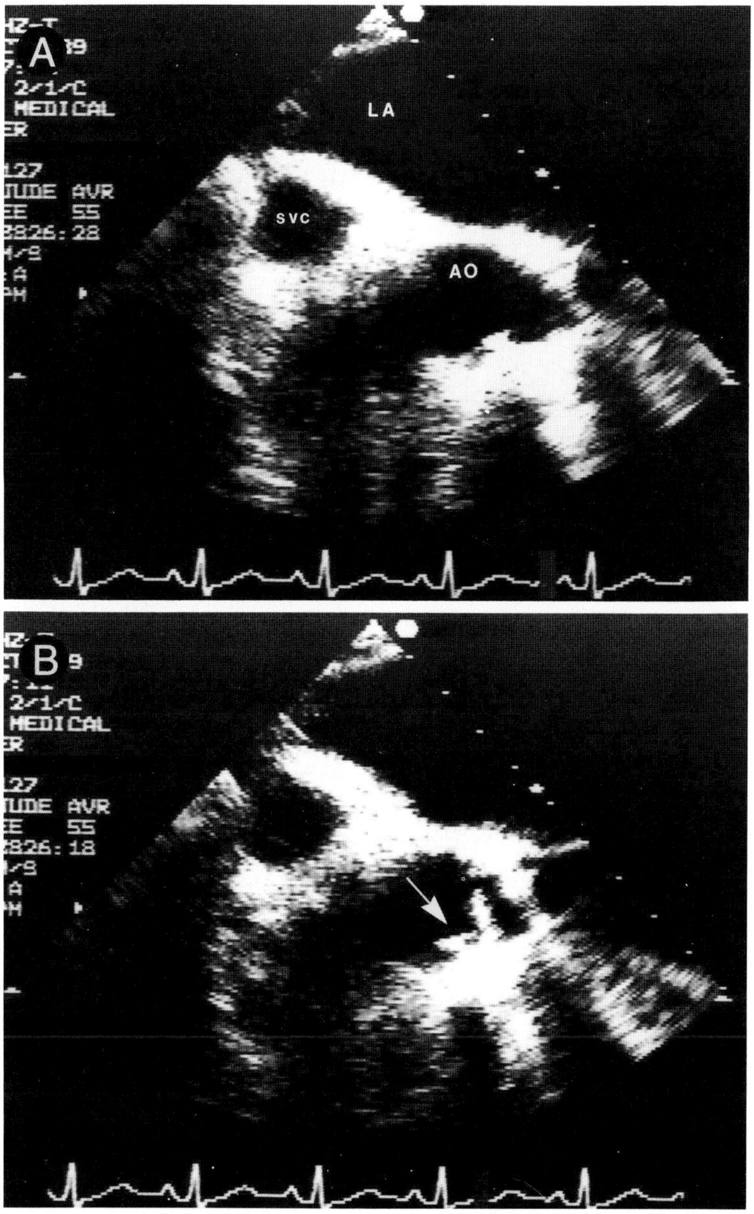

FIG 5–15.
In diastole **(A)** a portion of a closed St. Jude valve is seen in the aorta *(AO)*. During midsystole **(B)** the valve is only partially open, especially one disc *(arrow)* that has moved little when compared with its position in diastole. This patient was found at surgery to have a significant thrombus limiting the opening of both discs and producing clinically significant prosthetic aortic stenosis. *LA* = left atrium. *SVC* = superior vena cava. (From Dittrich HC, et al: *Am J Cardiol* 1990; 66:758–761. Used by permission.)

NEW APPLICATIONS

More recently, several investigators have begun to capitalize on the resolution of TEE to study pathophysiologic phenomena that have hitherto been controversial. Grigg et al.[38] recently studied 32 consecutive patients with hypertrophic cardiomyopathy and documented outflow tract gradients (82 ± 37 mm Hg). Analysis of mitral valve structure and function showed that the patients with obstructive hypertrophic cardiomyopathy had longer mitral valve leaflets, with contact between the anterior leaflet and septum and incomplete midmitral leaflet coaption at the level of the bend in the anterior leaflet. There was posteriorly directed mitral regurgitation associated with this abnormality. After surgical myectomy, when the interventricular septal thickness had decreased and the left ventricular outflow tract di-

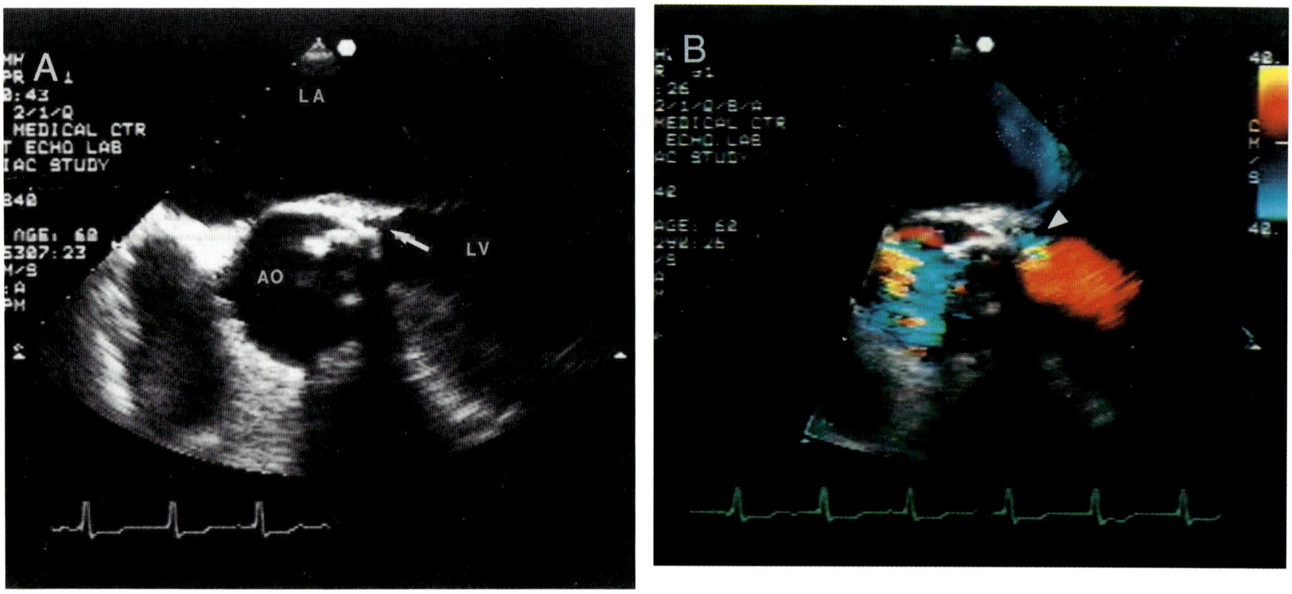

FIG 5–16.
A, a two-dimensional image shows a bioprosthesis in the aortic position. Note that the attenuation produced by the prosthetic material prevents evaluation of the valve leaflets. Shown is a potential space *(arrow)* between the prosthetic ring and the aorta *(AO).* **B,** color Doppler demonstrates diastolic flow representing paravalvular aortic insufficiency *(arrowhead). LA* = left atrium; *LV* = left ventricle.

ameter had increased, there was normalization of mitral leaflet motion and marked reduction or abolition of the mitral regurgitation. This is an interesting example of the use of two-dimensional valvular anatomy and motion as seen from the transesophageal window to study a hemodynamic phenomenon such as dynamic outflow tract obstruction. Although the significance of these findings as a cause or effect in the pathogenesis of dynamic outflow tract obstruction is still not entirely clarified, it seems to offer some useful insights into the phenomenon and may ultimately prove to be a useful tool in selecting patients who might benefit most from surgical myectomy. This example capitalizes on TEE's spatial resolution and superior image quality to address a clinical problem in a novel fashion, and it may prove to be more accurate if studied by using biplane technology.

As other technology develops such as the use of ultrasonic debridement of calcified aortic valves,[39] it is likely that the selection process for this procedure will be determined in large part by findings from TEE.

SUMMARY

This chapter discusses the utility and superiority of TEE for the assessment of native and prosthetic valve disease of all types. Clearly, this indication for TEE is well established and has provided important insight into the pathophysiology of valvular disorders.

REFERENCES

1. Seward JB, Khandheria B, Oh J, et al: Transesophageal echocardiography: Technique, anatomic correlations, implementation and clinical applications. *Mayo Clin Proc* 1988; 63:649–680.
2. Erbel R, Daniel W, Visser C, et al: Echocardiography in diagnosis of aortic dissection. *Lancet* 1989; 1:457–461.
3. Daniel WG, Erbel R, Kasper W, et al: Safety of transesophageal echocardiography. A multicenter survey of 10,419 examinations. *Circulation* 1991; 83:817–821.
4. Khandheria BK, Seward J, Bailey K, et al: Safety of transesophageal echocardiography: Experience with 2070 consecutive procedures (abstract). *J Am Coll Cardiol* 1991; 17:20.
5. Bansal RC, Shakudo M, Shah PM: Biplane transesophageal echocardiography: Technique, image orientation, and preliminary experience in 131 patients. *J Am Soc Echocardiogr* 1990; 3:348–366.
6. Flachskampf FA, Hoffmann R, Hanrath P: Experience with a transesophageal echotransducer allowing full rotation of the viewing plane. The omniplane probe (abstract). *J Am Coll Cardiol* 1991; 17:34.

7. Erbel R, Rohmann S, Drexler M, et al: Improved diagnostic value of echocardiography in patients with infective endocarditis by transesophageal approach: A prospective study. *Eur Heart J* 1988; 9:43–53.
8. Mügge A, Daniel W, Frank G, et al: Echocardiography in infective endocarditis: Reassessment of prognostic implications of vegetation size determined by the transthoracic and the transesophageal approach. *J Am Coll Cardiol* 1989; 14:631–638.
9. Shively BK, Gurule F, Roldan C,et al: Diagnostic value of transesophageal compared with transthoracic echocardiography in infective endocarditis. *J Am Coll Cardiol* 1991; 18:391–397.
10. Marks AR, Choong C, Chir M, et al: Identification of high-risk and low-risk subgroups of patients with mitral-valve prolapse. *N Engl J Med* 1989; 320:1031–1036.
11. Matsuzaki M, Toma Y, Kusukawa R: Clinical applications of transesophageal echocardiography. *Circulation* 1990; 82:709–722.
12. Daniel WG, Schroder E, Mügge A, et al: Transesophageal echocardiography in infective endocarditis. *Am J Card Imaging* 1988; 2:78–85.
13. Schluter M, Kremer P, Hanrath P: Transesophageal 2-D echocardiographic feature of flail mitral leaflet due to ruptured chordae tendineae. *Am Heart J* 1984; 108:609–610.
14. Dittrich HC, McCann H, Walsh T, et al: Transesophageal echocardiography in the evaluation of prosthetic and native aortic valves. *Am J Cardiol* 1990; 66:758–761.
15. Daniel WG, Mügge A, Martin R, et al: Improvement in the diagnosis of abscesses associated with endocarditis by transesophageal echocardiography. *N Engl J Med* 1991; 324:795–800.
16. Bansal RC, Graham B, Jutzy K, et al: Left ventricular outflow tract to left atrial communication secondary to rupture of mitral-aortic intervalvular fibrosa in infective endocarditis: Diagnosis by transesophageal echocardiography and color flow imaging. *J Am Coll Cardiol* 1990; 15:499–504.
17. Chow LC, Dittrich H, Dembitsky W, et al: Accurate localization of ruptured sinus of Valsalva aneurysm by real-time two-dimensional Doppler flow imaging. *Chest* 1988; 94:462–465.
18. Smith MD, Harrison M, Pinton R, et al: Regurgitant jet size by transesophageal compared with transthoracic Doppler color flow imaging. *Circulation* 1991; 83:79–86.
19. Yoshida K, Yoshikawa J, Yamaura Y, et al: Assessment of mitral regurgitation by biplane transesophageal color flow mapping. *Circulation* 1990; 82:1121–1126.
20. Klein AI, Obarski T, Stewart W, et al: Transesophageal Doppler echocardiography of pulmonary venous flow: A new marker of mitral regurgitation severity. *J Am Coll Cardiol* 1991; 18:518–526.
21. Labovitz AJ, Ferrara R, Kerr M, et al: Quantitative evaluation of aortic insufficiency by continuous wave Doppler echocardiography. *J Am Coll Cardiol* 1986; 3:1341–1347.
22. Perry GJ, Helmcke F, Nanda N, et al: Evaluation of aortic insufficiency by Doppler color flow mapping. *J Am Coll Cardiol* 1987; 9:952–958.
23. Drexler M, Erbel R, Rohmann S, et al: Diagnostic value of two-dimensional transesophageal versus transthoracic echocardiography in patients with infective endocarditis. *Eur Heart J* 1987; 8(suppl J):303–306.
24. Taams MA, Gussenhoven E, Cahalan M, et al: Transesophageal Doppler color flow imaging in the detection of native and Bjørk-Shiley mitral valve regurgitation. *J Am Coll Cardiol* 1989; 13:95–99.
25. Casale L, Goodman D, Buchbinder M, et al: Left atrial myxoma in a patient with rheumatic mitral stenosis: Implications for balloon valvuloplasty. *Am Heart J* 1991; 122:1474–1475.
26. Ballal RS, Mahan E, Nandan L, et al: Utility of transesophageal echocardiography in interatrial septal puncture during percutaneous mitral balloon commissurotomy. *Am J Cardiol* 1990; 66:230–232.
27. Kronzon I, Tunice P, Schwinger M, et al: Transesophageal echocardiography during percutaneous mitral valvuloplasty. *J Am Soc Echocardiogr* 1989; 1:380–385.
28. Kronzon I, Tunice P, Goldfarb A, et al: Echocardiographic and hemodynamic characteristics of atrial septal defects created by percutaneous valvuloplasty. *J Am Soc Echocardiogr* 1990; 3:64–71.
29. Hofmann T, Kaspar W, Meinertz T, et al: Determination of aortic valve orifice area in aortic valve stenosis by two-dimensional transesophageal echocardiography. *Am J Cardiol* 1987; 59:330–335.
30. Chandrasekeran K, Foley R, Weintraub A, et al: Evidence that transesophageal echocardiography can reliably and directly measure the aortic valve area in patients with aortic stenosis—a new application that is independent of LV function and does not require Doppler data (abstract). *J Am Coll Cardiol* 1991; 17:20.
31. Nellesen U, Schnittger I, Appleton C, et al: Transesophageal two-dimensional echocardiography and color Doppler flow velocity mapping in the evaluation of cardiac valve prostheses. *Circulation* 1988; 78:848–855.
32. Chan KL, Walley VM: Accuracy of transesophageal echocardiographic detection of cusp tears in degenerated bioprosthetic valves (abstract). *J Am Coll Cardiol* 1991; 17:371.
33. Chen YT, Kan M, Chen J, et al: Detection of prosthetic mitral valve leak: A comparative study using transesophageal echocardiography, transthoracic echocardiography, and auscultation. *J Clin Ultrasound* 1990; 18:557–561.
34. van den Brink RB, Visser C, Basart D, et al: Comparison of transthoracic and transesophageal color Doppler flow imaging in patients with mechanical prostheses in the mitral valve position. *Am J Cardiol* 1989; 63:1471–1474.

35. Mohr-Kahaly S, Kupferwasser I, Erbel R, et al: Regurgitant flow in apparently normal valve prostheses: Improved detection and semiquantitative analysis by transesophageal two-dimensional color-coded Doppler echocardiography. *J Am Soc Echo* 1990; 3:187–195.
36. Khandheria BK, Seward J, Oh J, et al: Value and limitations of transesophageal echocardiography in assessment of mitral valve prostheses. *Circulation* 1991; 83:1956–1968.
37. Dittrich HC, Nicod P, Hoit B, et al: Evaluation of Bjørk-Shiley prosthetic valves by real-time two-dimensional Doppler echocardiographic flow mapping. *Am Heart J* 1988; 115:133–138.
38. Grigg LE, Daniel L, Wigle E, et al: Clarification of the pathophysiology of hypertrophic obstructive cardiomyopathy by transesophageal echocardiography (abstract). *J Am Coll Cardiol* 1991; 17:35.
39. Freeman WK, Schwaff H, Orszulak T, et al. Ultrasonic aortic valve decalcifications: Serial Doppler echocardiographic follow-up. *J Am Coll Cardiol* 1990; 16:623–630.

Chapter 6

Detection of Cardiac and Paracardiac Masses

Andreas Mügge, M.D.

Christoph Stottmeister, M.D.

Klaus Bargheer, M.D.

Werner G. Daniel, M.D.

The diagnosis of cardiac mass lesions was almost restricted to necropsy until echocardiography became available. Since the initial ultrasonographic demonstration of an atrial myxoma by Effert and Domanig in 1959, the value of echocardiography for diagnosing cardiac mass lesions has become well established.[1] In particular, the two-dimensional technique that provides tomographic imaging can be considered the diagnostic procedure of choice for the assessment of abnormal masses in and around the heart.[2–8] In some patients, however, two-dimensional transthoracic echocardiography (TTE) may result in insufficient image quality because of emphysema, obesity, or chest deformities, and thus, no reliable diagnosis can be made. In addition, certain cardiac and paracardiac regions such as the left atrial appendage, the superior vena cava, and the thoracic aorta often cannot be visualized from the transthoracic approach.

During recent years, it has been shown that transesophageal echocardiography (TEE) using the unobstructed view from the esophagus to the heart provides an optimal image quality for most cardiac structures in virtually all patients.[9–12] Moreover, the close proximity of the esophagus to the heart allows the use of higher transducer frequencies to increase image resolution. Today, TEE is a well-established approach that has proved its usefulness in a variety of diseases such as detection of prosthetic valve malfunction,[13, 14] atrial septal abnormalities,[15, 16] aortic dissection,[17, 18] and congenital heart diseases such as discrete subvalvular aortic stenosis[19] and patent ductus arteriosus.[20] Although accompanied by minor discomfort, TEE can be easily performed in conscious patients at almost no risk.[21]

In this chapter we compare the diagnostic accuracy of TTE and TEE in the detection of cardiac and paracardiac masses. Three subgroups of patients studied at our institution will be discussed: (1) 80 patients with histologically proven infective endocarditis of 91 diseased valves, (2) 78 patients with 85 cardiac or extracardiac thrombi, and (3) 62 patients with cardiac or paracardiac tumors confirmed by other diagnostic techniques. Results of these studies demonstrate that TEE leads to a clinically relevant improvement of the diagnostic potential in patients in whom infective or noninfective mass lesions are suspected.

INFECTIVE VALVE-ATTACHED MASSES

Eighty consecutive patients were analyzed. In all patients, acute infective endocarditis was documented by clinical signs as well as by histologic findings. Histologic specimens were obtained during valve replacement (n = 62) and at necropsy (n = 18). In the 80 patients, a total of 91 valves were diseased (69 native valves [37 aortic, 30 mitral, and 2 tricus-

TABLE 6–1.

Detection of Vegetations by Transthoracic (TTE) and Transesophageal (TEE) Echocardiography in 80 Patients With 91 Histologically Proven Diseased Valves

		Vegetation Detected by TTE		Vegetation Detected by TEE	
Valve	*n*	"Definite"	"Possible"	"Definite"	"Possible"
Aortic valve	37	25 (68%)	8	35 (95%)	2
Mitral valve	30	20 (67%)	7	28 (93%)	2
Tricuspid valve	2	2 (100%)	—	2 (100%)	—
Prosthetic valve	22	6 (27%)	2	17 (77%)	2
Total (%)	91	53 (58%)	17 (19%)	82 (90%)	6 (7%)

pid] and 22 prosthetic valves [12 aortic position, 10 mitral position]). Echocardiography was performed 17 ± 2 days (mean ± SEM) before surgery or autopsy.

Comparison of TEE With TTE for Detection of Vegetations

Table 6–1 compares the diagnostic accuracy of TTE and TEE in the detection of histologically proven vegetations. A vegetation was considered to be "definite" when shaggy echoes in the M-mode study and a corresponding mass without restricted valve motion in the two-dimensional echocardiogram were found (Fig 6–1). A vegetation was defined as "possible" when the findings were suggestive of a vegetation but no clear differentiation from a pre-existing lesion with thickened or calcified leaflets was possible. TTE demonstrated definite vegetation in 53 (58%) of 91 diseased valves; 17 additional valves (19%) were considered to have possible vegetations. In native valves, TTE was able to visualize definite vegetations in 47 (68%) of 69 diseased valves, whereas a clear demonstration of vegetation was possible in only 6 (27%) of 22 diseased prosthetic valves. In contrast, TEE visualized definite vegetations in 82 (90%) of 91 diseased valves; 6 additional valves (7%) showed possible attached masses. In particular, in patients with prosthetic valve endocarditis, TEE showed a significantly higher detection rate for attached masses than did TTE (77% vs. 27%, $P < .05$; Fig 6–2). Overall, TTE and TEE findings were suggestive of infective endocarditis in 77% and 97% of diseased valves, respectively.

Echocardiography is the method of choice for the visualization of endocarditis-induced lesions.

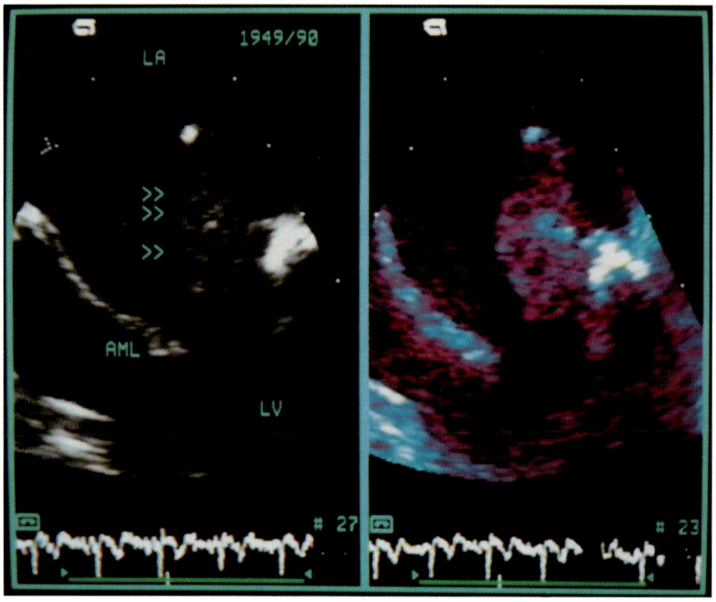

FIG 6–1.
TEE of a patient with a mobile vegetation attached to the posterior mitral valve and prolapsing into the left atrium *(arrows, left panel).* Enhanced display of vegetation was achieved by the use of the B color mode (*right* panel). *LA* = left atrium; *AML* = anterior mitral leaflet; *LV* = left ventricle.

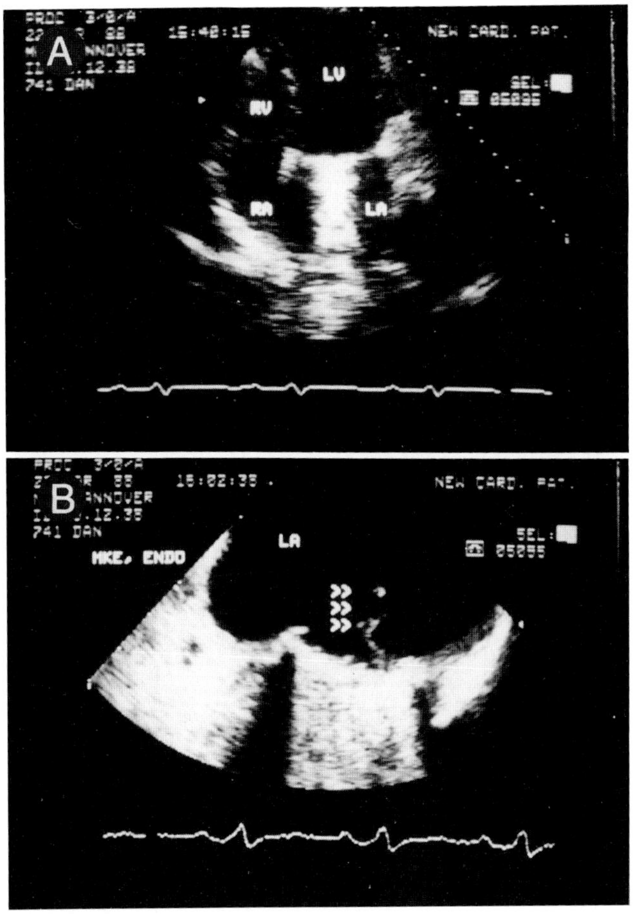

FIG 6–2.
TTE **(A)** and TEE **(B)** of a patient with a mechanical valve in the mitral position. Only TEE demonstrated mobile vegetation attached to the atrial side of the mitral valve prosthesis *(arrows)*. *LA/RA* = left/right atrium; *LV/RV* = left/right ventricle.

These lesions may consist of valve-attached infective masses (i.e., thrombotic/infectious material containing platelets, fibrin, erythrocytes, and granulocytes); endocarditis-induced valvular destructions (e.g., flail leaflet, ruptured chordae tendineae); and/or endocarditis-induced abscess formations. The term *vegetation* refers to the echocardiographic description of abnormal "shaggy" echoes paralleling valve motion without motion inhibition. It should be noted that echocardiography usually cannot differentiate between "true" valve-attached infective masses and endocarditis-induced valve destruction.[22] Thus, an echocardiographically detected vegetation may consist of both infective mass and destroyed leaflet. This lack of reliable differentiation between masses and other endocarditis-induced lesions, however, appears to be of minor clinical relevance regarding the echocardiographic diagnosis of endocarditis.[22]

The detection rate for valvular vegetations depends on the approach used. Whereas the use of M-mode echocardiography alone allows the detection of valvular vegetations in about 55% of cases, the combined use of M-mode and two-dimensional echocardiography increases the detection rate to about 70% to 75%.[22, 23] In the present series of patients with proven endocarditis, definite or possible vegetations were found in 77% of cases when transthoracic M-mode and two-dimensional echocardiography were used. This relatively low sensitivity of TTE in diagnosing endocarditis was due primarily to poor visualization of prosthetic valve-attached vegetations. Prosthetic valves, in particular mechanical devices, produce attenuation that obscures imaging of the region "behind" the occluder. For this reason, small vegetations are usually missed. Whereas the prolapsing part of a vegetation attached to a prosthetic valve in the aortic position may be visualized in the left ventricular outflow tract by the precordial approach, this is often impossible for vegetations attached to the atrial surface of a prosthesis in the mitral position[13, 22] (see Fig 6–2).

In contrast to TTE, the transesophageal approach allows the visualization of valve-attached vegetations with a high resolution; furthermore, TEE allows evaluation of the region "behind" the mitral valve prosthesis (see Fig 6–2). These advantages of TEE are a valuable addition to imaging modalities for the diagnosis of endocarditis. The use of TEE increases the detection rate of valve-attached infective masses up to 96%. A similar high detection rate using TEE was recently reported by Erbel and coworkers.[24] In our series, TEE failed to visualize valve-attached vegetations in only three cases; two of these patients had mechanical prostheses in both the aortic and mitral positions, while one patient had a device in the aortic position. In these three patients, the left ventricular outflow tract was partially obscured on the TEE image by heavy artifacts created by the mitral prosthesis and/or the cage of the aortic prosthesis, respectively. In all three patients, precordial echocardiography also failed to confirm the diagnosis of prosthetic valve endocarditis. The recent addition of biplane technology for TEE may compensate for an incomplete single-plane examination.[25] Although no systematic studies are available at the present time, one might expect that evaluation of prosthetic valves, including those devices in the aortic position, will be substantially enhanced by biplanar TEE imaging.

In addition to the detection of valve-attached vegetations, TEE is also known to improve the visu-

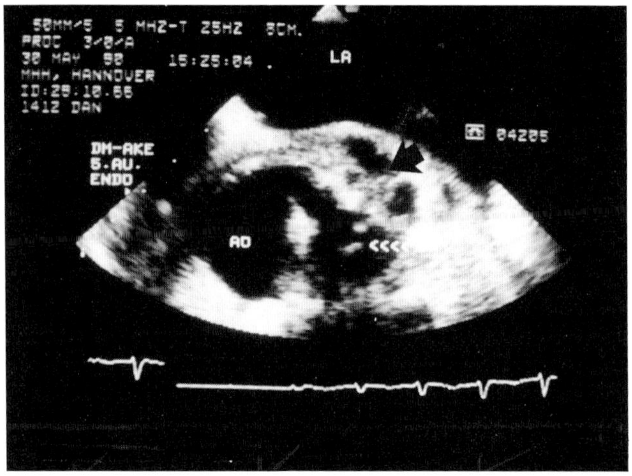

FIG 6–3.
TEE demonstrating abscess cavities *(large arrow)* in a patient with a mechanical device (Duromedics) in the aortic position. Blood cultures revealed *Staphylococcus aureus* septicemia. These abscess cavities could not be visualized by transthoracic echo. Subsequent cardiac surgery confirmed the diagnosis. *LA* = left atrium; *AO* = ascending aorta.

alization of endocarditis-associated abscesses (see Chapter 5). The identification of patients with endocarditis-associated abscesses is of particular interest since these patients have an increased risk of death. In a recent study from our laboratory, TEE identified 40 of 46 defined abscess areas, whereas TTE allowed the detection of only 13 areas[26] (Fig 6–3). In this series, sensitivity and specificity for the detection of abscesses associated with endocarditis were 28.3% and 98.6%, respectively, for TTE and 87.0% and 94.6% for TEE.

CARDIAC THROMBI OR THROMBI LOCALIZED IN GREAT THORACIC VESSELS

Seventy-eight consecutive patients were included in this study group. The diagnosis of cardiac thrombi or thrombus formation in the great thoracic vessels was documented in 56 patients by surgery (n = 36), autopsy (n = 2), or other commonly accepted diagnostic procedures such as computed tomography (n = 3), nuclear magnetic resonance (n = 4), or angiography (n = 11). In the remaining 22 patients, cardiac thrombi were visualized by echocardiography and arterial embolic events with subsequent embolectomy allowed for the presumptive diagnosis of thrombus formation. Seven of the 78 patients showed thrombus formation in more than one cavity. Ten patients experienced one or more episodes of pulmonary embolism; 26 patients, peripheral arterial embolism; and 10 patients, peripheral and cerebral arterial embolism. At the time of the echocardiographic study, 28 patients were in sinus rhythm, 47 had atrial fibrillation, and the remaining 3 patients had a pacemaker device.

Comparison of TEE and TTE for the Detection of Thrombi

The detection rates for intracardiac and extracardiac thrombi according to location are listed in Table 6–2. Almost all thrombi localized in the right atrium and ventricle were correctly detected by both TTE and TEE. Eight (31%) of 26 thrombi within the left atrial cavity were missed by the precordial technique, but all 26 were diagnosed by TEE. Failure of the precordial technique was due to insufficient image quality created by emphysema and mitral prosthesis–induced attenuation in 1 patient each, by flat mural thrombi in 3 patients (Fig 6–4), and by thrombi less than 10 mm in diameter in 3 patients.

A long thrombus straddling the interatrial septum through a patent foramen ovale or a small atrial septal defect was visualized in 3 patients by TEE (Fig 6–5). TTE had shown only isolated masses within both atria.

Twenty-nine patients had thrombus formation within the left atrial appendage (in 4 cases this was

TABLE 6–2.
Detection of 85 Cardiac or Extracardiac Thrombi in 78 Patients by Transthoracic and Transesophageal Echocardiography*

	Location†											
Echo Mode	RV	RA	LA	IAS	LAA	PA	SVC	IVC	Ao	MV	LV	Total
Transthoracic	1	4	18	3	—	—	—	1	—	1	6	34 (40%)
Transesophageal	1	5	26	3	29	2	3	1	2	6	3	81 (95%)
Total	1	5	26	3	29	2	3	1	2	6	7	85 (100%)

*From Mügge A, Daniel WG, Haverich A, et al: *Circulation* 1991; 83:70–78. Used by permission.
†RV = right ventricle; RA = right atrium; LA = left atrium; LAA = left atrial appendage; IAS = overriding thrombus in a patent foramen ovale/small atrial septal defect; PA = pulmonary artery; SVC = superior vena cava; IVC = inferior vena cava; Ao = descending aorta; MV = thrombus attached to a mitral valve prosthesis; LV = left ventricle.

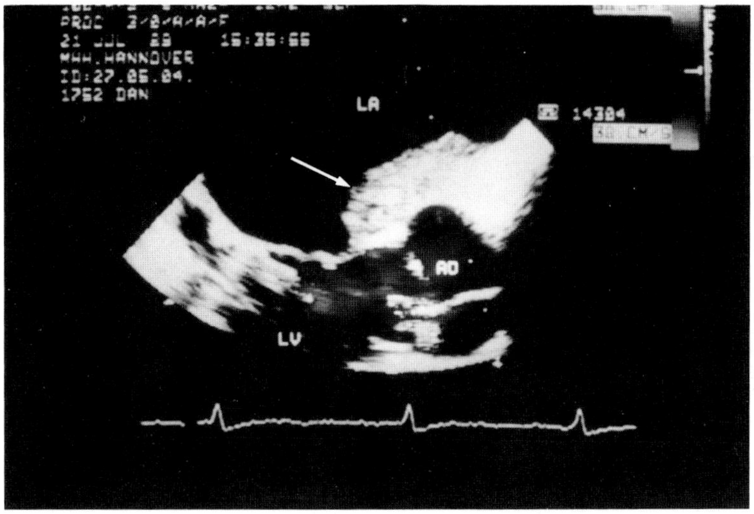

FIG 6–4.
TEE demonstrating a flat mural thrombus (*arrow*) within the left atrial cavity. Note the image is reversed, with right-sided structures to the viewer's right. LA = left atrium; *LV* = left ventricle; *AO* = aortic valve.

associated with a separate thrombus in the left atrial cavity). Whereas TEE visualized thrombi within the appendage in all cases (Fig 6–6), TTE failed in all instances. In some patients, echocardiographic differentiation between thrombi within the left atrial appendage and trabeculae may be difficult. In these patients, additional longitudinal views may be helpful to prove or exclude thrombus masses (Fig 6–7).

Thrombi confined to the great cardiac vessels were detected by TEE in all eight cases (Fig 6–8). In contrast, TTE failed to visualize thrombi within the descending aorta (attached to plaques), pulmonary artery, and superior vena cava (attached to a pacemaker wire or intravenous catheters).

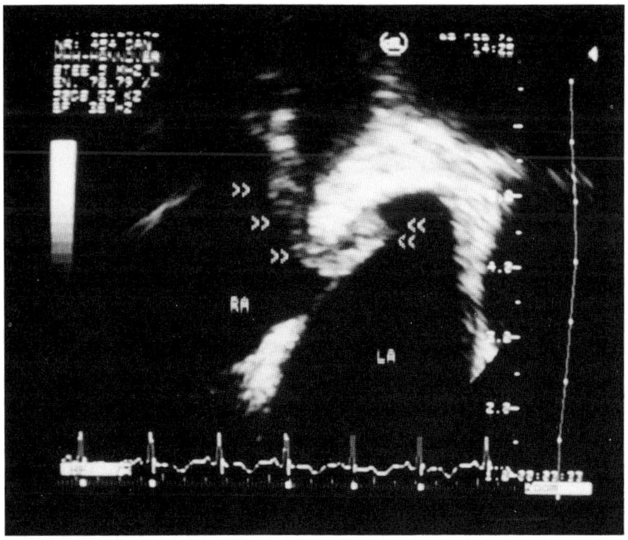

FIG 6–5.
TEE (longitudinal plane) demonstrating a thrombus straddling the interatrial septum through a patent foramen ovale *(arrows).* This patient had a history of deep venous thrombosis and recurrent pulmonary and arterial embolism. Based on TEE findings the diagnosis of paradoxical embolism was made, and the patient underwent emergency cardiac surgery. Note the inverted image display with the transducer at the bottom of the figure. *RA* = right atrium; *LA* = left atrium. (From Mügge A, Daniel WG, Haverich A, et al: *Circulation* 1991; 83:70–78. Used by permission.)

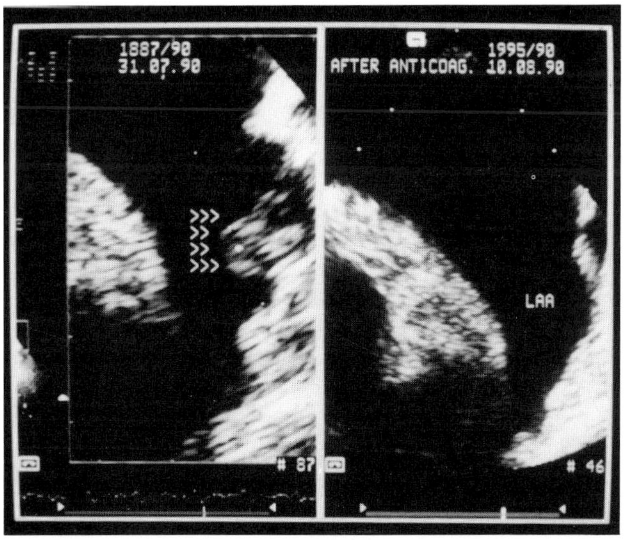

FIG 6–6.
TEE of a patient with a history of atrial fibrillation and recurrent transient ischemic attacks. Thrombotic masses were confined to the left atrial appendage *(left panel arrows).* After 11 days of anticoagulation (heparin, warfarin [Coumadine]), repeat TEE revealed dissolution of the thrombotic masses *(right panel).* After thrombus dissolution, no further embolic events occurred. *LAA* = left atrial appendage.

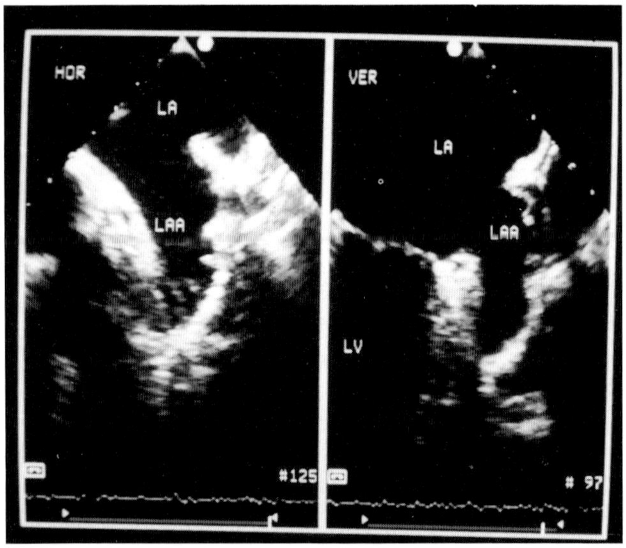

FIG 6–7.
TEE (transverse plane, *left panel;* longitudinal plane, *right panel*) in a patient with a bandlike structure within the tip of the left atrial appendage *(LAA).* This structure represents trabeculae and should not be mistaken for thrombus formation. The longitudinal plane may be helpful in differentiating thrombi from trabeculae or pectinate ridges within the left atrial appendage. *LA* = left atrium; *LV* = left ventricle.

Six patients were found to have thrombi attached to mitral valve prostheses. While TEE directly visualized thrombus formation in all cases, TTE findings were only indirectly suggestive of prosthetic malfunction (abnormal occluder motion, high transvalvular pressure gradient by Doppler), and visualization of thrombotic material was possible in only one case.

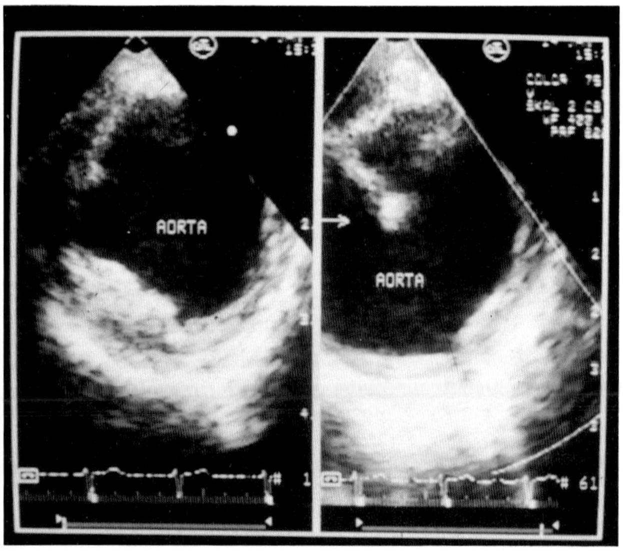

FIG 6–8.
TEE demonstrating extensive plaques within the descending thoracic aorta *(left panel).* The same patient also has a pedunculated mass attached to a plaque *(right panel, arrow)* that may represent thrombus formation and/or an intimal flap.

Seven patients after acute myocardial infarction showed a mural thrombus within the apical area of the left ventricle. Whereas TTE detected thrombi in 6 of 7 cases, monoplane TEE visualized an apical thrombus in only three instances.

In previous studies, the sensitivity of precordial echocardiography for the detection of atrial thrombi ranged between 38% and 61%.[7, 27–29] In the present series, TTE failed to detect thrombi within the left atrial cavity in about 31% of cases. This failure rate for TTE is remarkably high when one considers that TTE was generally accepted as the method of choice for the detection of atrial thrombi. In the current series, TTE missed small (<1 cm) mural thrombi and thrombi obscured by the shadowing of prosthetic devices. In these cases, the transesophageal approach, with its high resolution and unobstructed view, markedly improved the diagnostic potential of echocardiography. Thus, TEE appears to be the method of choice in the detection of atrial thrombi. It should be noted, however, that even with TEE (monoplane) a scan of the entire left atrium may not be possible in all patients. Although this was not observed in the present study, flat mural thrombi confined to the atrial roof may be difficult to visualize by transverse planes. This potential "blind spot" of monoplane TEE has been overcome by incorporation of the longitudinal plane into a biplane TEE probe; this allows assessment of the entire left atrium in virtually all patients.

An interesting subgroup of patients are those with thrombi confined to the left atrial appendage. In a few patients, thrombi within the left atrial appendage had been visualized by TTE.[27, 30, 31] In the vast majority of patients, however, a sufficient image quality of the left atrial appendage cannot be achieved, and therefore thrombi confined to this area were missed.[7, 28, 29, 32, 33] This is consistent with our findings that thrombotic material within the left atrial appendage was missed by TTE in all instances. In contrast to TTE, the left atrial appendage is freely accessible to ultrasound imaging from an esophageal transducer position, and thrombotic material within the left atrial appendage may be easily detected by this technique.[32, 33] Thus, TEE seems to be the method of choice for the detection of left atrial appendage thrombi. Occasionally, extensive trabeculae or pectinate ridges at the walls of the left atrial appendage are seen that may be confused with thrombi. In these cases, biplane views may clarify confusing echoes or irregularities (see Fig 6–7).

For the detection of mural left ventricular

thrombi by TTE, a sensitivity of about 90% has been reported.[8, 34, 35] Accordingly, six of seven thrombi localized in the apical region of the left ventricle were detected by TTE in the present series. In contrast, TEE visualized thrombi in only three instances. Thus, left ventricular thrombi may still be best diagnosed by TTE, with its multiple planes providing a much clearer visualization of the apical region in most patients. It remains to be seen whether biplane or the newer multiplane transducers will improve on the imaging of left ventricular thrombi, especially those at the apex.

Thrombi within the right heart are a rare finding and could be identified equally by both techniques in almost all patients. However, when thrombi are confined to the superior vena cava or pulmonary artery, TEE was clearly superior in demonstrating these masses. This might be of clinical relevance in patients with pacemaker devices and long-standing intravenous lines who are under intensive care or who are receiving long-term chemotherapy. In addition, TEE may also be a fast and reliable approach in the diagnosis of central pulmonary artery emboli.[36]

TEE allows a clear visualization of the interatrial septum. In three patients, a thrombus lodged in a patent foramen ovale or small septal defect could be identified by TEE. Although not studied systematically in the present investigation, biplanar TEE may further improve the delineation of atrial septal anatomy and demonstrate superior and inferior limbi of the atrial septum. This enhanced image by the additional longitudinal plane allowed for visualization of that part of the thrombus that was lodged between the two atrial limbi (see Fig 6–5). Although this condition is a rare finding, it elucidates the potential risk of paradoxical embolism in patients with a noncompetent atrial septum.

Extensive atherosclerotic plaques are a common finding in the arterial tree of older patients. TEE appears to be an ideal tool to visualize plaques within the thoracic aorta (see Fig 6–8). In two patients with peripheral arterial embolism, TEE showed pedunculated masses in the area of extensive atherosclerotic plaque of the descending thoracic aorta (see Fig 6–8). This undulating mass may represent an intimal flap or thrombotic material following rupture of an atherosclerotic plaque. It is reasonable to assume that these mobile masses caused arterial embolism. Although parts of the descending aorta can be visualized by precordial techniques, resolution and imaging quality are usually not sufficient to demonstrate these abnormalities. In contrast, TEE allows clear interrogation of the entire thoracic descending aorta including the aortic arch. In addition, biplanar TEE allows interrogation of the ascending aorta.[25] Although the detection of aortic plaques and thrombi does not lead to specific therapeutic consequences at the present time, knowledge of the precise location of this abnormality may be helpful preoperatively, e.g., to avoid this area for cross-clamping and cannulation maneuvers.[37] (See Chapter 7 for further discussion.)

CARDIAC AND PARACARDIAC TUMORS

Sixty-two consecutive patients were studied. A diagnosis of cardiac or paracardiac tumor was proved in all patients by surgery (n = 46), autopsy (n = 3), and/or other procedures such as computed tomography (n = 42) and nuclear magnetic resonance (n = 22).

Comparison of TEE and TTE for the Detection of Tumors

Table 6–3 summarizes the localization and etiology of cardiac and paracardiac tumors in 62 patients. Table 6–4 compares the tumor detection rate by TTE and TEE in these patients. Overall, TTE and TEE visualized tumor masses at least partially in 84% and 100% of cases, respectively. Whereas all 8 left-sided paracardiac tumors were correctly identified by both techniques, only 13 of 18 right-sided paracardiac masses were visualized by TTE. The 5 tumors that were missed by TTE but correctly identified by TEE were localized behind the sternum (Figs 6–9 and 6–10) lateral to the right ventricle (n = 3) and in the corner between the diaphragm and the heart (n = 1), or the tumor could not be differentiated from a

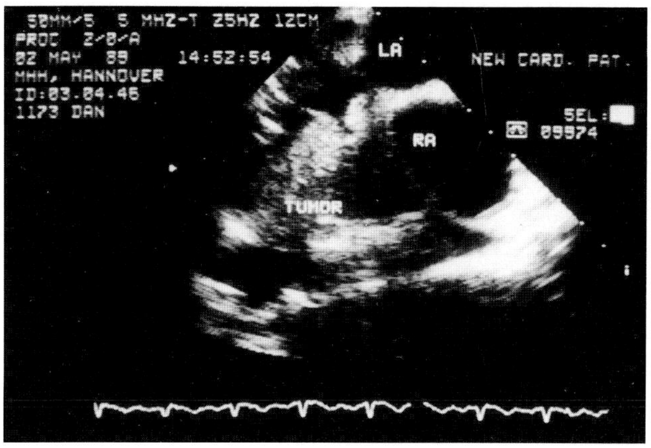

FIG 6–9.
TEE demonstrating a right paracardiac cystic mass (bronchial carcinoma) that was not clearly seen on the precordial views. *LA* = left atrium; *RA* = right atrium.

TABLE 6–3.
Etiology and Localization of Cardiac and Paracardiac Tumors in 62 Patients*

Localization†	Etiology/Histology	No. of Patients
Right paracardial	Malignant lymphoma	1
	Malignant thymoma	1
	Bronchial carcinoma	1
	Malignant histiocytoma	1
	Lupus erythematosus	1
	Metastasis of melanocarcinoma	1
	Malignant mesothelioma	1
	Lipoma	1
	Pericardial cyst	4
	Calcified hematoma	1
	Thrombosed RCA† aneurysm	1
& Penetration of PA	Bronchial carcinoma	1
& Penetration of PV	Bronchial carcinoma	1
& Penetration of RA	Malignant fibrosarcoma	1
& Penetration of RA + RV	Rhabdomyosarcoma	1
Left paracardial	Malignant lymphoma	1
	Epithelioid hemangioma	1
	Teratoma with a pseudocyst	1
	Malignant thymoma	1
	Lipoma	1
	Pericardial cyst	2
& Penetration of LV	Myofibroma	1
Right atrium	Rhabdomyosarcoma	1
	Myxoma	2
& IVC	Uterosarcoma	1
& IVC	Leiosarcoma	1
& IVC	Renal cell carcinoma	6
& IVC	Pheochromocytoma	1
& IVC/SVC	Renal cell carcinoma	1
& RV	Fibroleiomyoma	1
Left atrium	Myxoma	14
& RV	Rhabdomyosarcoma	1
Posterior left atrium	Bronchiogenic cyst	1
	Embryonic cyst	1
Right ventricle	Ectopic thyroid tissue	1
Left ventricle	Rhabdomyosarcoma	1
Descending aorta	Malignant histiocytoma	1
Para-ascending aorta	Malignant lymphoma	1
	Perforation with hematoma	1

*From Mügge A, Daniel WG, Haverich A, et al: *Circulation* 1991; 83:70–78. Used by permission.
†RCA = right coronary artery; PA = pulmonary artery; PV = pulmonary vein; RA = right atrium; RV = right ventricle, LV = left ventricle, IVC = inferior vena cava; SVC = superior vena cava.

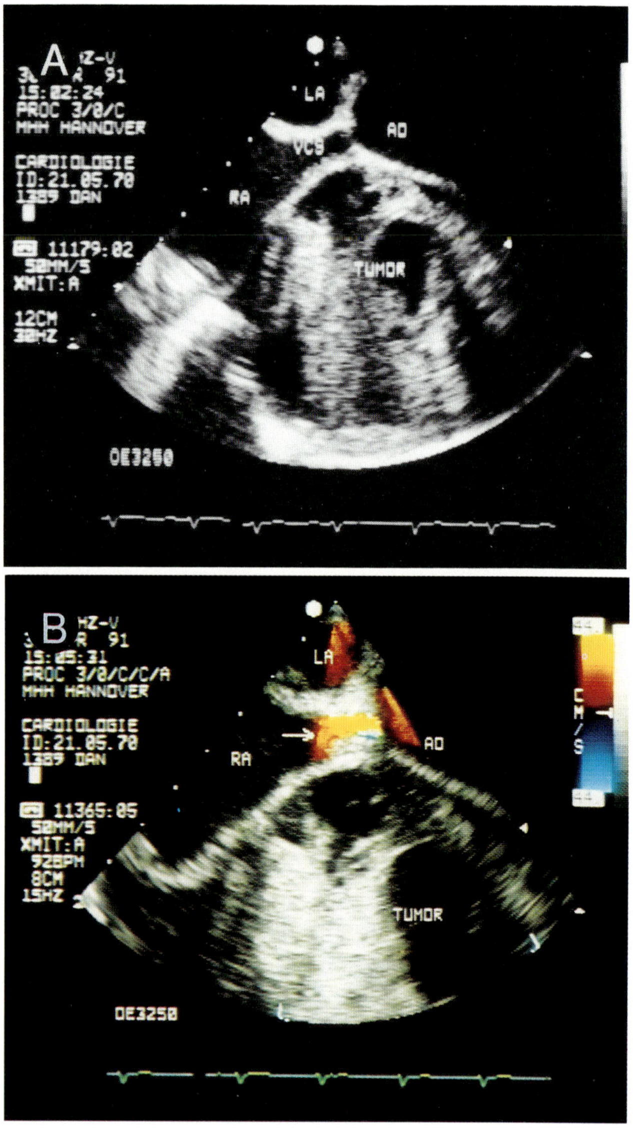

FIG 6–10.
A, TEE (longitudinal plane) of a patient with a large mass lesion (hematoma) behind the sternum and anterior to the great cardiac vessels. This tumor compressed the superior vena cava and resulted in accelerated flow as seen in **B** by color-coded Doppler *(arrow)*. *LA* = left atrium; *RA* = right atrium, *Ao* = ascending aorta; *VCS* = superior vena cava. (From Mügge A, Daniel WG, Haverich A, et al: *Circulation* 1991; 83:70–78. Used by permission.)

pericardial effusion by the precordial approach (n = 1). In two additional cases, TTE identified a right-sided paracardiac mass but missed tumor infiltration into the pulmonary artery (n = 1) or pulmonary vein (n = 1). In contrast, imaging from the esophagus could visualize this tumor infiltration.

Intracardiac tumors were detected correctly in almost all instances by both techniques. In one patient with a rhabdomyosarcoma infiltrating the atrium and right ventricle, only the tumor mass localized within the atrial cavity was identified by both techniques. In another patient with renal cell carcinoma involving the inferior and superior vena cava, the portion of tumor invading the superior vena cava was correctly identified by TEE but missed by TTE (Fig 6–11). In 16 patients, myxoma in the left (n = 14) and right (n = 2) atria were correctly diagnosed

TABLE 6–4.
Echocardiographic Detection of Cardiac and Paracardiac Tumors in 62 Patients*

Tumor Localization	No. of Patients	TTE†	TEE†
Right paracardial	14	9	14
& Penetration of the right heart	4	4‡	4
Left paracardial	7	7	7
& Penetration of the left heart	1	1	1
Right atrium†	3	3	3
& RV	1	1	1
& IVC	9	8	9
& IVC/SVC	1	1§	1
Left atrium	14	14	14
& Penetration of RV	1	1¶	1¶
Posterior left atrium	2	1	2
Right ventricle	1	1	1
Left ventricle	1	1	1
Descending aorta	1	0	1
Para-ascending aorta	2	0	2
Total	62	52 (84%)	62

*From Mügge A, Daniel WG, Haverich A, et al: *Circulation* 1991; 83:70–78. Used by permission.
†TTE = transthoracic echocardiography; TEE = transesophageal echocardiography; RV = right ventricle; IVC/SVC = inferior/superior vena cava.
‡Penetration of the pulmonary vein (n = 1) and the pulmonary artery (n = 1) not seen.
§Penetration of the SVC not seen.
¶Penetration of the RV not seen.

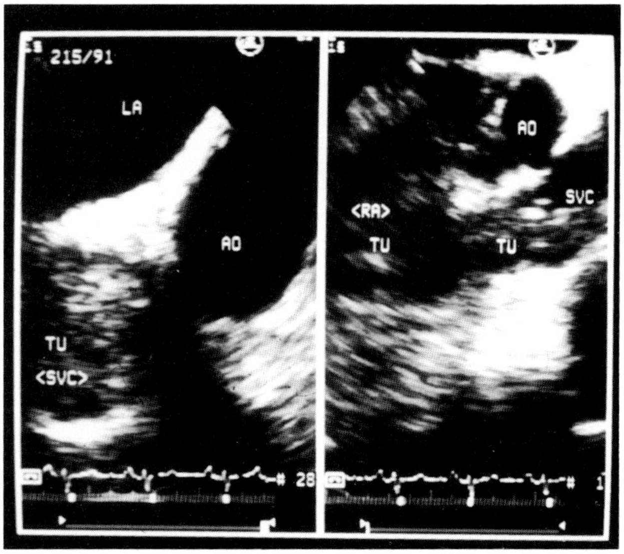

FIG 6–11.
TEE (transverse plane, *left panel;* longitudinal plane, *right panel*) demonstrating a tumor (renal cell carcinoma) involving the superior vena cava. The transverse plane allows visualization of the superior vena cava only at its level of entry into the right atrium. The longitudinal plane permits a long section through the superior vena cava and demonstrates the extent of tumor penetration into this great cardiac vein. *LA* = left atrium; *RA* = right atrium; *AO* = ascending aorta; *TU* = tumor; *SVC* = superior vena cava.

by both TTE and TEE (Fig 6–12). Although the detection rate for atrial myxoma was equal for both techniques, TEE revealed additional information in some patients, e.g., echolucent areas within the tumor in 2 instances. In addition, TEE clearly visualized the point of attachment to the septum in all patients with myxoma, whereas TTE failed in 3 cases due to insufficient imaging quality.

Para-aortic masses were diagnosed in three cases, in one case with invasion into the descending aorta. These masses were visualized exclusively by TEE (Fig 6–13) and missed by TTE.

The diagnosis of cardiac tumors was one of the first clinical applications of echocardiography.[38] Since then, the diagnosis of cardiac tumors, in particular atrial myxoma, by transthoracic M-mode and two-dimensional echocardiography has been well established.[4, 5, 28, 39–45] In our series, intracardiac tumors were identified equally by TTE and TEE in almost all patients. It should be noted that although echocardiography appears to be a very sensitive method in the detection of intracardiac tumors, it usually lacks information concerning the etiology of tumor masses. In our experience, differentiation between the most frequent intracardiac masses, thrombus and myxoma, may be difficult on the basis of tissue characteristics. In selected cases, however, additional echocardiographic findings such as the point of attachment, echo-lucent areas, or calcifications within the tumor mass may be helpful in differentiating thrombus from myxoma. In these patients,

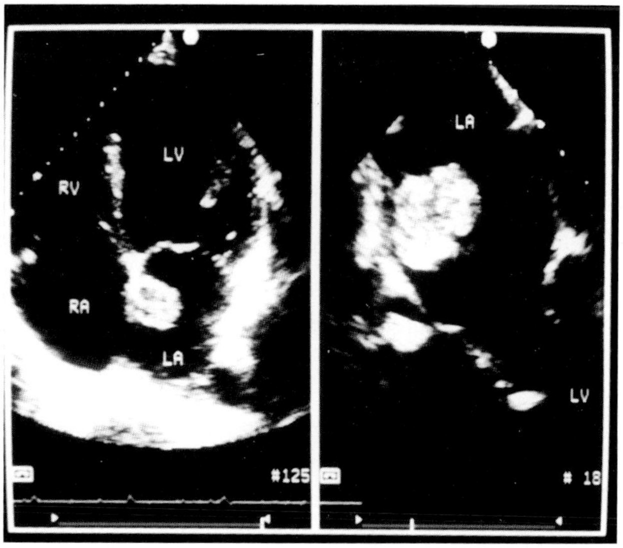

FIG 6–12.
Transthoracic (apical four-chamber view, *left panel*) and transesophageal *(right panel)* images of a patient with a mass (myxoma) within the left atrial cavity. Both techniques clearly visualized the tumor. *LA/RA* = left/right atrium; *LV/RV* = left/right ventricle.

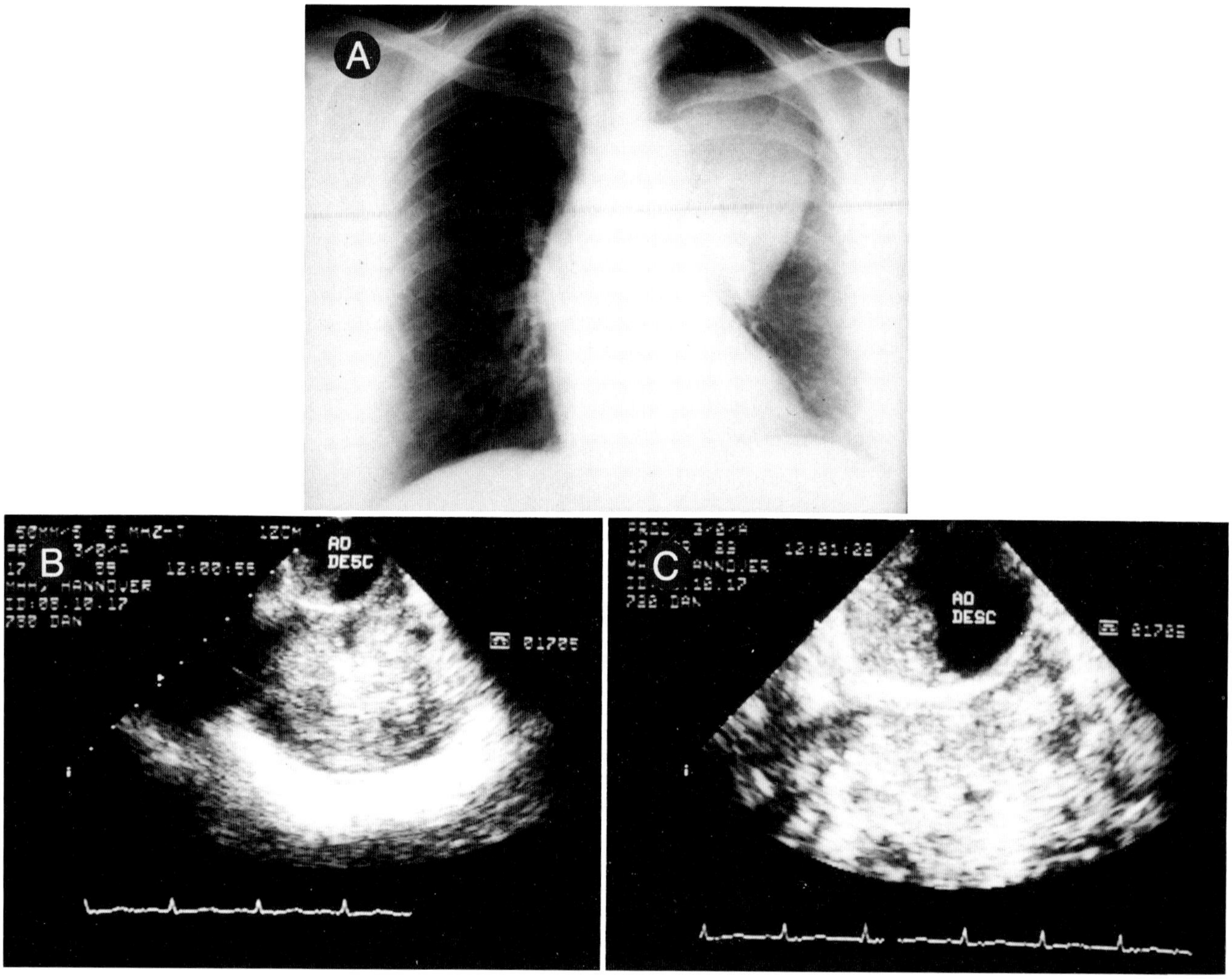

FIG 6–13.
Chest radiography and transesophageal images from a patient with a large para-aortic mass (malignant histiocytoma). The chest x-ray **(A)** demonstrates the mass on the left side of the heart. **B,** TEE visualizes a tumor (about 4.8 cm in diameter) located beside the descending thoracic aorta. **C,** magnification of the echocardiogram clearly demonstrates penetration of the lumen by the tumor mass. (From Mügge A, Daniel WG, Haverich A, et al: *Circulation* 1991; 83:70–78. Used by permission.)

TEE may be superior to the precordial approach for visualization of this additional information.[46, 47]

While the echocardiographic features of intracardiac masses have been described extensively, only a few reports have been published on the value of the technique for diagnosing paracardiac or pericardiac tumors.[2, 6, 46, 48–50] Paracardiac tumors adjacent to the left side of the heart are usually identified by both TTE and TEE. In contrast, paracardiac tumors on the right side were missed by TTE in about 28% of cases but could always be identified by TEE. Tumors localized anterior to the heart or in the corner between the heart and the diaphragm may be difficult to visualize by precordial techniques, although these masses are in the far field, TEE could identify them in all instances. In addition, TEE was superior in detecting para-aortic masses or masses penetrating the descending aorta. The close proximity allows an "ideal" investigation of the entire thoracic descending aorta from the esophagus.

Although TEE shows a high sensitivity in the detection of intracardiac and paracardiac tumors, this approach cannot displace other diagnostic techniques such as computed tomography or magnetic resonance imaging. This is because echocardiographic information concerning tumor extent and tissue characterization is often limited. In addition, primary tumors of the heart are less frequent than metastatic masses, which necessitates excluding tumor manifestation more distant from the heart. Nevertheless, TEE may be superior to the transthoracic approach as an initial screening procedure in patients with suspected cardiac or paracardiac tumors.

SUMMARY

TEE has now been clearly established as a superior imaging modality for intracavitary thrombi, especially those located in posterior structures such as the left atrium. In addition, TEE can define much smaller valvular vegetations than could be visualized with TTE. Importantly, TEE has expanded the use of ultrasound in defining cardiac and paracardiac tumors and masses. The latter group were heretofore visualized almost always by other modalities such as computed tomography.

This chapter presents our experience in imaging these cardiac and paracardiac mass lesions and also reviews the current literature involving TEE in these abnormalities. It is clear that TEE provides important information in the assessment of all types of cardiac and paracardiac lesions.

REFERENCES

1. Bogren HG, DeMaria AN, Mason DT: Imaging procedures in the detection of cardiac tumors, with emphasis on echocardiography: A review. *Cardiovasc Intervent Radiol* 1980; 3:107–125.
2. Chandraratna PAN, Aronow WS: Detection of pericardial metastases by cross-sectional echocardiography. *Circulation* 1981; 63:197–199.
3. DePace NL, Soulen RL, Kotler MN, et al: Two-dimensional echocardiographic detection of intraatrial masses. *Am J Cardiol* 1981; 48:954–960.
4. Fyke FE, Seward JB, Edwards WD, et al: Primary cardiac tumors: Experiences with 30 consecutive patients since the introduction of two-dimensional echocardiography. *J Am Coll Cardiol* 1985; 5:1465–1473.
5. Kutalek SP, Panidis IP, Kotler MN, et al: Metastatic tumors of the heart detected by two-dimensional echocardiography. *Am Heart J* 1985; 109:343–349.
6. Mancuso L, Potrolo F, Bondi F, et al: Echocardiographic recognition of mediastinal masses. *Chest* 1988; 93:144–148.
7. Shrestha NK, Morena FL, Narciso FV, et al: Two-dimensional echocardiographic diagnosis of left atrial thrombus in rheumatic heart disease. *Circulation* 1983; 67:341–347.
8. Stratton JR, Lighty GW, Pearlman AS, et al: Detection of left ventricular thrombus by two-dimensional echocardiography: Sensitivity, specificity, and causes of uncertainty. *Circulation* 1982; 66:156–166.
9. Frazin L, Talano JV, Stephanides L, et al: Esophageal echocardiography. *Circulation* 1976; 54:102–108.
10. Mitchell MM, Sutherland GR, Gussenhoven EJ, et al: Transesophageal echocardiography. *J Am Soc Echocardiogr* 1988; 1:362–377.
11. Schlüter M, Langenstein BA, Polster J, et al: Transesophageal cross-sectional echocardiography with phased array transducer system: Technique and initial clinical results. *Br Heart J* 1982; 48:67–72.
12. Seward JB, Khandheria BK, Oh JK, et al: Transesophageal echocardiography: Technique, anatomic correlation, implementation, and clinical applications. *Mayo Clin Proc* 1988; 63:649–680.
13. Mügge A, Daniel WG, Grote J, et al: Assessment of anatomical abnormalities in prosthetic valve malfunction by transesophageal echocardiography, in Erbel R, et al (eds): *Transesophageal Echocardiography*. Berlin, Springer-Verlag, 1989, pp 107–114.
14. Nellessen U, Schnittger I, Appleton CP, et al: Transesophageal two-dimensional echocardiography and color Doppler flow velocity mapping in the evaluation of cardiac valve prostheses. *Circulation* 1988; 78:848–855.
15. Daniel WG, Hausmann D, Mügge A, et al: Echocardiographic diagnosis of atrial septal defects: When should we use the transesophageal approach? *Circulation* 1990; 82(suppl 3):31.
16. Mügge A, Daniel WG, Klöpper JW, et al: Visualization of patent foramen ovale by transesophageal color-coded Doppler echocardiography. *Am J Cardiol* 1988; 62:837–838.
17. Erbel R, Engberding R, Daniel WG, et al: Echocardiography in diagnosis of aortic dissection. *Lancet* 1989; 1:457–460.
18. Mügge A, Daniel WG, Laas J, et al: False-negative diagnosis of proximal aortic dissection by computed tomography or angiography and possible explanations based on transesophageal echocardiographic findings. *Am J Cardiol* 1990; 65:527–529.
19. Mügge A, Daniel WG, Wolpers HG, et al: Improved visualization of discrete subvalvular aortic stenosis by transesophageal color coded Doppler echocardiography. *Am Heart J* 1989; 117:474–475.
20. Mügge A, Daniel WG, Lichtlen PR: Imaging of patent ductus arteriosus by transesophageal color coded Doppler echocardiography. *J Clin Ultrasound* 1991; 19:128–129.
21. Daniel WG, Erbel R, Kasper W, et al: Safety of transesophageal echocardiography. A multicenter survey of 10,419 examinations. *Circulation* 1991; 83:817–821.
22. Mügge A, Daniel WG, Frank G, et al: Echocardiography in infective endocarditis: Reassessment of prognostic implications of vegetation size determined by the transthoracic and the transesophageal approach. *J Am Coll Cardiol* 1989; 14:631–639.
23. Daniel WG, Schröder E, Mügge A, et al: Transesophageal echocardiography in infective endocarditis. *Am J Card Imaging* 1988; 2:78–85.

24. Erbel R, Rohmann S, Drexler M, et al: Improved diagnostic value of echocardiography in patients with infective endocarditis by transesophageal approach: A prospective study. *Eur Heart J* 1988; 1:43–53.
25. Seward JB, Khandheria BK, Edwards WD, et al: Biplanar transesophageal echocardiography: Anatomic correlations, image orientation, and clinical applications. *Mayo Clin Proc* 1990; 65:1193–1213.
26. Daniel WG, Mügge A, Martin RP, et al: Improvement in the diagnosis of abscesses associated with endocarditis by transesophageal echocardiography. *N Engl J Med* 1991; 324:795–800.
27. Chiang CW, Pang SC, Lin FC, et al: Diagnostic accuracy of two-dimensional echocardiography for detection of left atrial thrombus in patients with mitral stenosis. *J Ultrasound Med* 1987; 6:525–529.
28. Roudant R, Gosse P, Aouizerate E, et al: The diagnosis of intraatrial masses with two-dimensional echocardiography: Experience with 64 patients. *Echocardiography* 1987; 4:431–436.
29. Schweizer P, Bardos P, Erbel R, et al: Detection of left atrial thrombi by echocardiography. *Br Heart J* 1982; 45:148–156.
30. Bansal RC, Heywood JT, Applegate PM, et al: Detection of left atrial thrombi by two-dimensional echocardiography and surgical correlation in 148 patients with mitral valve disease. *Am J Cardiol* 1989; 64:243–246.
31. Herzog CA, Bass D, Kane M, et al: Two-dimensional echocardiographic imaging of left atrial appendage thrombi. *J Am Coll Cardiol* 1984; 3:1340–1344.
32. Aschenberg W, Schlüter M, Kremer P, et al: Transesophageal two-dimensional echocardiography for the detection of left atrial appendage thrombus. *J Am Coll Cardiol* 1986; 7:163–166.
33. Mügge A, Daniel WG, Hausmann D, et al: Diagnosis of left atrial appendage thrombi by transesophageal echocardiography: Clinical implications and follow-up. *Am J Card Imaging* 1990; 4:173–179.
34. Takamoto T, Kim D, Urie PM, et al: Comparative recognition of left ventricular thrombi by echocardiography and cineangiography. *Br Heart J* 1985; 53:36–42.
35. Visser CA, Kan G, Meltzer RS, et al: Long-term follow-up of left ventricular thrombus after acute myocardial infarction. *Chest* 1984; 86:532–536.
36. Wittlich N, Erbel R, Todt M, et al: Detection of pulmonary artery thrombi by transesophageal echocardiography in patients with pulmonary embolism. *Eur Heart J* 1989; 10(suppl):21.
37. Tunick PA, Kronzon I: Protruding atherosclerotic plaque in the aortic arch of patients with systemic embolization: A new finding by transesophageal echocardiography. *Am Heart J* 1990; 120:658–660.
38. Effert S, Domanig E: Diagnostik intraaurikulärer Tumoren und grosser Thromben mit dem Ultraschall-Echoverfahren. *Dtsch Med Wochenschr* 1959; 84:6–8.
39. Ennker J, Daniel WG, Doehring W, et al: Surgical experience with left atrial myxomas. *Herz* 1983; 8:227–233.
40. Felner JM, Knopf WD: Echocardiographic recognition of intracardiac and extracardiac masses. *Echocardiography* 1985; 2:3–55.
41. Kronzon I, Rosenzweig B, Dack S: Diagnosis of a large left atrial myxoma: The role of two-dimensional echocardiography. *J Clin Ultrasound* 1982; 10:39–41.
42. Panidis IP, Kotler MN, Mintz GS, et al: Clinical and echocardiographic features of right atrial masses. *Am Heart J* 1984; 107:745–758.
43. Perry LS, King JF, Zeft HJ, et al: Two-dimensional echocardiography in the diagnosis of left atrial myxoma. *Br Heart J* 1981; 5:667–671.
44. Salcedo EE, Adams KV, Lever HM, et al: Echocardiographic findings in 25 patients with left atrial myxoma. *J Am Coll Cardiol* 1983; 1:1162–1166.
45. St. John Sutton MG, Mercier LA, Giuliani ER, et al: Atrial myxomas: A review of clinical experience in 40 patients. *Mayo Clin Proc* 1980; 55:371–376.
46. Mügge A, Daniel WG, Haverich A, et al: Diagnosis of noninfective cardiac mass lesions by two-dimensional echocardiography. Comparison of the transthoracic and transesophageal approach. *Circulation* 1991; 83:70–78.
47. Thier W, Schlüter M, Krebber HJ, et al: Cysts in left atrial myxoma identified by transesophageal cross-sectional echocardiography. *Am J Cardiol* 1983; 51:1793–1795.
48. Chandraratna PAN, Littmann BB, Serafini A, et al: Echocardiographic evaluation of extracardiac masses. *Br Heart J* 1978; 40:741–749.
49. Daniel WG, Döhring W, Frank G, et al: Non-invasive diagnosis of a pericardial cyst: Combined use of M-mode echocardiography and computed tomography. *Eur Heart J* 1980; 1:201–204.
50. Engberding R, Schulze-Waltrup N, Grosse-Heitmeyer W, et al: Transthorakale und transösophageale 2-D-Echokardiographie in der Diagnostik peri- und parakardialer Tumoren. *Dtsch Med Wochenschr* 1987; 112:49–52.

Chapter 7

Evaluation of Aortic Disease

Mark M. Mitchell, M.S., M.D.

Transesophageal echocardiography (TEE) is useful not only in examination of the heart but also for examination of the thoracic aorta.[1, 2] TEE has been found particularly useful in the diagnosis and management of thoracic aortic aneurysms, dissections, congenital abnormalities, and embolic disease.[1–4]

Conventional transthoracic (body surface) echocardiography (TTE) can provide images of the aortic root, proximal aortic arch, and arch vessels and sometimes useful images of a portion of the descending thoracic aorta that is adjacent to the atrioventricular groove.[5] Thus, almost the entire thoracic aorta can be visualized. However, there are problems. Although image quality is typically excellent in young children, images are generally of poorer quality in adults and are unobtainable in more than 30% of patients with obesity or pulmonary emphysema.[2]

TEE provides excellent-quality images of the aortic root, distal aortic arch, and descending thoracic aorta. The quality and resolution of TEE images is typically superior to those obtained by TTE due to the proximity of the transducer to the structures of interest, the applicability of higher carrier frequency transducer arrays (5 to 7.5 MHz as opposed to 2.5 to 3.5 MHz), and the lack of intervening chest wall structures.[6] Even in patients where TTE imaging of the aorta is possible, TEE provides improved diagnostic capability despite the fact that TEE usually cannot provide images of some portion of the proximal aortic arch because of anatomic interposition of the air column in the trachea and/or the left mainstem bronchus.[2, 4, 7] In practice, TEE and TTE are complementary techniques, and the whole thoracic aorta can be reliably imaged by a combination of TTE and TEE.[2]

It is interesting to compare TEE with the other imaging modalities used to examine the thoracic aorta, computer-aided tomographic (CAT) scanning, magnetic resonance imaging (MRI), angiography, and plain radiographs. TEE has the advantage of being portable. The echo machine can be brought to the patient in the clinic, intensive care unit, trauma unit, or operating room, whereas CAT, MRI, and angiography require that the patient be moved to special locations that are not always optimal for continuing care of a critically ill or injured patient. CAT and MRI also significantly limit access to the patient during the time that the scanning is being done. MRI cannot be used on patients with metallic prosthetic valves or pacemakers because of the potentially hazardous strong magnetic fields.[8] In tracheally intubated and sedated or anesthetized patients, TEE can be used to continuously monitor the progression of the patient's aortic disease on a minute-to-minute basis, even intraoperatively, whereas the other imaging modalities are typically employed as one-time diagnostic tests or at best give episodic "snapshots" of the patient's disease. These advantages of TEE are of course most important in acute situations such as aortic dissection.

Plain radiographs of the chest have the advantage of being the least expensive of these procedures, but they also provide the least information. Neither plain radiography nor CAT and MRI provide any information about aortic blood flow, wall motion, or the status of the aortic valve, whereas color flow mapping plus pulsed Doppler with TEE and angiography with fluoroscopy or cinemagraphic exposures do. Adequate examination with CAT and angiography requires the use of contrast agents that are potentially hazardous.[8] The x-ray– or photographic-based technologies generally provide somewhat higher resolution images than are available with TEE.

Aortic angiography has generally been considered the "gold standard" in aortic diagnosis.[8] Aortography demonstrates filling and flow in the aortic lumen, separates true from false channels, and allows definition of entry and exit intimal tears. However, both false-negative and false-positive findings can occur as a result of unusual intimal tearing, equal simultaneous opacification of various channels, or thrombosis of false channels, and in some cases a thickened aortic wall may be confused with a false channel.[9, 10]

Aortic angiography is the most invasive of the procedures used to image the aorta. Although TEE is less invasive and safer than angiography, it is more invasive than MRI and CAT.[6, 11] Passage of the TEE probe into the esophagus does produce some stress and discomfort for the patient. But this is surprisingly well tolerated, even in patients with acute aortic dissections.[2, 4, 12, 13] The use of TEE does require access to the patient's oropharynx and consideration of airway management and may be contraindicated in patients with esophageal varices or strictures, problems with swallowing, or incompletely evaluated penetrating chest trauma.[6]

STANDARD TEE VIEWS OF THE AORTA

The standard anatomic views for examination of the thoracic aorta are relatively straightforward because the descending aorta and aortic root are basically simple cylindrical structures and the transducer is constrained to the interior of the esophagus, which is roughly parallel to the descending aorta. The acoustic window through which TEE can image the structures of the heart, aorta, and to some limited extent the lungs, noncardiac mediastinal structures, and upper abdominal organs (transverse colon, liver, omentum) has as its cephalad limit the point at which the transducer passes behind the trachea and/or the left main-stem bronchus and as its caudad limit the point at which it descends below the fundus of the stomach and no longer remains in the vicinity of the diaphragm. With current technology, the features of the thoracic aorta are examined with either a transversely or longitudinally oriented transducer array.

As shown in Figure 7–1, the course of the esophagus begins in the midline as an extension of the posterior portion of the oropharynx and descends in the midline on the anterior surface of the vertebral column until it veers somewhat to the left as it reaches the cardiac sphincter and joins the fundus of the stomach. The aorta begins at the aortic valve annulus about midway in the anteroposterior dimension and swings anteriorly and then posteriorly as it crosses from the right to left of the midline and becomes the transverse aortic arch. It then descends along to the left of and slightly anterior to the vertebral column until after it penetrates below the diaphragm. Therefore, as shown in Figure 7–2, we find the transverse aortic arch directly anterior to the esophagus and the descending aorta moving progressively more to the left and posteriorly as we advance the TEE probe more caudad, until finally the aorta is posterior to the probe in the fundus of the stomach where the displacement between the

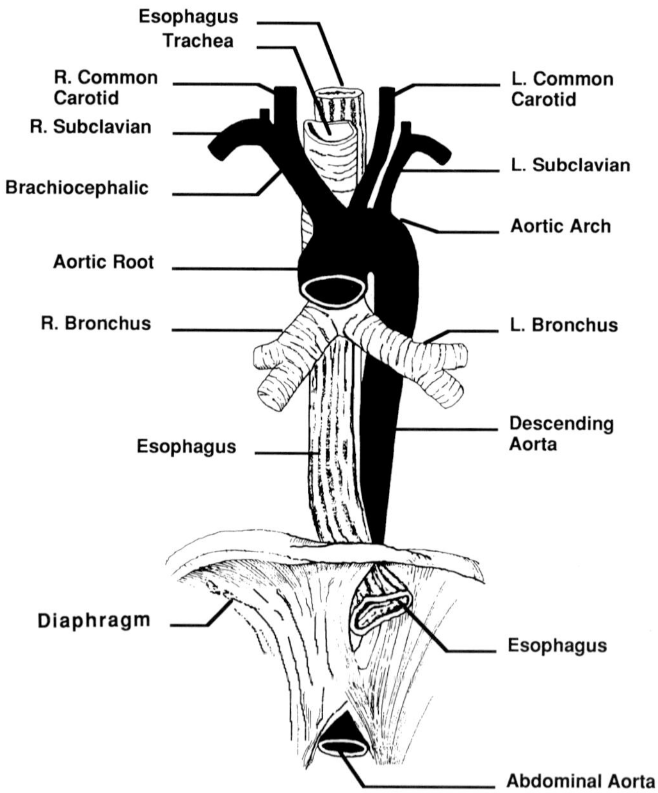

FIG 7–1.
TEE anatomy showing the anatomic relationships of the thoracic aorta and its major branches, the esophagus, the trachea and major bronchi, and the diaphragm.

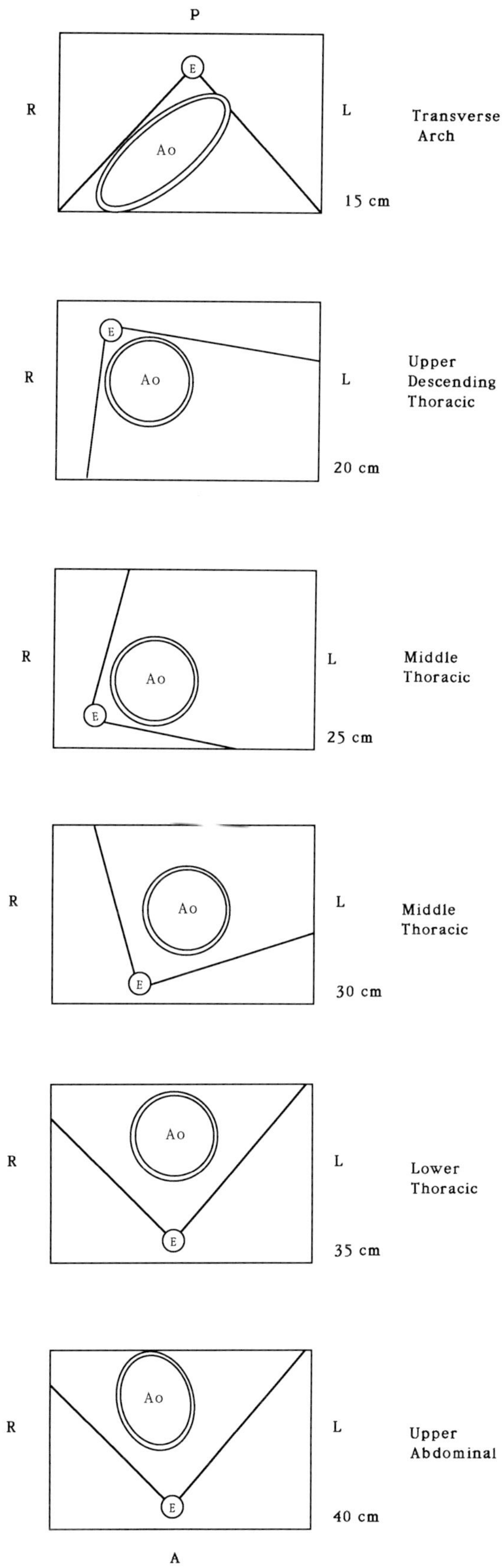

esophagus and aorta becomes progressively larger and eventually the aorta can no longer be imaged.[14]

Transverse Images

When a conventional TEE probe is used with transverse imaging, there are four standard views of the thoracic aorta. These are views of the aortic root above the aortic valve, the transverse and distal aortic arch, the midthoracic aorta, and the distal thoracic or proximal abdominal aorta from the fundus of the stomach.

Aortic Root Above the Aortic Valve

The aortic root at the level of the aortic valve cusps is seen in Figure 2–14,A). Figure 2–15,A shows the aortic root at the level of the coronary ostia. The right coronary artery is often difficult to visualize at its origin. Figure 7–3 shows the aortic root at the level of the pulmonary arteries. Attempts to image more cephalad are usually unsuccessful due to interposition of the trachea and/or the left mainstem bronchus. In this view, flow in the aortic lumen is almost perpendicular to the ultrasound beam, which limits the utility of this view for Doppler assessment.

Notice in Figure 7–3 that there is a segment between the aorta and main pulmonary artery that is not clearly defined. This "dropout" is often but not consistently seen and is of uncertain etiology, but it is not an anatomic communication or window. The normal adult aortic root diameter is 30 to 35 mm.[2]

At the Transverse and Distal Aortic Arch

Figure 2–21,A shows the transverse aortic arch. The left subclavian artery and other arch vessels are sometimes seen in images from the transverse plane, but they are more reliably identified from longitudinal images (see below).

In the Midthoracic Region

Figure 2–19,F shows a transverse section of the descending thoracic aorta in the midthoracic region. It should have a smooth, well-defined intimal surface with a circular cross section. The normal diameter for an adult will be about 18 to 25 mm, and it will

FIG 7–2.
Orientation of the aorta relative to the esophagus at various levels of transverse scan planes. The distances shown are from the incisor teeth. *Ao* = aorta; *E* = esophagus; *A* = anterior; *P* = posterior; *R* = right; *L* = left.

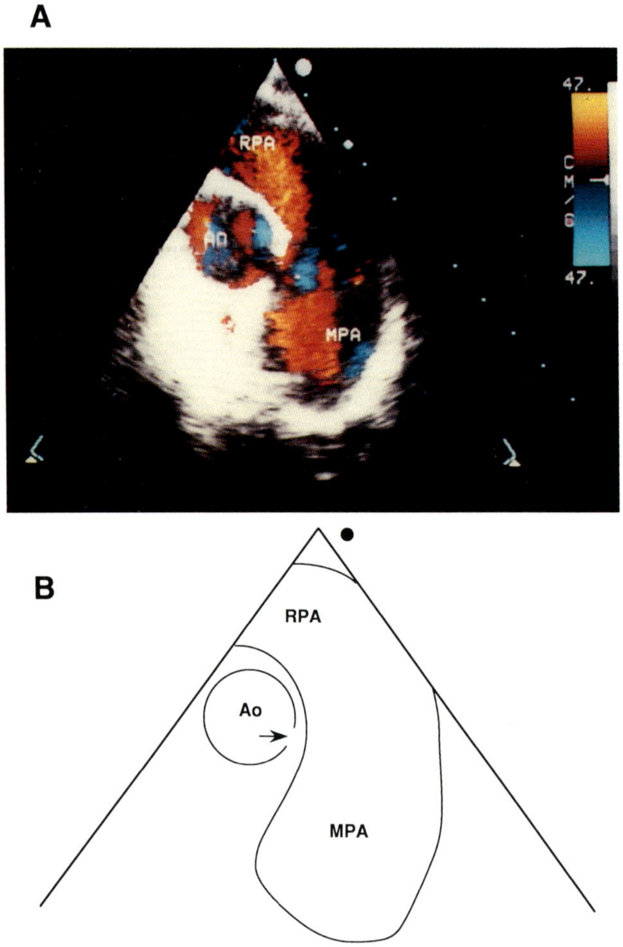

FIG 7–3.
Aortic root at the level of the pulmonary arteries. The color flow Doppler image shows the ascending aorta *(Ao)*, main pulmonary artery *(MPA)*, and right pulmonary artery *(RPA)*. The left pulmonary artery is not well visualized because the trachea or the left main bronchus is situated between it and the TEE transducer. The *arrow* in the line interpretation indicates a region of echo dropout that is often found in this view (see the text).

taper smoothly, becoming smaller as more caudal sections are imaged.[2] The takeoff of intercostal arteries are occasionally seen, but usually these are not well defined. Backflow of blood into the lumen of the descending aorta from collateral perfusion of intercostal arteries can be seen in cross-clamped isolated aortic segments during repair of aortic dissections as shown in Figure 7–4.

From the Fundus of the Stomach

With the transducer in the fundus of the stomach, it becomes displaced from the aorta, which is finally lost from view. This looks similar to Figure 2–19,F except that the aortic lumen is further from the apex of the two-dimensional image and may be somewhat elliptical because the TEE probe is deflected from parallel to the axis of the aorta by the confines of the fundus of the stomach. This is about the same probe insertion depth at which a nearly apical short axis view of the left ventricle can be obtained if the probe is rotated to the left and flexed.[15] Sometimes portions of the liver, portal veins, colon, and omentum (in patients with ascites) can also be seen at this level.

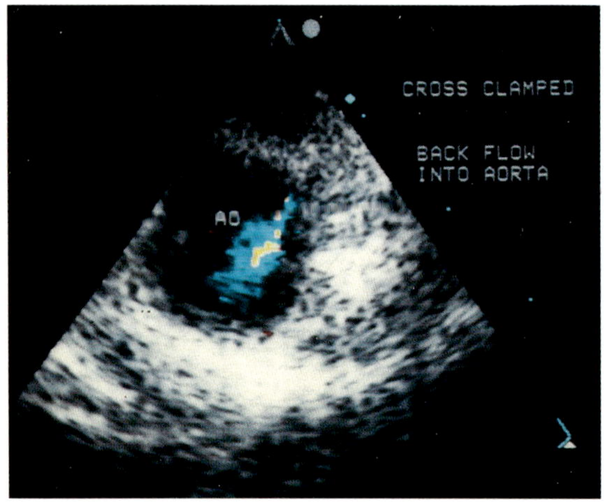

FIG 7–4.
Descending thoracic aorta with backflow from the intercostal arteries. Color flow Doppler indicates the location of an intercostal artery by collateral back-bleeding into a segment of the descending thoracic aorta that is isolated by cross-clamps above and below the image plane during surgical repair of a traumatic aortic disruption.

Longitudinal Images

When a biplane or longitudinal-plane TEE probe is used, standard views are also seen from the same four regions as with transverse imaging.

At the Aortic Root, Including the Aortic Valve

Figure 2–16 shows the aortic valve and aortic root in a longitudinal view. Although this view is perpendicular to that seen with a transverse transducer orientation, flow through the valve is often still almost perpendicular to the ultrasound beam. This limits the utility of these views for Doppler assessment. In some patients with vascular disease and in older patients, the aortic root may be oriented more anteriorly, as in Figure 2–16. This places the aortic root lumen more nearly parallel to the ultrasound beam and is more favorable for Doppler examination.

At the Aortic Arch

Figure 2–21,B–D shows the transverse aortic arch from the longitudinal plane. These views demonstrate the origins of the great vessels. A segment of the proximal aortic arch is still usually inaccessible to TEE, even with a longitudinal probe, because the trachea or the left main-stem bronchus is still interposed between the transducer and the proximal aortic arch, but in most patients more of the arch is seen with longitudinal than with transverse imaging, and in some patients all of the aortic arch is seen with longitudinal arrays.

In the Midthoracic Region

Figure 7–5 shows a segment of the descending thoracic aorta in the midthoracic region. Cephalad is to the right, and caudad is to the left. Careful rotational adjustment of the probe will allow examination of the entire lumen of the descending thoracic aorta.

From the Fundus of the Stomach

The descending thoracic aorta seen from the fundus of the stomach looks about the same as from the midthoracic region, shown in Figure 7–5, but with more distance between the apex of the image (location of the transducer) and the lumen. As with transverse views, the imaging section may also become somewhat oblique to the axis of the aorta at this level.

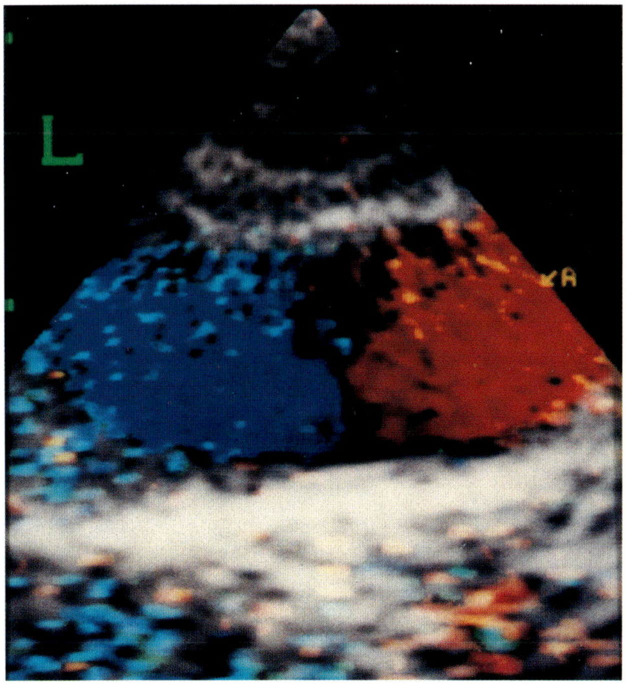

FIG 7–5.
Longitudinal view of the descending thoracic aorta *(A)* in the midthoracic region with color flow Doppler indicating the direction of flow. Note that this view corresponds to image G of Figure 2–18.

Supplementation by Surface Views of the Aortic Arch

TTE imaging can be used to supplement TEE examination of the aortic arch and major vessels and provide information about that portion of the arch not seen by TEE.[2, 5, 16] Figure 7–6 shows such a view in a child. Hyperextension of the neck and the use of a physically small surface transducer (even in adults) may facilitate this examination from the su-

A

B

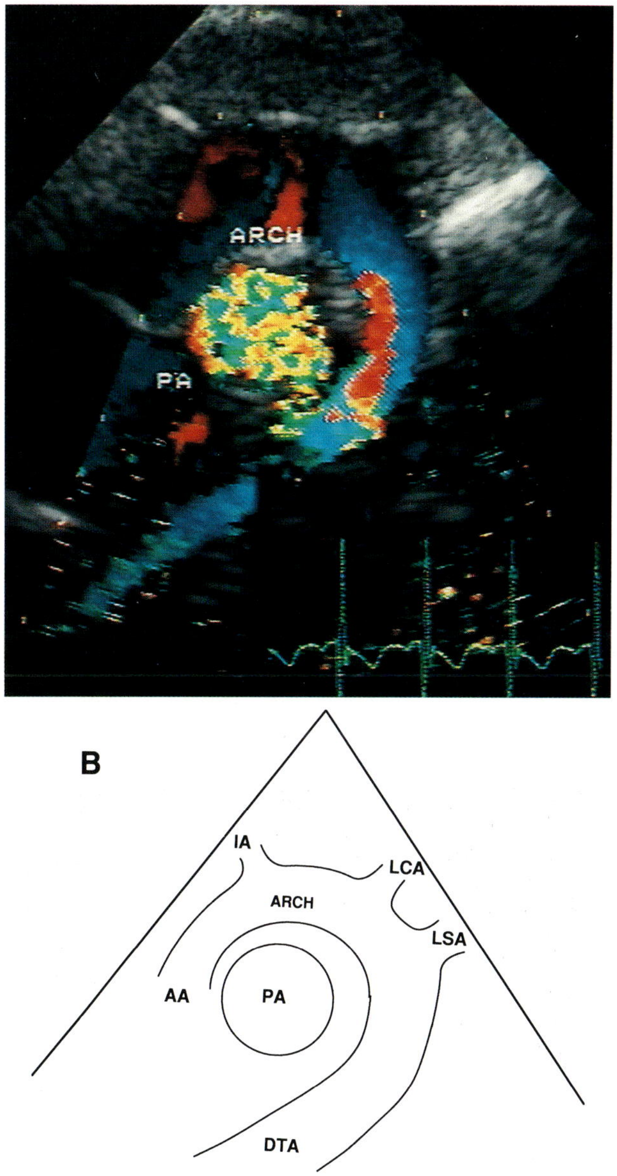

FIG 7–6.
The aortic arch *(ARCH)* from near the aortic annulus *(AA)* to the descending thoracic aorta *(DTA)* and the major arch vessels as imaged by TTE in a suprasternal view. The pulmonary artery *(PA)* is also seen, and the blood flow pattern is shown by color Doppler. *IA* = innominate artery, *LCA* = left carotid artery, *LSA* = left subclavian artery.

prasternal notch and/or parasternal first intercostal space. Of course, maintaining these images for continuous monitoring of an acute process is unreasonable, and obtaining them during surgery may be precluded by interference with the surgical field.

Normal Blood Flow in the Thoracic Aorta

Color flow patterns are observable and useful in both longitudinal and transverse orientations. Color flow Doppler can be used to aid in the location and identification of vascular structures. In examination of the aorta, it will be especially useful in situations where the image quality is substandard. It can also be used to detect abnormal flow patterns suggesting or confirming aortic pathology or to confirm that there is a normal flow pattern within the aorta.

Transverse

Blood flow in both the ascending and the descending aortas is perpendicular to the imaging plane for TEE with transverse transducer orientation, so the major velocity component of the aortic flow is not detectable by Doppler or color Doppler techniques. But in the descending aorta blood flow has a gentle swirling motion in the counterclockwise direction, as seen in Figure 7–7. This flow is called a left-handed swirl by hydraulic engineers since the motion follows the direction of the curve of the fingers of a relaxed left hand if the abducted thumb is pointed along the axis of the major flow.

At the level of the transverse aortic arch, blood flow is from the patient's right to his left and posterior toward the TEE transducer, so a significant component of the flow velocity is detectable by Doppler.

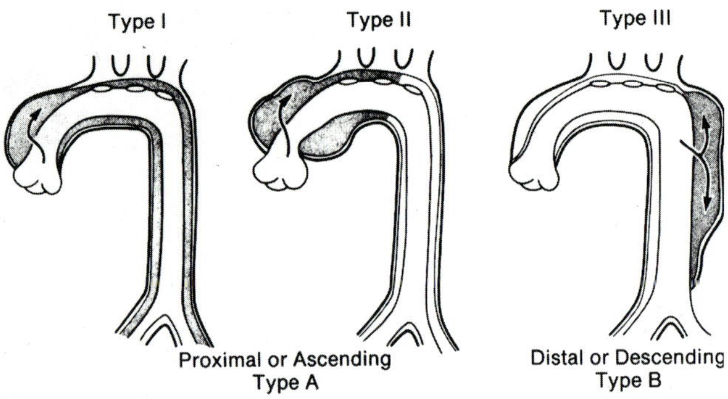

FIG 7–8.
The classification of thoracic aortic dissections is based on anatomic location. The DeBakey classification consists of types I, II, and III, and the Stanford classification consists of types A and B. DeBakey type III and Stanford type B originate distal to the left subclavian artery and extend caudad. (From Benumof JL: Anesthesia for emergency thoracic surgery, in *Anesthesia for Thoracic Surgery*. Philadelphia, WB Saunders Co, 1987. Used by permission.)

Since flow velocities are high in the aorta, there is predictable aliasing with color flow Doppler.

Longitudinal

For TEE with a longitudinally oriented transducer, a view as in Figure 7–5 is seen in the descending thoracic aorta. With color flow Doppler, the angles between the ultrasound beam and the major blood flow produce a pattern with blue toward the diaphragm and red toward the head.

When the aortic arch is viewed with a longitudinal array, flow is almost perpendicular to the transducer as it goes from right to left and posteriorly. Again, flow rates are high enough that there will

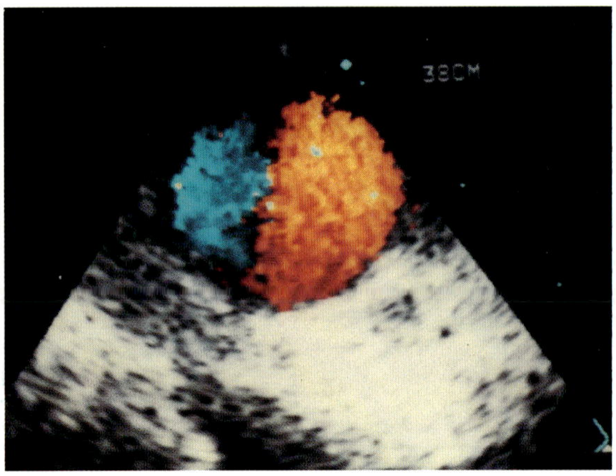

FIG 7–7.
The color Doppler flow pattern in the descending thoracic Aorta indicates a swirling motion. The tip of the TEE probe is 38 cm from the patient's lips.

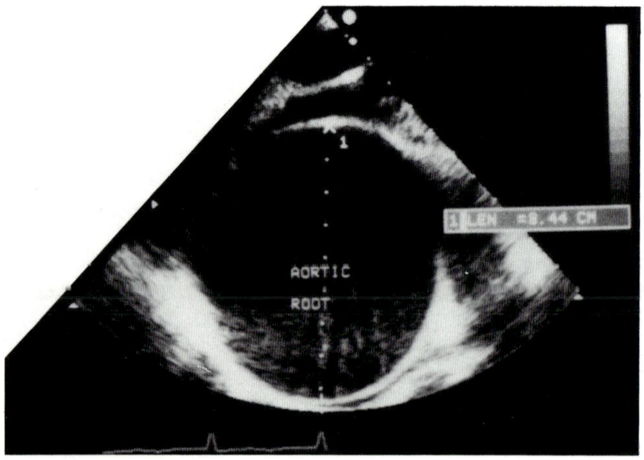

FIG 7–9.
Dilated aortic root in a patient with Marfan's syndrome. The intraluminal diameter is in excess of 8 cm, and there is significant aortic valve incompetence.

typically be aliasing of the small component of the velocity toward the transducer when color flow Doppler is used.

ABNORMAL FINDINGS

The following discussion presents a few interesting abnormal findings that can be discovered by using TEE. This is not intended as an exhaustive catalog.

Aortic Dissection or Disruption

Aortic dissections and disruptions are most often due to atherosclerotic disease or trauma.[2, 4, 6, 13, 16–18] Aortic dissections are classified by type as indicated in Figure 7–8.[19] Identification of the type of dissection is critical to proper surgical management since a DeBakey type III or Stanford type B dissection is preferentially approached through a left thoracotomy, whereas all other types must be approached through a median sternotomy.[20] Patients with Marfan's syndrome are predisposed to aortic dissections due to cystic medial necrosis.[3, 21, 22] Patients with Takayasu's aortitis can also present with aortic aneurysms and damaged aortic valves.[23] Figure 7–9 shows an aneurysmally dilated aortic root in a patient with Marfan's syndrome. Figures 7–10 and 7–11 show examples of TEE findings in patients with aortic dissections. Figure 7–12 shows a DeBakey type III traumatic com-

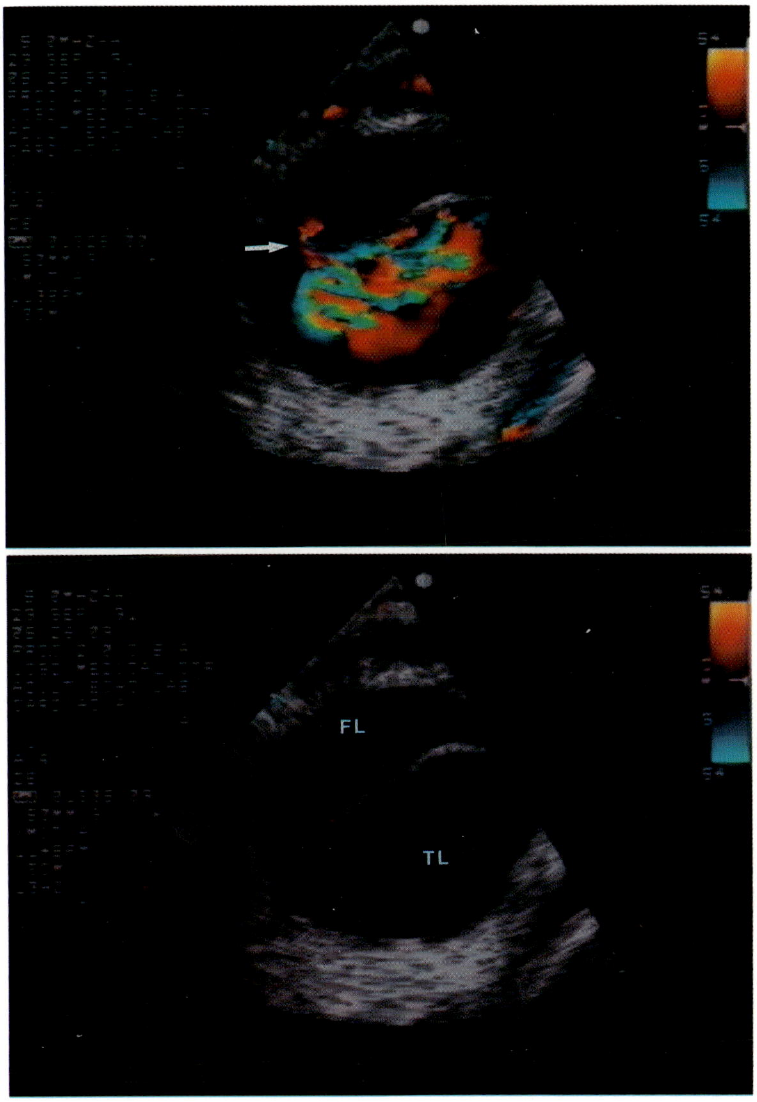

FIG 7–10.
Aortic dissection. Color flow Doppler identifies the intimal tear *(arrow)* in the flap dividing a false lumen *(FL)* from the true lumen *(TL)* in the descending aorta.

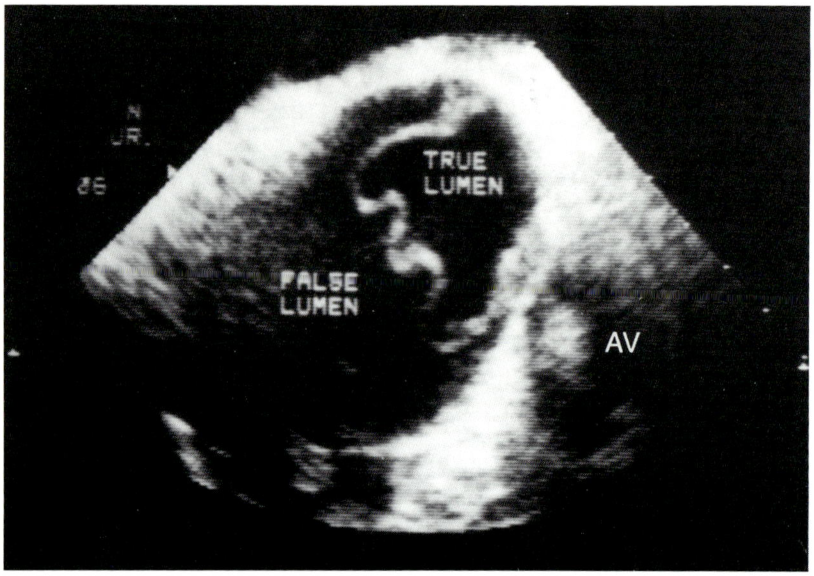

FIG 7–11.
Aortic dissection. A large intimal flap is seen to separate a false lumen from the true lumen in a DeBakey type I aortic dissection. There was also involvement of the aortic valve *(AV)* with acute aortic insufficiency.

plete disruption of the descending thoracic aorta with echocardiographic evidence of blood flow outside of the confines of the expected aortic lumen and loss of a well-defined intimal surface. Continuity of blood flow was maintained only by retropleural tissues. Figure 7–13 shows an intimal tear in the distal aortic arch near the left subclavian artery that was detected only by color flow Doppler. No intimal abnormalities could be seen with two-dimensional imaging alone or by CAT scan. Aortic angiography was suggestive but equivocal. Our experience suggests that the presence of any color flow Doppler evidence of intra-aortic flow turbulence should be considered as evidence of intimal damage.

In a recently published European cooperative study the sensitivity of TEE for aortic dissection was 99% with a specificity of 98% as compared with 83% and 100%, respectively, for CAT scan and 88% and 94%, respectively, for aortography.[13] This study employed only monoplane TEE, and this accounted for one false-negative finding in a patient with a DeBakey type II dissection. Use of biplane TEE has

A

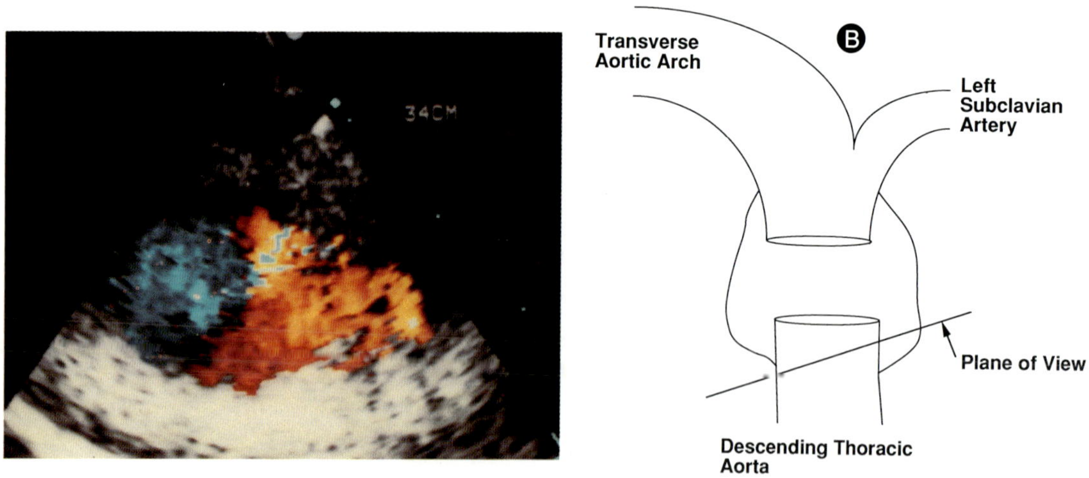

FIG 7–12.
Aortic disruption. **A,** a transverse view of the descending thoracic aorta shows flow outside the confines of the expected aortic lumen. With color Doppler turned off, the intimal surface was very ill defined at this level despite good image quality. **B,** drawing of the imaging plane.

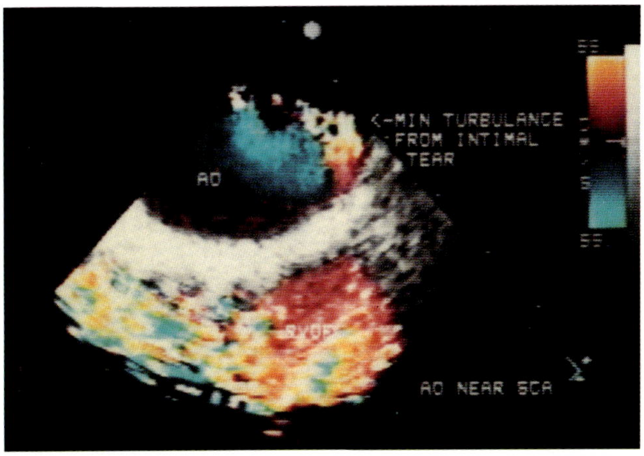

FIG 7-13.
An intimal tear in the distal aortic arch *(Ao)* near the left subclavian artery *(SCA)* is seen with color flow Doppler. No abnormality was detectable with two-dimensional imaging alone.

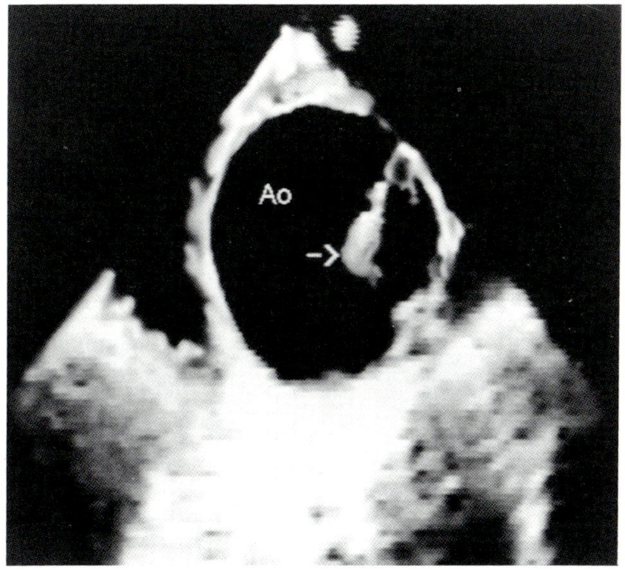

FIG 7-14.
Mobile intra-aortic mass. This pedunculated intraluminal mass *(arrow)* was found incidentally in the aorta *(Ao)* of a patient with atherosclerotic cardiovascular disease who was presenting for coronary artery bypass grafting. The patient had no prior or subsequent history of embolic disease.

substantially eliminated this problem and raises the sensitivity of TEE still higher.[24] In some institutions TEE is the diagnostic imaging modality of choice when aortic dissection is suspected, and surgical intervention may proceed without aortography or CAT scan.[6]

Atheromatous Disease

In TEE examination of the aorta of patients with atherosclerotic vascular disease, it is common to find echo-bright thickenings of the aortic luminal surface that intrude into the lumen. These findings are presumed to represent atherosclerotic plaques.[25-31] These plaques can ulcerate and become the nidus for intraluminal thrombus formation and the sources of systemic arterial emboli.[31] Figure 7-14 shows a pedunculated, mobile intraluminal mass. Such lesions have been found in about 1% of patients with recent strokes and are a presumed source of emboli[31] (see Chapter 4). But they have also been found in about 1% of patients with known cardiovascular disease who have not had embolic episodes, and the clinical significance of their presence is not completely appreciated.[32]

Congenital Variations

TEE and adjunct TTE can be useful in diagnosing and describing congenital variations in the anatomy of the aorta and major arch vessels.[33-35] As an example, Figure 7-15 shows a right aortic arch. The descending thoracic aorta is found to the right of the right atrium at the level of a four-chamber view instead of to the left of the left atrium as is usual.

SUMMARY

TEE is useful in the examination of the thoracic aorta, especially for aortic aneurysms, dissection and

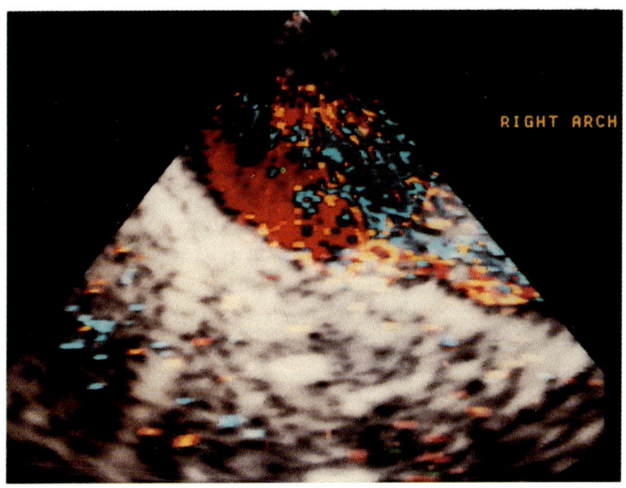

FIG 7-15.
Right-sided aortic arch (compare with Fig 2-21). The transverse arch comes from the patient's left to become the descending aorta located to the right of the esophagus and spinal column.

disruptions, congenital abnormalities, and embolic disease. Although TEE is usually blind to a portion of the transverse aortic arch, a combination of TEE and TTE can provide reliable imaging of the entire thoracic aorta. TEE has the advantage of being less invasive than aortic angiography. TEE allows better continued access to the patient during intensive care than MRI or CAT scan does, and it has more portability than these other imaging modalities. TEE can often be used for continuous monitoring of patients in acute situations. The use of standard anatomic views is an important aid to the interpretation of TEE images of the thoracic aorta. Color Doppler flow mapping in conjunction with TEE provides useful information about aortic blood flow patterns and may aid in the detection, identification, and evaluation of structural abnormalities.

REFERENCES

1. Gussenhoven EJ, Taams MA, Roelandt J, et al: Oesophageal echocardiography. *Int J Card Imaging* 1987; 2:231–239.
2. Erbel R, Borner N, Steller D, et al: Detection of aortic dissection by transesophageal echocardiography. *Br Heart J* 1987; 58:45–51.
3. Doerr W: Thoracic aortic aneurysms. *Thorac Cardiovasc Surg* 1987; 35:111–121.
4. Engberding R, Bender F, Grosse-Heitmeyer W, et al: Identification of dissection or aneurysm of the descending thoracic aorta by conventional and transesophageal echocardiography. *Am J Cardiol* 1987; 59:717–719.
5. Mintz GS, Kotler MN, Segal BL, et al: Two dimensional echocardiographic recognition of the descending thoracic aorta. *Am J Cardiol* 1979; 44:232–238.
6. Mitchell MM, Sutherland GR, Gussenhoven EJ, et al: Transesophageal echocardiography: State-of-the-art technologies. *J Am Soc Echocardiogr* 1988; 1:362–377.
7. Khandheria BK, Tajik AJ, Taylor CL, et al: Aortic dissection: Review of value and limitations of two-dimensional echocardiography in a six-year experience. *J Am Soc Echocardiogr* 1989; 2:17–24.
8. Goldman A, Kotler M, Scanlon M, et al: The complementary role of magnetic resonance imaging, Doppler echocardiography, and computed tomography in the diagnosis of dissecting thoracic aneurysms. *Am Heart J* 1986; 111:970–981.
9. Jamison N: Misleading aortographic finding in acute aortic dissection explained. *J R Soc Med* 1984; 77:427.
10. Shuford W, Sybers R, Weens H: Problems in the aortographic diagnosis of dissecting aneurysms of the aorta. *N Engl J Med* 1969; 280:225.
11. Daniel W, Erbel R, Kasper W, et al: Safety of transesophageal echocardiography: A multicenter survey of 10,419 examinations. *Circulation* 1991; 83:817–821.
12. Gussenhoven EJ, Taams MA, Roelandt JRTC, et al: Transesophageal two-dimensional echocardiography: Its role in solving clinical problems. *J Am Coll Cardiol* 1986; 8:975–979.
13. Erbel R, Daniel W, Visser C, et al: Echocardiography in diagnosis of aortic dissection. *Lancet* 1989; 3:457–461.
14. Seward JB, Khandheria BK, Oh JK, et al: Transesophageal echocardiography: Technique, anatomic correlation, implementation, and clinical applications. *Mayo Clin Proc* 1988; 63:649–680.
15. Orihashi K, Hong Y, Sisto D, et al: The anatomical location of the transesophageal echocardiographic transducer during a short-axis view of the left ventricle. *J Cardiothorac Anesthesia* 1990; 4:726–730.
16. Kasper W, Meinertz T, Kersting F, et al: Diagnosis of dissecting aortic aneurysm with suprasternal echocardiography. *Am J Cardiol* 1978; 42:291–294.
17. Goldman ME, Guarino T, Mindich BP: Localization of aortic dissection intimal flap by intraoperative two-dimensional echocardiography. *J Am Coll Cardiol* 1985; 6:1155–1159.
18. Mohr-Kahaly S, Erbel R, Steller D, et al: Aortic dissection detected by transesophageal echocardiography. *Int J Card Imaging* 1986; 2:31–35.
19. Benumof JL: Anesthesia for emergency thoracic surgery, in *Anesthesia for Thoracic Surgery*. Philadelphia, WB Saunders Co, 1987.
20. Prandi L, Colombi P, La Vecchia L: Diagnosis and surgical management of patients with aneurysms of the thoracic aorta with various causes. *Br Heart J* 1986; 55:81–91.
21. Pruzinsky M, Katz N, Green C, et al: Isolated descending thoracic aortic aneurysm in Marfan's syndrome. *Am J Cardiol* 1988; 61:1159–1160.
22. Liu M, Louie E, Levitsky S: Color flow Doppler assessment of aortic regurgitation complicated by aneurysmal dilation and dissection of the ascending aorta in the Marfan syndrome. *Am Heart J* 1988; 115:1118–1119.
23. Iga K, Hori K, Kobashi Y, et al: Successful surgical treatment of acute aortic regurgitation caused by Takayasu's aortitis. *J Thorac Cardiovasc Surg* 1990; 99:946–948.
24. Seward JB, et al: Biplane transesophageal echocardiography: Anatomic correlations, image orientation, and clinical application. *Mayo Clin Proc* 1990; 65:1193–1213.
25. Gagliardi JM, Batt M, Khodja RH, et al: Mural thrombus of the aorta. *Ann Vasc Surg* 1988; 2:201–204.
26. Karalis DG, Chandrasekaran K, Victor MF, et al: The recognition and embolic potential of intraaortic atherosclerotic debris. *Circulation* 1990; 82(suppl 3):246.
27. Nader RG, Barr F, Rubin R, et al: Aortic degenerative changes and thrombus formation: An unusual cause

of massive myocardial infarction with normal coronary arteries. *Am J Med* 1989; 86:718–722.

28. Orihashi K, Leehn L, Hong Y, et al: Abnormal findings of the descending thoracic aorta in patients undergoing coronary artery bypass surgery examined by transesophageal echocardiography (abstract). *Anesthesiology* 1990; 73:431.
29. Rudas G, Bors S: Aortic thrombosis diagnosed by ultrasound. *Pediatr Radiol* 1988; 18:77–78.
30. Sadony V, Walz M, Lohr E, et al: Unusual cause of recurrent arterial embolism: Floating thrombus in the aortic arch surgically removed under hypothermic cardiocirculatory arrest. *Eur J Cardiothorac Surg* 1988; 2:469–471.
31. Tunick PA, Kronzon I: Protruding atherosclerotic plaque in the aortic arch of patients with systemic embolization: A new finding seen by transesophageal echocardiography. *Am Heart J* 1990; 120:658–660.
32. Mitchell M, Frankville D, Weinger M, et al: Detection of thoracic aortic atheroma with transesophageal echocardiography in patients without symptoms of embolism. *Am Heart J* 1991; 122:1768–1771.
33. Enderlein M, Silverman N, Stanger P, et al: Usefulness of suprasternal notch echocardiography for diagnosis of double aortic arch. *Am J Cardiol* 1986; 57:359–361.
34. Murdison K, Andrews B, Chin A: Ultrasonographic display of complex vascular rings. *J Am Coll Cardiol* 1990; 15:1645–1653.
35. Celano V, Pieroni D, Gingell R, et al: Two-dimensional echocardiographic recognition of the right aortic arch. *Am J Cardiol* 1983; 51:1507–1512.

Chapter 8

Applications in Congenital Heart Disease

George R. Sutherland, F.E.C.S., F.R.C.P.

Oliver F. W. Stümper, M.D.

The use of the transesophageal approach was introduced in adult patients with acquired heart disease in an attempt to circumvent ultrasonic attenuation caused by the chest wall and lungs, which frequently restricts precordial echocardiographic imaging in this age group. Frazin et al. initially attempted this by using an M-mode technique, but it was not until the introduction of transesophageal two-dimensional phased-array imaging by Hanrath et al. (using a 2.5-MHz phased-array transducer mounted at the tip of an endoscope) that the technique appeared to be of potential clinical value. Although a number of publications on the use of this probe appeared in the literature, interest in the technique remained limited because image quality was poor and only morphologic information could be obtained. It was not until the introduction of the second generation of transesophageal probes in 1986–1987, which provided the combination of high-resolution imaging of morphology (centered around 5.0 MHz) and the definition of intracardiac flow patterns by color flow mapping and pulsed Doppler studies, that transesophageal imaging began to generate much interest. Over a remarkably short period of time, this ultrasound approach has been shown to be of major value in the assessment of mitral valve disease, mitral prosthetic dysfunction, infective endocarditis, the assessment of intracardiac sources of emboli, and the evaluation of thoracic aorta pathology.[1] In addition to diagnostic studies, the transesophageal approach has been employed to monitor left ventricular function and interventional procedures in both the operating suite and the catheterization laboratory.

With the introduction of dedicated pediatric transesophageal probes in 1989,[2] transesophageal echocardiography (TEE) has become available for studying congenital heart defects in even small children.[3, 4] To determine what role TEE might play in pediatric cardiology, we reviewed our experience with 247 TEE examinations performed as part of a prospective study in 213 children during a 24-month period. The studies were carried out in three clinical situations: for the primary diagnosis of congenital heart disease, for monitoring either in cardiac surgery during the perioperative period or during interventional cardiac catheterization procedures, and for assessment of surgical results in the late follow-up period. The transesophageal information obtained in each of these clinical situations was correlated with information derived (where appropriate) from prior transthoracic echocardiographic studies, intraoperative epicardial ultrasound, cardiac catheterization, and surgical inspection. The age at investigation ranged from 0.2 to 14.8 years (mean age, 4.8 years) and the weight from 3.7 to 52 kg (mean weight, 17.2 kg). Recently, some investigators have reported successful studies in still smaller children including premature infants.[5, 6] However, since transesophageal studies in children must be considered a semi-invasive procedure with inherent life-threatening potential complications, it is our opinion that children weighing less than 4 kg should be studied only where TEE is likely to provide important clinical information unobtainable by any other diagnostic technique.

TECHNICAL ASPECTS OF PERFORMING TEE IN CHILDREN

In the majority of the 213 children, the studies were performed under general anesthesia administered for either cardiac catheterization or cardiac surgery. However, in selected cases, studies were carried out on a day-care admission basis by using either general anesthesia or appropriate intravenous sedation. Endocarditis prophylaxis was not given in any child. This remains our standard policy. We did not experience any evidence of bacterial endocarditis resulting from these 247 procedures, nor have we in a further 257 studies carried out without antibiotic prophylaxis in a series of adolescent and adult patients with congenital heart disease. (See Chapter 3 for a detailed discussion of this topic.) Probe insertion was successful in all but 1 child. Three children referred for a transesophageal study were excluded on the basis of either severe coagulation disorder (2 patients) or severe spinal deformity (1 patient). Important complications were encountered during 3 studies (1.2% of the total pediatric cases). These included self-terminating short-lived arrhythmias in 2. No deaths occurred. There was no incidence of esophageal perforation. Signs of minor esophageal bleeding (streaking of the probe with blood) were encountered in only 1 patient. This very low complication rate would suggest that in trained hands and with appropriate care being taken in probe manipulation, TEE in children over 4 kg in body weight is a safe technique.

TEE IN THE PRIMARY DIAGNOSIS OF CONGENITAL HEART DISEASE IN THE PEDIATRIC AGE GROUP

With the natural reduction in ultrasound windows that occurs in later childhood, the transthoracic and subcostal approaches are frequently compromised. In children with complex congenital heart disease associated with cardiac malposition, malrotation, or thoracic cage abnormalities, a comprehensive assessment of intracardiac morphology from the precordium may be limited. In such cases the transesophageal approach offers an alternative and potentially better acoustic window. The technique usually (but not invariably) provides excellent image quality since it is not restricted by either the thoracic cage or interposed lung tissue. Such primary diagnostic studies are best combined with diagnostic cardiac catheterization studies in order that both can be carried out during the one anesthetic.

Atrial Appendage Juxtaposition

Esophageal imaging allowed visualization of both atrial appendages in every patient studied. Thus, by observing the unique morphologic characteristics of either atrial appendage, the direct diagnosis of the atrial situs is provided.[7] Similarly, TEE is, in our experience, the definitive diagnostic technique in identifying juxtaposition (either right or left) of the atrial appendages.[8] Although both of these morphologic entities are of somewhat limited clinical importance, their definition may be of value when planning a number of surgical procedures (such as a Fontan operation).

Anomalous Venous Connections

In the preoperative definition of the venous connections to the heart, the transesophageal approach proved to be largely superior to the transthoracic ultrasound approach in the documentation of anomalous systemic and pulmonary venous connections.[9] In particular, our experience showed that anomalous superior vena cavae connections or partial anomalous pulmonary venous connections were consistently better defined from within the esophagus than from the precordium. The correct morphology of the systemic veins could be documented in all patients studied, and the site of drainage of all four pulmonary veins could be defined in 92% of all cases. When compared with surgical inspection (which is considered the gold standard in the definition of venous connections to the heart), TEE had a sensitivity and specificity of 100% in the detection of anomalous venous connections. In addition, the technique contributed additional important morphologic information when compared with angiocardiography. Thus, TEE should be considered a most valuable diagnostic adjunct in the preoperative evaluation of children in whom anomalous venous connections are either suspected or must be excluded (since their presence would considerably alter the surgical approach).

Abnormalities of the Interatrial Septum

Transesophageal cross-sectional imaging also allows a much improved assessment of the integrity of the atrial septum. It can consistently define the number of atrial septal defects present and their individual morphologies (Fig 8–1). In particular, sinus venosus or multiple atrial septal defects are more readily identified by combined transesophageal cross-sectional imaging and color flow mapping.[10, 11] In children with suspected superior sinus venosus atrial septal defects in whom precordial or subcostal imaging is nondiagnostic, transesophageal imaging in the transverse plane will consistently define the morphology that characterizes the defect and the associated abnormalities of drainage of the right-sided pulmonary veins. Such detailed studies will normally obviate the need for diagnostic cardiac catheterization. It has been our experience that the addition of scanning in the longitudinal plane has added nothing to the definition of these defects. The transesophageal evaluation of patients with deficiencies of the fossa ovalis (secundum-type atrial septal defects) provides a new insight and understanding of the complex anatomy of the atrial septum. In particular, the anterosuperior rim of the defect can be better defined by esophageal scanning than by precordial or subcostal imaging. In view of the recent development of transcatheter techniques that use occlusive devices for closure of these defects, TEE definition of the precise defect morphology and the relationship of the defect margins to other important atrial structures (the coronary sinus or the orifices of the cavae, etc.) should become important in appropriate patient selection.[12]

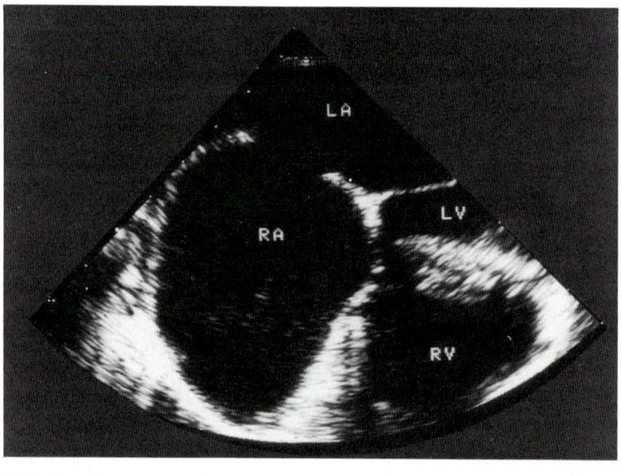

FIG 8–1.
Transverse plane transesophageal image of a secundum atrial septal defect. The margins of the defect are well delineated and are shown to lie within the secundum atrial septum. The defect measures 1.8 cm in this plane. Further scanning in the transverse plane confirmed normal drainage of all four pulmonary veins to the left atrium *(LA)*. A left superior vena cava was excluded. In such cases, scanning in the longitudinal plane is required for accurate sizing of the defect prior to consideration of umbrella device defect closure. Any attempt at device closure should subsequently be monitored by biplane transesophageal echocardiography. (*LV* = left ventricle; *RA* = right atrium; *RV* = right ventricle.)

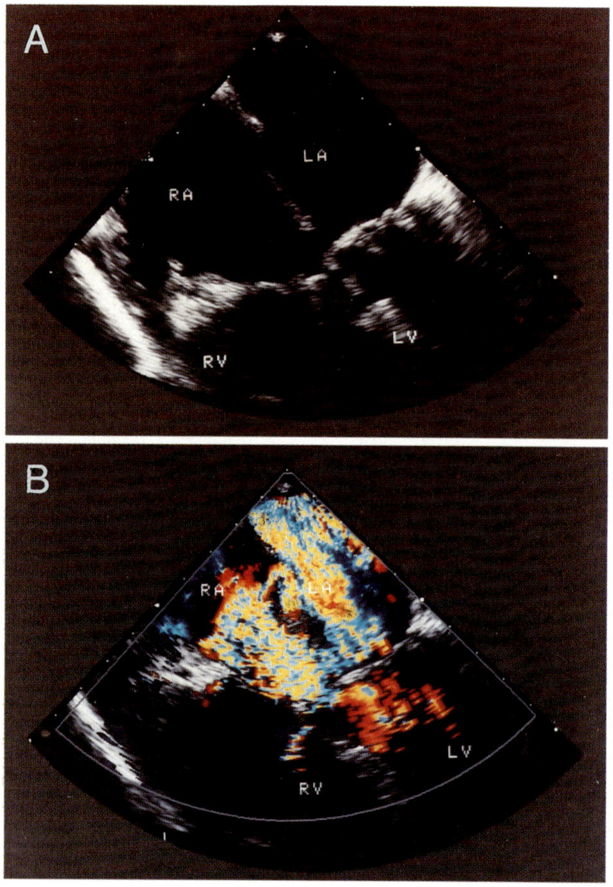

FIG 8–2.
A, transverse plane image of a partial atrioventricular septal defect. The defect is well defined as being roofed superiorly by the secundum atrial septum and inferiorly by the common atrioventricular valve. Note the close-packed chordae closing what is a potential ventricular component to the defect. In addition, note the slight bulge of the patent foramen ovale into the left atrium. **B,** color Doppler image from the same patient. This color flow map demonstrates regurgitation from both the left and right component of the common atrioventricular valve. Note also the communication across the primum atrial septum. In addition, there is a small left to right shunt through the foramen ovale. Transesophageal imaging in the transverse plane will normally give the optimal morphologic and hemodynamic information on these defects. The complexity of the intracardiac shunting is well appreciated using this technique. (*LA* = left atrium; *LV* = left ventricle, *RA* = right atrium; *RV* = right ventricle.)

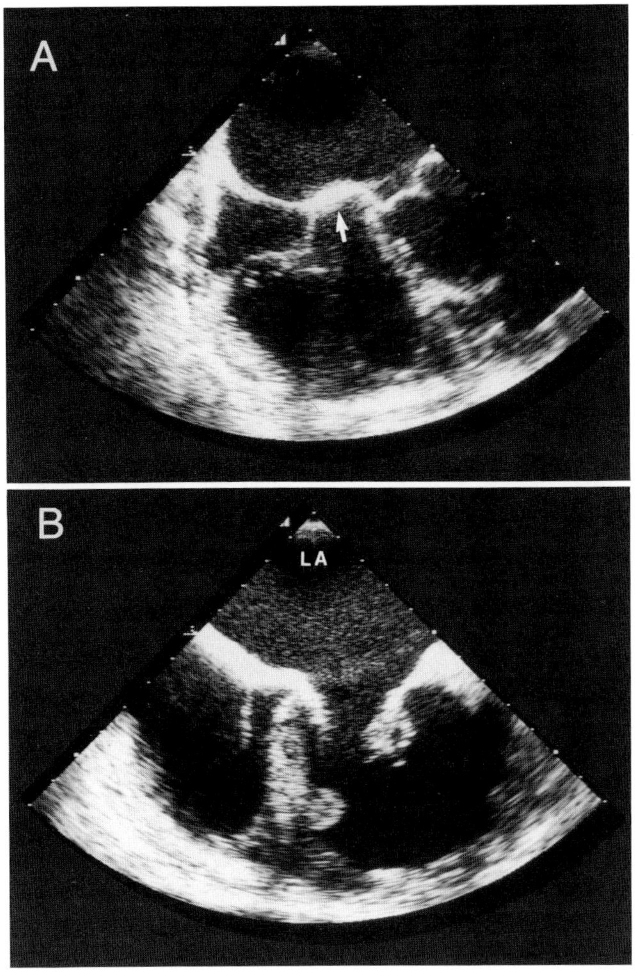

FIG 8–3.
A, transverse plane systolic image of a patient with atrioventricular discordance and an intact ventricular septum. The transverse plane view demonstrates well the abnormal orientation of the atrial septum as compared to the ventricular septum which is a consistent feature of this abnormal atrioventricular connection. In addition, the abnormal reversed implantation of the atrioventricular valve septal leaflets into the base of the atrial septum is well seen. The right-sided atrioventricular valve implants into the base of the primum septum while the left atrioventricular valve (the morphologic tricuspid valve) is inserted lower into the crest of the ventricular septum. The valves are separated by an extensive atrioventricular septum *(arrow)*. **B,** transverse plane image of the same patient taken in diastole. This demonstrates the opening of the left-sided atrioventricular valve (the tricuspid valve) with the chordae implanting only on to the septum, again confirming the morphology of this valve and this ventricle. Note the spontaneous contrast in the left atrium *(LA)* which was a reflection of the low cardiac output in this patient due to failure of the systemic (morphologic right) ventricle.

Atrioventricular Valve Morphology

In the assessment of the complexities of morphology and function of either atrioventricular valve (Figs 8–2 and 8–3) and its subvalvar apparatus in complex congenital heart disease, transesophageal studies can frequently contribute additional valuable information when compared with precordial ultrasound studies (see Fig 8–2). The mechanism of valvular regurgitation and the site and number of regurgitant jets are often better defined (see Fig 8–2). However, the major contribution of the technique in the evaluation of these lesions lies in the ability of the high resolution of transesophageal imaging to definitively exclude chordal straddling.[13] In addition, in patients with either tricuspid or mitral atresia it better differentiates an imperforate valve from an absent connection.

Ventricular Outflow Evaluation

The technique also offers an improved insight into the spectrum of lesions producing left ventricular outflow obstruction.[14] Multiple insertions of so-called fibromuscular membranes are better defined, as is any involvement in the obstructive lesion of the anterior leaflet of the mitral valve or its subvalvular apparatus. In contrast, in our experience, relatively little additional information (compared with precor-

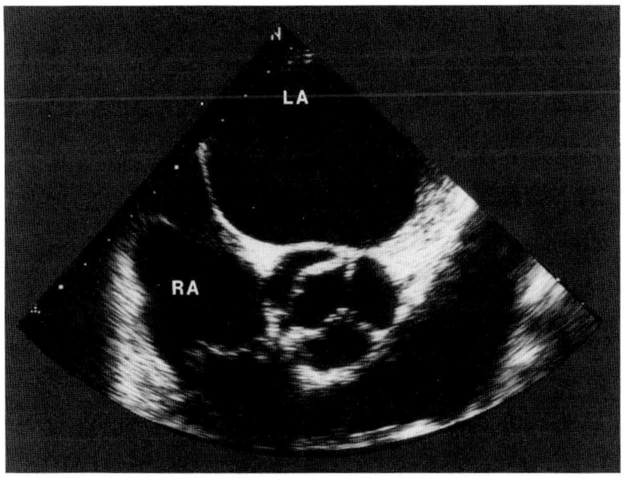

FIG 8–4.
Longitudinal axis image taken in systole from a patient with a morphologically tricuspid but functionally bicuspid aortic valve. This morphology is clearly demonstrated in this image. One advantage of the longitudinal plane is that it is possible using the lateral steering mechanism to obtain a cross-sectional image of the aortic valve in the majority of patients. This can give valuable new information on valve morphology and function. (*LA* = left atrium; *RA* = right atrium.)

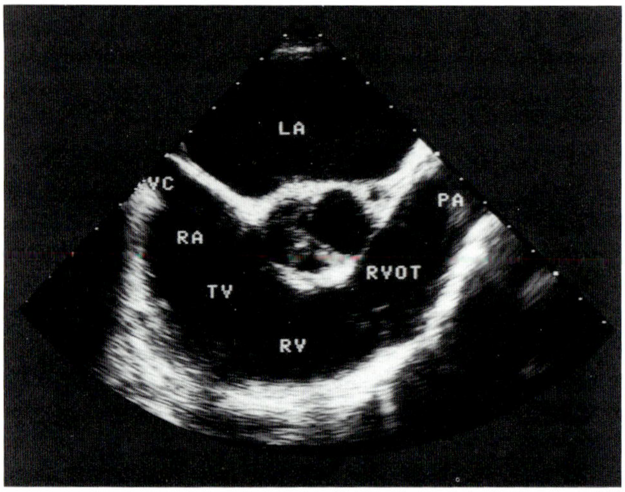

FIG 8–5.
Transesophageal image taken in the long axis to demonstrate the appearances of the normal inflow and outflow tract *(RVOT)* of the right ventricle *(RV)*. It is this longitudinal scan plane that reveals the most information on the morphology of pulmonary valve or sub pulmonary obstruction. This region is poorly characterized by transverse axis scanning. (*LA* = left atrium; *PA* = pulmonary artery; *RA* = right atrium; *SVC* = superior vena cava; *TV* = tricuspid valve.)

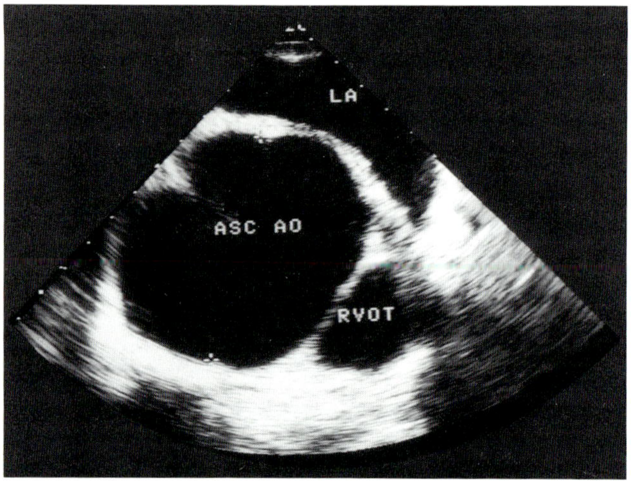

FIG 8–7.
Transverse axis scan from a patient with Marfan's syndrome. The transverse scan of the ascending aorta *(ASCAO)* shows gross dilatation of this vessel with a dimension of 6.6 cm. This patient had developed acute chest pain but with no evidence of dissection. As a result of this acute dilatation of the aortic root imaged on transesophageal echocardiography, he was referred for acute aortic surgery. (*LA* = left atrium; *RVOT* = right ventricular outflow tract.)

dial imaging) is obtained by transverse-plane transesophageal imaging of lesions involving the ventricular septum, the right ventricular outflow tract, or the thoracic aorta.[4] Longitudinal-plane imaging cannot scan the ventricular septum and has no place in the evaluation of ventricular septal defects, whereas the longitudinal approach has major benefits in the evaluation of lesions involving the aortic valve (Fig 8–4), the right ventricular outflow tract (Fig 8–5), the left pulmonary artery, the arterial duct (Fig 8–6), and the thoracic aorta (Fig 8–7).

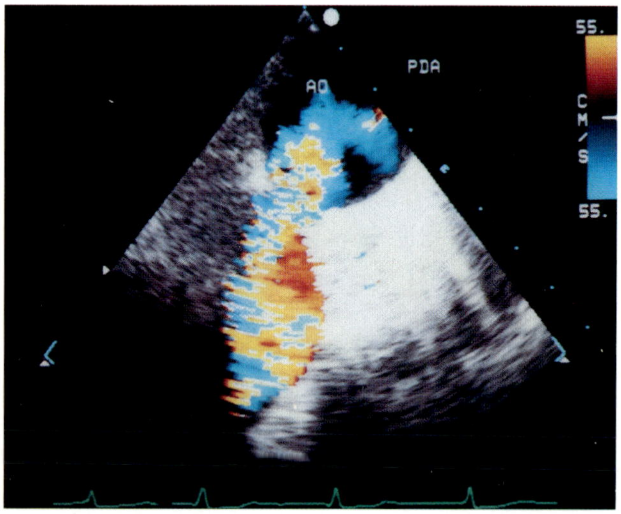

FIG 8–6.
Patent ductus arteriosis. Transverse view of the descending thoracic aorta *(AO)* just distal to the aortic arch, demonstrating flow into the left pulmonary artery through a large patent ductus arteriosis *(PDA)*. The use of color flow Doppler mapping facilitates identification of the PDA. (Courtesy of Mark Mitchell, M.D., University of California, San Diego.)

MONITORING DURING CARDIAC SURGERY AND INTERVENTIONAL CARDIAC CATHETERIZATION IN CHILDREN

TEE in Cardiac Surgery

In theory, TEE would appear to be the ultimate monitoring technique in surgery for congenital heart disease in the pediatric age group because it does not interfere with the surgical procedure or invade the sterile operative field. However, to date, both the image quality and the range of scan planes that can be obtained by direct epicardial ultrasound studies are, in our experience, much superior to those obtained from a single-plane transesophageal study.[15] This limitation of intraoperative transesophageal imaging is only partially overcome by the addition of scanning in the longitudinal plane. Further advantages of epicardial imaging include, first, its wide availability (no special probes are required, and standard ultrasound machines can be used); second, epicardial imaging is less demanding in manpower (if the surgeon performs the scan); and third, it is possible to perform studies in virtually all children (even neonates). Transesophageal imaging, as a result of the limited scan planes available, is also limited by its inability to obtain information from behind prosthetic material that lies in its path. Epicardial imaging, as a direct consequence of the wide variety of scanning positions available, can allow the interrogation of both sides of any intracardiac prosthetic material. A further advantage of TEE lies in its ability to allow the continuous monitoring of both ventricular function and volume status before and after bypass.

In the postbypass exclusion of residual hemodynamic lesions, the transesophageal approach has been shown to be superior to the epicardial approach in the assessment of surgical repairs involving the atrioventricular valves.[16] Following closure of ventricular septal defects, transesophageal studies were recently reported by Roberson et al. to be superior to direct epicardial imaging in the evaluation of surgical results.[17] Our own experience, however, is substantially different. Following prosthetic patch closure of ventricular septal defects, a large area of ultrasound shadowing in the right ventricle may prevent the acquisition of meaningful color flow mapping information and thus makes the exclusion of residual shunting by transesophageal studies unreliable. The degree of prosthetic flow masking is variable and is directly related to the prosthetic patch material. Dacron patches are virtually impenetrable by ultrasound, whereas biologic patches will be partially (but variably) penetrated. Thus, we currently recommend the use of contrast echocardiographic studies using epicardial imaging as the intraoperative technique for use in the rapid identification and semiquantitation of residual shunting following ventricular septal defect closure.[18]

Following Fontan-type procedures even minor residual hemodynamic lesions may be detrimental. Intraoperative ultrasound studies are perhaps their most rewarding in this context because they provide a detailed assessment of the immediate surgical results and an accurate identification of even minor residual lesions. They therefore open up the possibility of immediate reoperation on a second period of bypass. In our experience, epicardial ultrasound techniques proved to be a most valuable tool in the majority of such cases studied.[19] However, problems were encountered when epicardial scanning was used to assess patch integrity following total cavopulmonary connections. This was due to the presence of prosthetic material causing flow masking within the right atrial cavity. These limitations could be circumvented by the (additional) use of intraoperative transesophageal studies.[20] Thus, in the intraoperative setting, epicardial and TEE studies should be considered complementary rather than mutually exclusive techniques for use in the evaluation of surgical repairs (Table 8–1). The decision to use one or other (or both) technique should be based on the

TABLE 8–1.

A Comparison of Intraoperative Transesophageal and Epicardial Echocardiography in the Assessment of Intracardiac Morphology and Hemodynamics During the Surgical Correction of Congenital Heart Disease*†

	Epicardial Echocardiography		Transesophageal Echocardiography	
	Morphological Condition	Function	Morphological Condition	Function
Systemic venous return	+++	++	++	+
Pulmonary venous return	++	+	+++	+++
Atrial septum	+++	++	+++	+++
Tricuspid valve	++	++	+	++
Mitral valve	+++	++	+++	+++
Ventricular septum	+++	+++	+	+[1]
Ventricular chambers	+++	++	+	+++
LVOT	+++	+++	+++	+
RVOT	+++	+++	−(+)[2]	−
Thoracic aorta	++	++	+	−
Pulmonary arteries	++	++	+[2]	+[2]

*From Stümper O, Kaulitz R, Sreeram N, et al: *J Am Soc Echocardiogr* 1990; 3:392–401. Used by permission.
†LVOT = left ventricular outflow tract; RVOT = right ventricular outflow tract; − = inadequate; + = adequate; ++ = good; +++ = excellent; [1] = inadequate after prosthetic patch closure of ventricular septal defects; [2] = largely dependent on the size of the acoustic window.

consideration of a combination of factors. These should include the weight of the patient, the lesion, and the surgical correction planned. In selected cases, a combination of both techniques would appear to provide the maximal information.

In the early postoperative setting, with the chest closed, precordial ultrasound studies may be limited in the diagnostic information that can be derived due to the presence of wound dressings, suction tubes, and entrapped air.[21] In such cases, the transesophageal approach can allow detailed information to be obtained, and a full assessment of the repair can be undertaken. This is especially true of repairs at the atrial or atrioventricular junction level. Following atrial correction procedures for complete transposition or Fontan-type procedures for complex congenital heart disease, transesophageal studies would appear to be the diagnostic technique of choice in early postoperative evaluation. In addition, the technique can allow the continuous monitoring of systemic ventricular function and ventricular filling characteristics following repair of complex congenital heart disease. Thus, TEE has an important role to play in the diagnosis and management of early postoperative complications. Recently, Zahn and associates reported their experience with the technique in the early postoperative evaluation of children who have undergone an arterial switch procedure for complete transposition.[22]

TEE in Interventional Procedures

Although TEE has been used successfully in the monitoring of aortic and mitral valvuloplasty in the adult patient population,[23] so far no reports have addressed which role it may play in monitoring of the wide spectrum of catheter intervention procedures currently used in children with congenital heart disease. Our initial experience suggests that such studies can be performed without interfering with or prolonging the procedure. In fact, the amount of radiation received and the dose of contrast material used to monitor the results of the intervention were substantially limited in our series. The technique provides real-time imaging information on the intervention, which is of value in guiding the procedure, in the immediate exclusion of complications, and in the assessment of immediate hemodynamic changes.[24] In particular, balloon catheter placement across either a semilunar or an atrioventricular valve is greatly enhanced when compared with standard radiographic monitoring. Entrapment of the guidewire or catheter within the subvalvular apparatus is readily documented and should allow subsequent repositioning in order to prevent immediate complications. During aortic valvuloplasty, the development of aortic incompetence can be readily detected and its mechanism readily defined, thus allowing correct decisions to be made as to the advisability of subsequent balloon inflations. During aortic or pulmonary angioplasty procedures, intimal dissection can be reliably identified or excluded. Finally, transesophageal studies would appear to be the monitoring technique of choice during balloon dilatations of obstructed venous pathways that have occurred following a Mustard procedure. In contrast, the monitoring of device closure of a ductus arteriosus was, in our experience, not enhanced by single-plane transesophageal imaging. Further applications for transesophageal monitoring of interventional procedures include the device closure of atrial septal defects, recently reported in a series of adult patients by Hellenbrand and associates,[25] closure of ventricular septal defects,[26] and the monitoring of coil embolization of coronary artery fistulas and blade septostomies.

POSTOPERATIVE FOLLOW-UP OF CONGENITAL HEART DISEASE IN CHILDREN

A high proportion of children with surgically corrected congenital heart disease require close follow-up. Precordial ultrasound studies play an integral part in this patient population. However, in clinical practice, these studies are frequently restricted in the range of information that can be derived. Both the presence of fibrous tissue adhesions and the natural reduction of the precordial and subcostal ultrasound windows often preclude a complete assessment of the surgical repair. Frequently, little information can be obtained from precordial studies in patients following an atrial baffle procedure (Mustard or Senning) for complete transposition, following Fontan-type procedures, or after prosthetic valve replacement. In these patients the alternative transesophageal ultrasound approach has proved to be the most rewarding.[27]

Following Mustard procedures, the technique provides a detailed and complete assessment of atrial baffle morphology and function in all patients studied.[28] The entire systemic and pulmonary venous pathways can be interrogated with ease. Pathway obstructions or baffle leakage, the two most common postoperative sequelae, can be readily identified or definitively excluded. In addition, transesophageal pulsed-wave Doppler studies would appear to be of value in the exclusion of individual pulmonary venous obstruction. Moreover, these studies may provide a most valuable tool in the assessment of systemic ventricular function following a Mustard procedure.[29] In view of the range of information to be derived in this group of patients, transesophageal studies should, in our opinion, become an integral part in the follow-up of every Mustard procedure. In most cases they should obviate the need for routine follow-up cardiac catheterization.

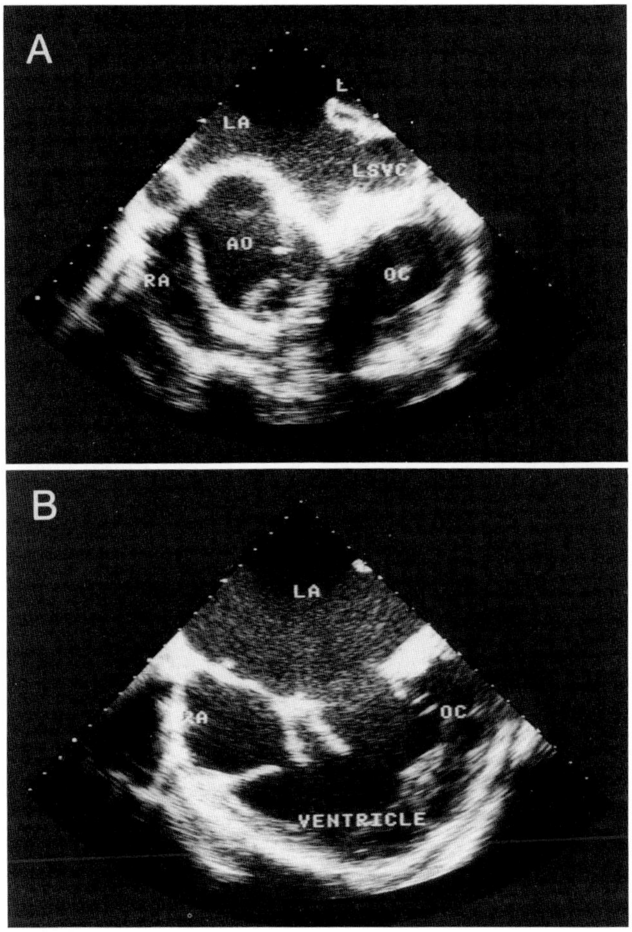

FIG 8–8.
A, transverse plane image demonstrating the characteristic position of a left superior vena cava *(LSVC)* in a patient with a double inlet left ventricle. A left superior vena cava will characteristically be positioned between the left upper pulmonary vein (*L*) and the left atrial appendage. Where such a structure is visualized, its drainage site must be determined. A complete scan of the left atrium *(LA)* and coronary sinus must be performed to determine this. (*AO* = aortic outflow; *RA* = right atrium.) **B,** transverse plane scan of the inlet of the main ventricular chamber in the same patient with double inlet left ventricle. Note the clear confirmation in this patient that both atrioventricular valves drain to the morphologic left ventricle and do not drain to the outlet chamber *(OC)*. There also is spontaneous contrast in the dilated left atrium. This again is a reflection of the low cardiac output in this patient. Precordial echocardiography in this case had suggested the diagnosis to be atrioventricular discordance. It has been our experience that where doubt exists, the distinction between double inlet left ventricle and atrioventricular discordance may definitively be made by transesophageal echocardiography.

Following Fontan-type procedures transesophageal ultrasound can provide a detailed assessment of the function of the Fontan connection, the rapid exclusion or exact localization of residual atrial shunting, and the assessment of any atrioventricular valve regurgitation. Right atrial thrombus formation or the occurrence of spontaneous atrial contrast (indicative of abnormally low velocities of flow within the atrium—a prethrombotic state) can be better documented by transesophageal imaging studies than by transthoracic studies.[30] In our experience, the technique proved to be far superior to transthoracic ultrasound studies in evaluation of the morphology and function of posterior Fontan connections and Glenn shunts. In addition, transesophageal pulsed-wave Doppler studies are a most sensitive tool in the definition of even minor obstructions to pulmonary blood flow. Combined pulsed Doppler interrogation of pulmonary arterial and pulmonary venous flow patterns following various modifications of the procedure show that the principal determinant force in driving the Fontan circulation lies in the systemic venous pressure. Variations of pulmonary arterial flow patterns are reflections of the effects of the function of any incorporated right-heart chamber and intrathoracic pressure changes occurring with respiration. Only major pressure changes within the left heart are transmitted retrogradely through the pulmonary vascular bed. Pulmonary venous flow patterns were found to be independent of the Fontan procedure employed.[30]

As with adult patients who have undergone prosthetic valve replacement, transesophageal imaging is the technique of choice in the postoperative evaluation of children with prosthetic valve dysfunction. Paravalvular leakage, endocarditis lesions, or atrial thrombus formation can all be defined with an improved accuracy when compared with transthoracic ultrasound studies. (See Chapter 5 for a detailed discussion.)

LIMITATIONS OF TEE STUDIES IN CHILDREN

Although the atrial and atrioventricular cardiac structures are usually assessed in more detail from within the esophagus than from the precordium (Figs 8–3 and 8–8), other areas of the heart are less well visualized. Major limitations include the inability of single-plane transesophageal imaging to (1) reliably assess the morphology of the right ventricular outflow tract, (2) define the presence or degree of arterial override above a ventricular septal defect, or (3) reliably determine the integrity of the apical muscular or outlet portions of the ventricular septum (Figs 8–9 and 8–10). In addition, in some children the ventriculoarterial junction cannot be assessed accurately. The ascending aorta is only partially visualized by the transverse-plane technique, and definition of coarctation of the descending aorta is poor. A patent ductus arteriosus may be missed on both transverse-plane cross-sectional imaging and color flow mapping because of the interposition of the bronchial tree between the transducer and the area of interest. Similarly, the proximal part of the left pulmonary artery is frequently difficult to visualize when using the transverse-plane approach, although a more peripheral segment can frequently be demonstrated to lie anterior to the descending aorta.

The hemodynamic evaluation of congenital heart disease by transesophageal pulsed Doppler ultrasound is limited to the assessment of pulmonary venous flow patterns, ventricular inflow patterns, and the flow patterns within the pulmonary arteries. Although continuous-wave Doppler facilities have recently become available on pediatric transesophageal probes, the additional value of this modality must be considered to be limited because the transverse-plane esophageal approach is poorly aligned to the majority of intracardiac flows. Continuous-wave interrogation from within the esophagus may be of greater value when using the longitudinal-plane approach.

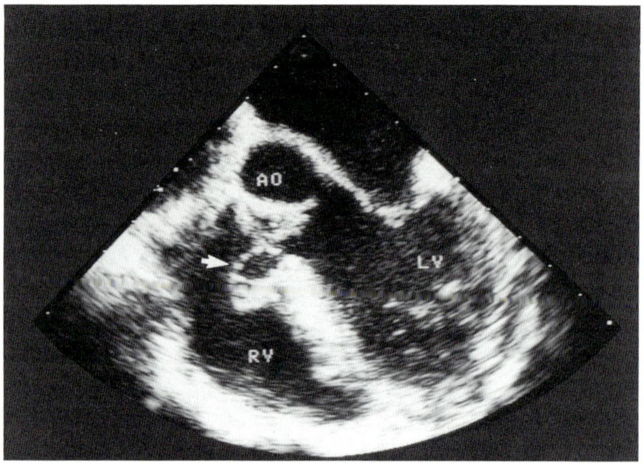

FIG 8–10.
Transverse plane transesophageal image taken from a patient in whom a perimembranous ventricular septal defect was partially walled off by the development of a tricuspid valve pseudoaneurysm *(arrow)*. Color flow mapping clearly showed the presence of flow into the pseudoaneurysm and then into the right ventricle *(RV)*. The whole morphology was better defined by transesophageal imaging compared to the precordial findings. *AO* = aorta; *LV* = left ventricle.

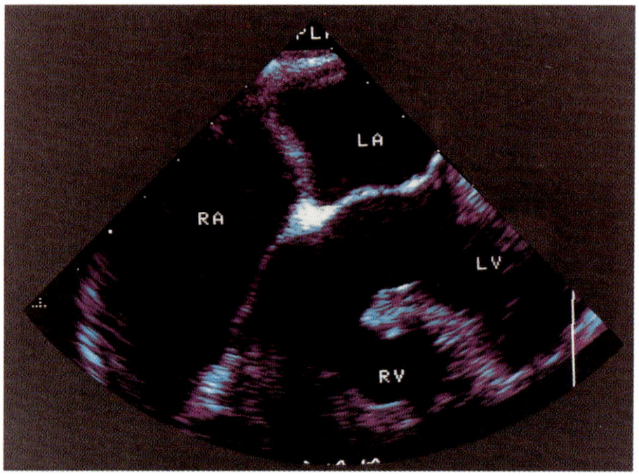

FIG 8–9.
Transverse plane image from a patient with a large unrestrictive perimembranous ventricular septal defect. Such large defects are readily seen on transverse plane scanning and are normally also visualized in longitudinal plane scanning. It has been our experience that smaller ventricular septal defects are poorly visualized by the longitudinal plane and indeed may occasionally be missed by transverse plane scanning. Large apical muscular ventricular septal defects may be missed using either plane. In addition, transesophageal echocardiography may give a false-positive appearance of small perimembranous ventricular septal defects as there frequently is an area of dropout in the membranous septum using transverse plane transoesophageal imaging. (*LA* = left atrium; *LV* = left ventricle; *RA* = right atrium; *RV* = right ventricle.)

CURRENT INDICATIONS FOR TEE IN CHILDREN

In view of the advantages and limitations, it becomes evident that transesophageal studies in children should be contemplated only in selected cases. The potential risks of general anesthesia or heavy sedation for such studies has to be weighed against the clinical need to obtain definitive diagnostic and/or monitoring information. From our experience, transesophageal studies are of additional diagnostic value in children with either suspected or documented cardiac lesions involving either the systemic or pulmonary venous return to the heart, the atrial chambers, the atrioventricular junction, or the left ventricular outflow tract. In addition, transesophageal studies are indicated in those patients in whom the precordial ultrasound information is suboptimal and in whom a definitive diagnosis is essen-

TABLE 8–2.
Current Indications for Transesophageal Studies in Children With Congenital Heart Disease

Primary diagnosis
Anomalous systemic venous connections
Anomalous pulmonary venous connections
Atrial arrangement, atrial isomerism
Juxtaposition of the atrial appendages
Atrial septal defects
Atrioventricular junction abnormalities
Left ventricular outflow tract obstruction
Monitoring
Perioperative
Surgical repair at the atrial level
Atrioventricular valve repair/replacement
Mustard/Senning procedure
Fontan-type procedures
Continuous monitoring during the early postoperative period
Diagnosis and management of early postoperative complications
Interventional catheterization
Guidance of balloon catheter position
Exclusion of immediate complications
Assessment of immediate hemodynamic results/changes
Dilatations of venous pathway obstructions
Device closure of atrial septal defects
Follow-up
Mustard/Senning procedures
Fontan-type procedures
Atrioventricular valve repair/replacement
Suspected residual or acquired atrial lesions

tial. A list of what we consider to be "established" indications for a transesophageal study in the pediatric age group is given in Table 8–2. Currently, with only single-plane pediatric transesophageal imaging probes being commercially available, we feel that such studies are rarely indicated for the investigation of children with isolated congenital lesions involving only the ventricular septum, the right ventricular outflow tract, the semilunar valves, or the great arteries. In our opinion, in all these lesions, more and better ultrasound information can be obtained from the precordium, and a transesophageal study rarely will provide any additional data. A good case in point is the tetralogy of Fallot: little additional information will be gained from an esophageal study either before or after correction. In fact, transesophageal information, because of its incompleteness, may be falsely reassuring and may miss major residual lesions.

FUTURE DIRECTIONS

Biplane transesophageal transducers have already been introduced for use in adult patients,[31] and miniaturized prototypes are being developed for use in children. The provision of an additional longitudinal-axis scan plane allows, among others, for a much improved assessment of the thoracic aorta and the right ventricular outflow tract (Figs 8–11 and 8–12).[32] In addition, only the use of this longitudinal scan plane provides an accurate assessment of the vertical dimension (major axis) of atrial septal defects and thus would appear to be mandatory in the patient selection for transvenous defect closure.[33] We have now studied some 58 patients with simple or complex congenital heart lesions using either pediatric or adult biplane probes. The benefits of longitudinal plane scanning are listed in Table 8–3. Given a comparable image quality, these biplane transducers are likely to become the new standard in transesophageal imaging in congenital heart disease until multiplane technology ultimately becomes feasible (see Chapter 12). In addition to biplane pediatric transducers, dedicated neonatal transducers are now being tested that should allow the safe investigation of premature infants. These latter probes may become a versatile monitoring technique in the critically ill neonate or in the early postoperative period.

Transesophageal pulsed-wave Doppler studies may open up a whole new field of hemodynamic studies in children with congenital heart disease. The possibility to acquire both high-quality individ-

TABLE 8–3.
Biplane TEE: Advantages of Longitudinal vs. Transverse Plane in the Assessment of Congenital Heart Disease

Structure	New Information†
Vena cavae	Left SVC*
Atria	Pulmonary venous connections
	Secundum atrial septal defects* (including Device closure)
	Anterior Fontan connections*
	Anterior conduits*
Atrioventricular valves	A-V valve morphology*
	A-V valve regurgitation*
	Chordal insertion
Ventricles	Muscular outlet septum
Outflow tracts	RVOT*
	LVOT*
Semilunar valves	Aortic valve*
	Pulmonary valve
Great vessels	Ascending aorta (Marfan)
	A-P window
	Distal main LPA*
	PDA

*Important new information.
† A-P = aorto-pulmonary; A-V = atrioventricular; LPA = left pulmonary artery; LVOT = left ventricular outflow tract; PDA = patent ductus arteriosus; RVOT = right ventricular outflow tract; SVC = superior vena cava.

ual pulmonary vein flow patterns together with ventricular inflow patterns and apex cardiograms and their subsequent integration and correlation is likely to provide new insights into systolic and diastolic ventricular function in both preoperative and postoperative congenital heart lesions.

With the current improvements in and increased availability of alternative imaging techniques such as magnetic resonance imaging, detailed correlative studies are required to define the role of pediatric transesophageal ultrasound in the assessment of complex congenital heart disease.

TEE ASSESSMENT OF THE ADOLESCENT AND ADULT WITH CONGENITAL HEART DISEASE

Whereas transesophageal imaging has a developing and (at the time of writing) slightly contentious role in the assessment of congenital heart disease in pediatric patients, the same does not apply to similar studies in the adolescent and adult age groups. In these older patients transesophageal studies can be carried out in the outpatient clinic in the same manner as in adult patients with acquired heart disease. There is no need for general anesthesia for such studies, but because of the complexity (and hence duration) of the studies, appropriate short-acting sedation with an intravenous agent is often given.

The normal range of currently available adult transesophageal probes (including biplane probes) can be used for such studies. However, we would not recommend that these be carried out in adolescents under the age of 16 years without the use of heavy sedation. Whereas we do not routinely give secretion-drying agents to our adult patients prior to a routine outpatient transesophageal study, we have found that adolescent patients frequently produce copious secretions during such studies, and thus we now advise routine premedication with an appropriate drying agent in this age group. As with the pediatric patients, we do not give routine antibiotic pro-

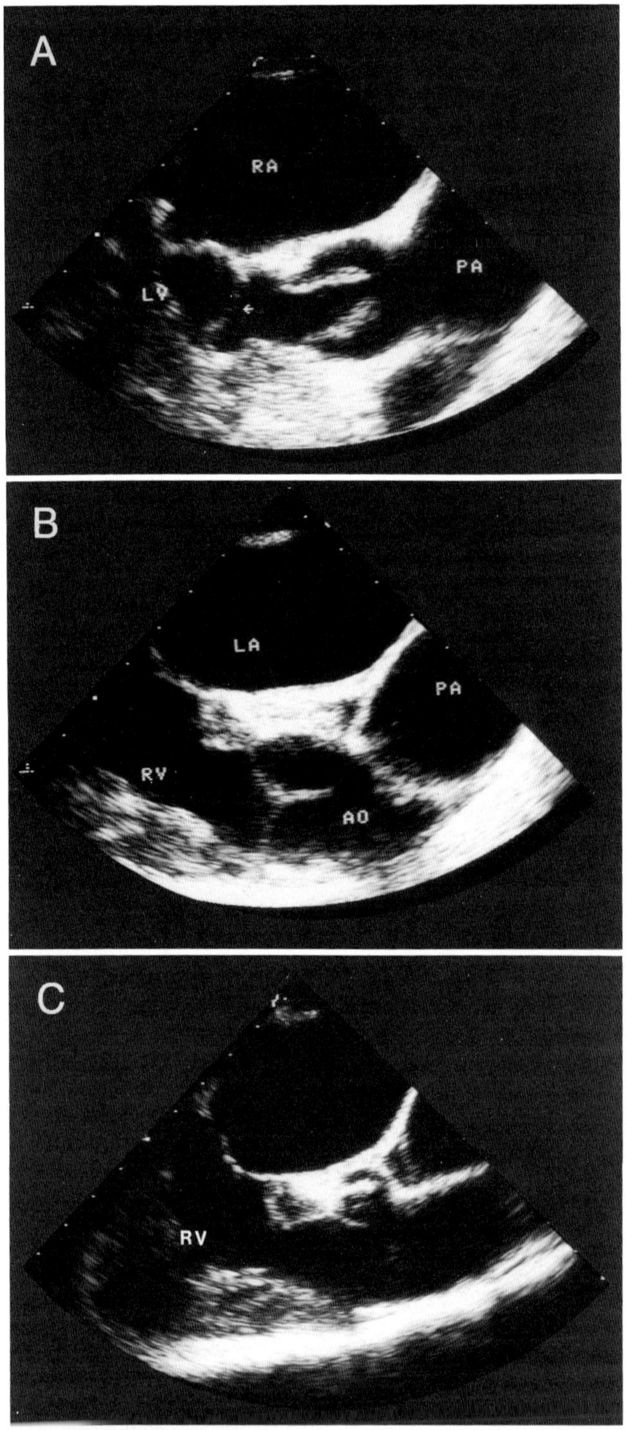

FIG 8–11.
A, longitudinal plane image from a patient with atrioventricular discordance, ventriculo-arterial discordance, and subpulmonary and pulmonary valve obstruction. This image demonstrates the left ventricular *(LV)* outflow tract with a subpulmonary obstructive fibromuscular membrane *(arrow)* and a thickened doming bicuspid pulmonary valve. Note the associated post stenotic dilatation of the main pulmonary artery *(PA)*. **B,** this image was obtained by rotating the probe to the patient's left from the imaging position demonstrated in **A.** In this image, we now see the unobstructed right ventricular *(RV)* outflow tract and the aortic valve. **C,** With further rotation to the patient's left, the whole of the inflow of the morphologic right ventricle, the shape of the ventricle and the right ventricular outflow tract giving rise to the aorta is well seen. It is our impression that such a transesophageal longitudinal plane scan in patients with complex abnormality of the outflow tracts in atrioventricular discordance will demonstrate best the obstruction at subvalve or valvar level and determine its precise etiology. (*RA* = right atrium; *LA* = left atrium; *AO* = aorta.)

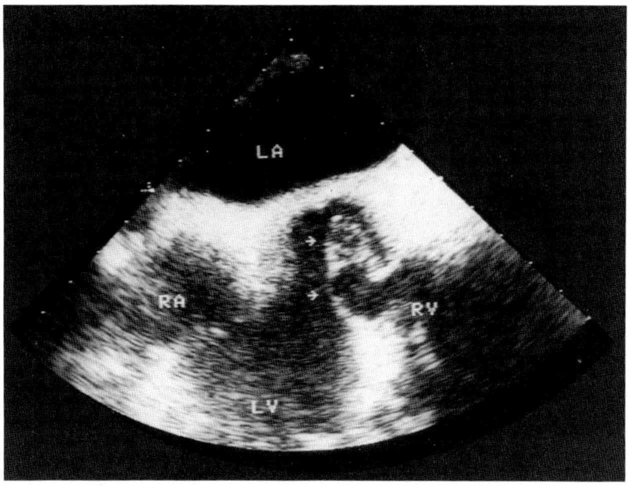

FIG 8–12.
A transverse axis scan in a patient with atrioventricular discordance and subpulmonary obstruction. In this rare case, it will be seen that the subpulmonary obstruction is caused by a true aneurysm of the membranous septum (*arrows*) which bulges into the upper pulmonary area. This morphology was better appreciated by transverse axis scanning rather than longitudinal scanning. (*LA* = left atrium; *LV* = left ventricle; *RA* = right atrium; *RV* = right ventricle.)

phylaxis to cover these studies. Where the patient is cyanotic or in a low-output state as a result of poor systemic ventricular function, we would advise the use of transcutaneous monitoring of oxygen saturation during the procedure.

Whereas in the pediatric age group the image quality obtained from the use of the dedicated pediatric probes may frequently be inferior to that obtained from the precordium due to the reduced number of elements which can be mounted on the smaller transducer head, in the adolescent and adult age group, the reverse usually holds true. Precordial ultrasound imaging in this age group is frequently difficult, and even where image quality is good, depth penetration for color information presents problems. Thus, little information may be derived on structures and flows within the atria or the systemic or pulmonary veins. Transesophageal imaging circumvents these problems. In our experience, both in the Thoraxcentre (Rotterdam) and currently in Edinburgh, the evaluation of congenital heart disease has become the second most common clinical reason for referral for a transesophageal study in the adult population. As indicated previously, we have undertaken 257 such investigations on an outpatient basis in adolescents and adults with congenital heart disease. These studies were carried out without complication in every case, although in 4% of cases the study had to be terminated earlier than the operator would have wished due to patient intolerance of the procedure. The majority of such studies were carried out in patients who had had a prior correction of a complex cardiac lesion.

With the proper integration of such studies into clinical practice, a new and unique diagnostic window is available to the cardiologist.[34] At present, where patient selection is appropriate (i.e., the lesions to be studied are likely to be better interrogated from the esophagus), such studies have, in our experience, proved to be complementary to cardiac catheter information and give a greater yield of information than either CT scanning or the current generation of magnetic resonance imagers. This is likely to remain the case for the foreseeable future.

SUMMARY

This chapter reviews the use of TEE in congenital heart disease, pointing out the benefit in complex problems such as atrioventricular discordance and pathology involving the right ventricular outflow tract. A comparison of epicardial and transesophageal echocardiography during surgery for correction of congenital heart defects is made, indications for TEE in congenital disease are discussed, and the additional benefits of biplane imaging in many of these patients are pointed out. From this information, it is clear that TEE plays a very important role in the diagnosis and care of patients with many forms of congenital heart disease.

REFERENCES

1. Gussenhoven EJ, Taams MA, Roelandt JRTC, et al: Transesophageal two-dimensional echocardiography: Its role in solving clinical problems. *J Am Coll Cardiol* 1986; 8:975–979.
2. Kyo S, Koike K, Takanawa E, et al: Impact of transesophageal Doppler echocardiography on pediatric cardiac surgery. *Int J Card Imaging* 1989; 4:41–42.
3. Ritter Sb, Hillel Z, Narang J, et al: Transesophageal real time Doppler flow imaging in congenital heart disease: Experience with the new pediatric transducer probe. *Dynamic Cardiovasc Imaging* 1989; 2:92–96.
4. Stümper O, Elzenga NJ, Hess J, et al: Transesophageal echocardiography in children with congenital heart disease—an initial experience. *J Am Coll Cardiol* 1990; 16:433–441.
5. Sahn DJ, Moises V, Cali G, et al: Important roles of transesophageal color Doppler flow mapping studies in infants with congenital heart disease (abstract). *J Am Coll Cardiol* 1990; 15(suppl A):204.
6. Ritter SB, Thys D: Transesophageal color flow imaging in infants and children with congenital heart disease (abstract). *Clin Res* 1990; 38:450.

7. Stümper O, Sreeram N, Elzenga NJ, et al: The diagnosis of atrial situs by transesophageal echocardiography. *J Am Coll Cardiol* 1990; 16:442–446.
8. Stümper O, Rijlaarsdam M, Vargas-Barron J, et al: The assessment of juxtaposed atrial appendages by transoesophageal echocardiography. *Int J Cardiol* 1990; 29:365–371.
9. Stümper O, Vargas-Barron J, Rijlaarsdam M, et al: The assessment of anomalous systemic and pulmonary venous connections by pediatric transesophageal echocardiography (abstract). *J Am Coll Cardiol* 1991; 17(suppl A):256.
10. Kronzon I, Tunick PA, Freedberg RS, et al: Sinus venosus type atrial septal defect is frequently missed by conventional echocardiography and is better detected by transesophageal echocardiography (abstract). *J Am Coll Cardiol* 1990; 15(suppl A):74.
11. Tucillo B, Stümper O, Hess J, et al: Transesophageal echocardiographic evaluation of atrial morphology in children with congenital heart disease. *Eur Heart J* 1991; 12(suppl):283.
12. Morimoto K, Matsuzaki M, Tohma Y, et al: Diagnosis and quantitative evaluation of secundum type atrial septal defects by transesophageal Doppler echocardiography. *Am J Cardiol* 1990; 66:85–91.
13. Sreeram N, Stümper O, Kaulitz R, et al: The comparative value of surface and transesophageal ultrasound in the assessment of congenital abnormalities of the atrioventricular junction. *J Am Coll Cardiol* 1990; 16:1205–1214.
14. Stümper O, Elzenga NJ, Sutherland GR: Obstruction of the left ventricular outflow tract in childhood—improved diagnosis by transoesophageal echocardiography. *Int J Cardiol* 1990; 28:107–109.
15. Stümper O, Kaulitz R, Sreeram N, et al: Intraoperative transesophageal versus epicardial ultrasound in surgery for congenital heart disease. *J Am Soc Echocardiogr* 1990; 3:392–401.
16. Muhiudeen I, Roberson D, Silverman N, et al: Intraoperative transesophageal echocardiography in infants and children with regurgitant valvar lesions (abstract). *J Am Soc Echocardiogr* 1990; 3:213.
17. Roberson D, Muhiudeen I, Silverman N, et al: Intraoperative transesophageal echocardiography in infants and children with cardiac shunt lesions (abstract). *J Am Soc Echocardiogr* 1990; 3:213.
18. Stümper O, Fraser AG, Elzenga NJ, et al: Assessment of ventricular septal defect closure by intraoperative epicardial ultrasound. *J Am Coll Cardiol* 1990; 16:1672–1679.
19. Stümper O, Sutherland GR, Sreeram N, et al: The role of intraoperative ultrasound in patients undergoing a Fontan-type procedure (abstract). *Br Heart J* 1990; 64:86.
20. Fyfe DA, Kline CH, Greene RM, et al: Transesophageal echocardiography after modified Fontan operations in infants and children (abstract). *Int J Card Imaging* 1990; 5(suppl):20.
21. Sreeram N, Kaulitz R, Stümper O, et al: Comparative roles of intraoperative epicardial and early postoperative transthoracic echocardiography in the assessment of surgical repair for congenital heart defects. *J Am Coll Cardiol* 1990; 16:913–920.
22. Zahn E, Musewe N, Dyck J, et al: Transesophageal echocardiographic evaluation of the arterial switch in the early post-operative period (abstract). *Circulation* 1990; 82(suppl 3):439.
23. Cyran SE, Kemball TR, Schwartz DC, et al: Evaluation of balloon aortic valvuloplasty with transesophageal echocardiography. *Am Heart J* 1988; 115:460–462.
24. Stümper O, Hess J, Sutherland GR: Paediatric transesophageal echocardiography—the value of a new diagnostic technique (abstract). *Int J Card Imaging* 1990; 5:19.
25. Hellenbrand WE, Fahey JT, McGowan FX, et al: Transesophageal echocardiographic guidance of transcatheter closure of atrial septal defect. *Am J Cardiol* 1990; 66:207–213.
26. van der Velde ME, Sanders SP, Perry SB, et al: Transesophageal echocardiographic guidance for transcatheter device closure of ventricular septal defects (abstract). *J Am Coll Cardiol* 1991; 17:19.
27. Stümper O, Kaulitz R, Elzenga NJ, et al: The value of transoesophageal echocardiography in children with congenital heart disease. *J Am Soc Echocardiogr* 1991; 4:323–330.
28. Kaulitz R, Stümper O, Geuskens R, et al: The comparative values of the precordial and transesophageal approaches in the ultrasound evaluation of atrial baffle function following an atrial correction procedure. *J Am Coll Cardiol* 1990; 16:686–694.
29. Kaulitz R, Stümper O, Fraser AG, et al: The potential value of transoesophageal evaluation of individual pulmonary vein flow after an atrial baffle procedure. *Int J Cardiol* 1990; 28:299–308.
30. Stümper O, Sutherland GR, Geuskens R, et al: Transesophageal echocardiography in the evaluation and management of the Fontan circulation. *J Am Coll Cardiol* 1991; 17:1152–1160.
31. Omoto R, Kyo S, Matsumura M, et al: Biplane color transesophageal Doppler echocardiography (color TEE): Its advantages and limitations. *Int J Card Imaging* 1989; 4:57–58.
32. Stümper O, Fraser AG, Ho SY, et al: Transoesophageal echocardiography in the longitudinal axis: Correlation between anatomy and images and its clinical implications. *Br Heart J* 1990; 64:282–288.
33. Kobayashi T, Musewe N, Benson L, et al: Biplane transesophageal echocardiographic evaluation of the atrial septal defect in children: Implications for percutaneous device occlusion (abstract). *Circulation* 1990; 82(suppl 3):402.
34. Sreeram N, Sutherland GR, Geuskens R, et al: The role of transoesophageal echocardiography in adolescents and adults with congenital heart disease. *Eur Heart J* 1991; 12:231–241.

PART III

Applications in Surgery and Intensive Care

Chapter 9

A Practical Guide to Intraoperative Transesophageal and Epicardial Echocardiography

Gerald I. Cohen, M.D.

William J. Stewart, M.D.

Allan L. Klein, M.D.

Ernesto E. Salcedo, M.D.

Intraoperative echocardiography (IOE) provides substantial benefits to the patient with cardiovascular disease and to the work of both the surgeon and cardiologist. The most dramatic example of this benefit is in the patient who has IOE during valve repair surgery. When compared with prosthetic valves, repair reduces operative risk and complications and preserves ventricular function.[1–5] IOE allows the surgeon to evaluate and refine operative technique by giving immediate feedback on operative results and provides the echocardiographer and anesthesiologist with important hemodynamic and physiologic information.[1, 6]

This chapter presents a practical guide to intraoperative transesophageal echocardiography (TEE) and epicardial imaging and the merits of both approaches based on the Cleveland Clinic experience. The impact of echo findings on decision making in the operating room is emphasized. This overview will provide an introduction to the newcomer to IOE and help the experienced echocardiographer adjust his skills to the environment of cardiac surgery.

PREOPERATIVE ECHOCARDIOGRAPHY

With either transesophageal or epicardial echocardiography, impediments to ultrasound penetration such as fat, lung, and bone are not interposed, and excellent image quality is obtained.[7, 8] Nevertheless, one should not negate the value of preoperative transthoracic echocardiography (TTE). In particular, the time to decide whether surgery is needed and what surgery should be done is before the patient enters the operating room. Goal-directed transthoracic imaging may provide crucial information not obtainable intraoperatively. For example, a true short-axis study of the mitral and aortic valves to demonstrate leaflet morphology and the origin and direction of valvular insufficiency by using color Doppler may be more readily obtained during TTE than TEE. The transthoracic study is often capable of evaluating the heart from more acoustic windows than TEE. TTE provides more time than does IOE to obtain a complete study using all ultrasound modalities including continuous-wave Doppler. In the awake patient, the hemodynamic information obtained is more relevant to day-to-day life than during anesthesia, mechanical ventilation, or thoracotomy. In some patients, loading conditions change on entering the operating room, which may cause disparate preoperative and intraoperative findings, especially the severity of valve regurgitation or the gradient across a stenotic valve.[6] Furthermore, intraoperative echocardiography should not be a substitute for high-quality hemodynamic and angiographic appraisal obtained during preoperative cardiac catheterization.

When the type of surgery that is needed is not clearly indicated during TTE, a transesophageal study on an ambulatory basis may also be necessary.[8–11] Structural details of the posterior aspect of the heart, valves, and aorta are more vivid, and mitral and tricuspid regurgitation are better assessed than during TTE. Transesophageal and transthoracic imaging complement each other in that they have the opposite side of the heart as their near-field. Furthermore, the transducers are located on opposite sides of structures that cause shadowing, such as intracardiac calcification and valve prostheses.[12]

INTRAOPERATIVE ECHOCARDIOGRAPHY

Clinical Correlation and Preparation

On entering the operating room, the echocardiographer assumes the identity of consultant to the cardiovascular surgeon and anesthesiologist. Ideally, time should be apportioned to examine the patient's chart to become familiar with the clinical history and previous echocardiographic and angiographic studies. Ultimately, the echocardiographer joins the surgical team in affirming what procedures must be performed. This is best served by diligent attention to detail, compulsive records of the patient's symptoms and history, and a thorough knowledge of cardiovascular hemodynamics.

Insertion of the Transesophageal Probe

Insertion of the transesophageal probe into the anesthesized patient requires caution and experience. After induction of general anesthesia and endotracheal intubation with an occlusive air-filled balloon, the stomach contents are emptied by suction with a nasogastric tube, which is subsequently removed. A moderate amount of water-soluble gel is inserted in the pharynx to lubricate the probe and facilitate its passage. With the control knobs unlocked, the shaft of the probe straight, and the mandible clasped with the left thumb behind the incisors, the probe is positioned in the center of the oropharynx, and the jaw is lifted. The probe is advanced in a blind fashion under light, gentle pressure into the esophagus. It is dangerous to jab or force entry of the transesophageal probe. If the probe cannot be advanced easily, its tip is repositioned in the oropharynx and its insertion reattempted. Guidance with a gloved finger may be needed to keep the probe in the midline, especially if the probe is deflected by the endotracheal tube to the side of the hypopharynx or into the pyriform sinus. If insertion continues to be difficult, laryngoscopic guidance may be necessary. As soon as the transducer passes the crucial triage point at 18 to 20 cm from the teeth, it should be easy to advance the probe toward the stomach at the 40- to 50-cm mark. The patient's ventilation is then rechecked.

Probe insertion is much easier before the metal anesthetic shield is attached onto the table over the patient's head. The TEE probe is usually inserted after induction of anesthesia and left within the esophagus until repeat imaging after cardiopulmonary bypass. Because the same echo machine can be used for other patients within the hospital while the TEE probe is idle during cardiopulmonary bypass, it is useful to have multiple TEE probes that will fit the same machine.

Technique of Epicardial Echocardiography

Epicardial imaging is performed by using standard transthoracic transducers, usually 3.5 MHz for adult patients. After scrubbing and gowning, the echocardiographer prepares the probe with the help of an ungowned person who will subsequently be required to adjust the control knobs of the echo machine. The transducer is covered by two plastic sheaths containing sterile gel. Apical and posterior cardiac imaging is not possible because the transducers are too large to fit in the space between the parietal pericardium and the heart without causing significant distortion of the chambers or causing arrhythmias. We have identified four standard epicardial transducer positions (Fig 9–1): the parasternal-equivalent, aortopulmonary sulcus, subcostal-equivalent, and aorta–superior vena cava views.[7, 13, 14] The complete IOE study includes all long-axis views from all four transducer positions; short-axis views from parasternal-equivalent and subcostal-equivalent views are also important to visualize the medial vs. lateral relationships of aortic and mitral valve structures.

Comparison of Transesophageal and Epicardial Echocardiography

TEE and epicardial imaging are complementary, but each has certain advantages and disadvantages.[1, 6, 13, 14] Epicardial imaging offers excellent images of the anterior aspect of the heart from a greater number of planes than does TEE. During epicardial echocardiography, the transducer can be positioned anywhere over the entire exposed surface

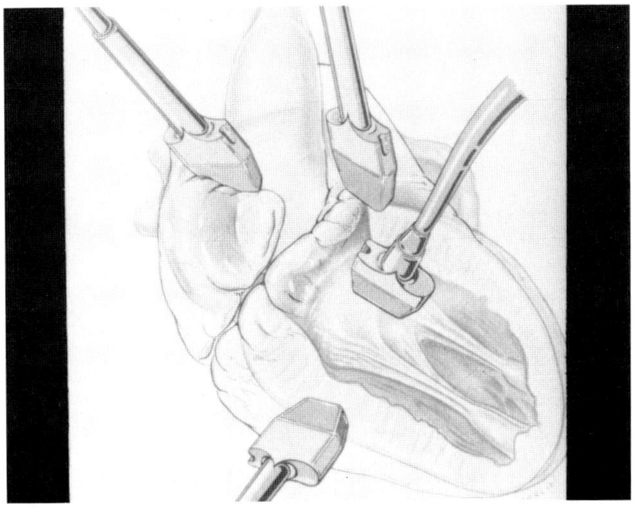

FIG 9–1.
The four standard transducer positions used in epicardial echocardiography. (From Stewart WJ, Currie PJ, Agler DA, et al: *Dynamic Cardiovasc Imaging* 1987; 1:179–186. Used by permission.)

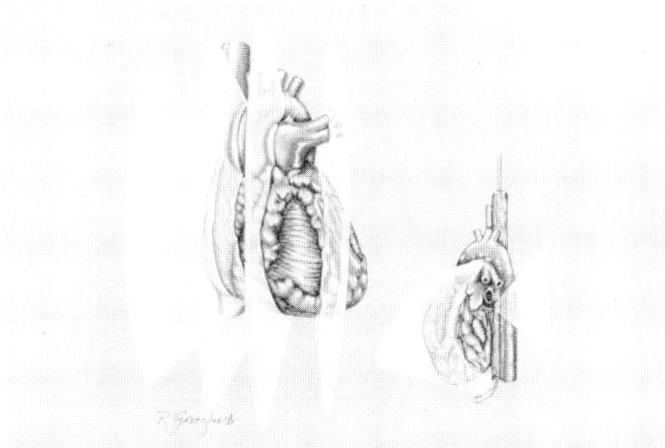

FIG 9–2.
The longitudinal image planes obtainable during biplane TEE. (From Cohen GI, Chan KL: *Am J Cardiol* 1990; 66:1007–1012. Used by permission.)

of the heart. Epicardial imaging can be used in neonates or individuals with esophageal disease. Furthermore, continuous-wave Doppler is readily employed during epicardial echocardiography. However, the posterior aspect of the heart is less well seen than with TEE, and care must be taken to avoid compromising the sterile field. Transducer contact at sites of bypass graft anastomosis should be avoided. The sheaths that cover the transducer are expensive. A learning curve must be followed to obtain proficiency.

TEE also has its advantages and disadvantages.[9] Although both transesophageal and epicardial echocardiography in the operating room are limited by time constraints, TEE is more conveniently performed and does not interrupt surgery as much.[15, 16] Recently, biplane TEE, with the addition of longitudinal image planes aligned parallel to the esophagus (Fig 9–2), has become the industry standard.[17–23] However, the number of views even by multiplane TEE are limited by the probe's position in the esophagus and stomach. This also limits the versatility of continuous-wave Doppler examination. Thus, measurement of left ventricular outflow tract gradients[24, 25] is more readily obtained during epicardial imaging than during TEE. Care must be taken to avoid dislodgement of the endotracheal tube during TEE. Risks are very small but include trauma to the oropharynx or esophagus and the remote possibility of perforation.[26, 27] Routine administration of antibiotics prior to cardiovascular surgery further minimizes the remote possibility of endocarditis from TEE.[28] Finally, despite the premium on time and the liability of delay of the operative process, the policy for intraoperative echocardiography at the Cleveland Clinic Foundation is to do a complete diagnostic study, whether a TEE or epicardial technique or both are used. On numerous occasions, we have found unexpected and important abnormalities that were missed during the preoperative workup or that occurred as a complication of the surgery itself.

INTRAOPERATIVE ECHOCARDIOGRAPHY IN MITRAL VALVE DISEASE

The most common indication for IOE in our institution is to assess patients undergoing repair of the mitral valve. Other indications in order of frequency include assessment of aortic valve disease, congenital heart disease, tricuspid valve disease, hypertrophic cardiomyopathy, and ventricular function (Fig 9–3).

Mitral Valve Anatomy

Echocardiography prior to cardiopulmonary bypass provides an understanding of key features of mitral anatomy and pathophysiology. It is essential to understand the anatomy of the normal mitral valve. The mitral apparatus includes the annulus, leaflets, chordae, and papillary muscles. The valve is a "curtain" of tissue extending from the annulus into the left ventricle. The posterior leaflet is usually divided into three portions, the lateral, middle (usually the largest), and medial scallops. Chordae extend from the margins of both leaflets and converge

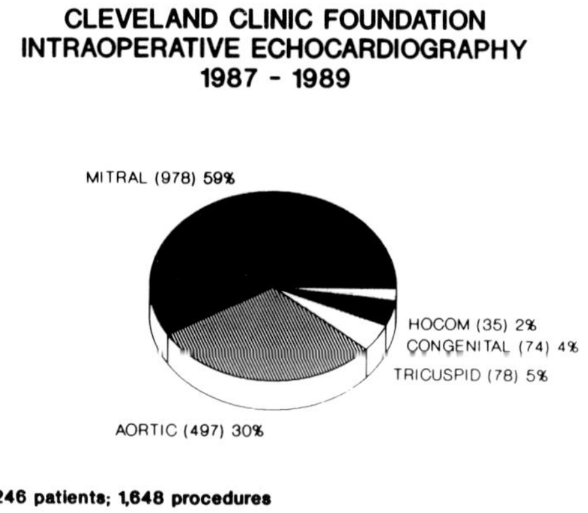

FIG 9–3.
Frequency of lesions evaluated in 1,246 patients studied by IOE at the Cleveland Clinic Foundation from 1987 to 1989.

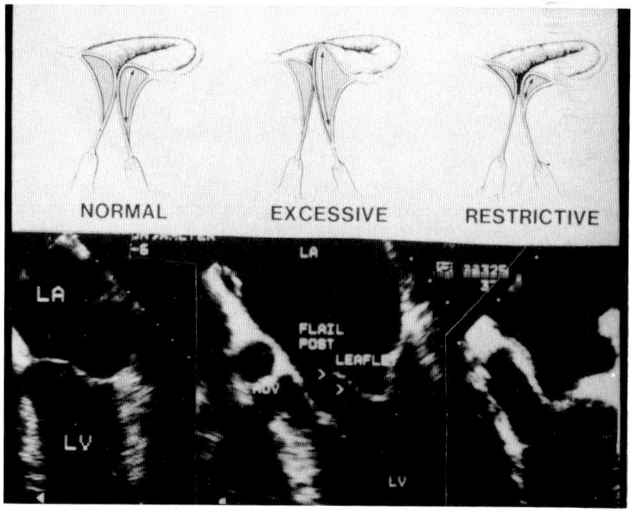

FIG 9–4.
Mitral regurgitation can be classified into problems associated with excessive, normal, or restricted leaflet motion as determined by two-dimensional echocardiography. (In part from Cosgrove DM, Stewart WJ: *Curr Probl Cardiol* 1989; 14:353–416. Used by permission.)

toward the papillary muscles. Most chordae are termed "rough-zone" chordae because they insert into the thickened distal portion of the leaflets. There are also basal chordae that insert into the base of the posterior leaflet and very thick strut chordae that insert into the anterior leaflet. Fan-shaped chordae are present at the medial and lateral commissures.

Valve competence depends on the integrity of the entire subvalvular and valvular apparatus. The anterior leaflet is semicircular or triangular and is long relative to the broader and shorter posterior leaflet, with its wider attachment to the annulus. On average, 14 primary chordae insert into the posterior leaflet and 9 into the anterior leaflet. Each papillary muscle provides chordae to roughly half of each leaflet. The posteromedial papillary muscle is more vulnerable to ischemia, infarction, and rupture because of its single blood supply from the posterior descending artery, while both the circumflex and left anterior descending coronary arteries supply the anterolateral papillary muscle.[29, 30]

Two-Dimensional Studies Before Cardiopulmonary Bypass

A methodical and complete echocardiographic examination prior to cardiopulmonary bypass is important in order to obtain maximum diagnostic information. Mitral leaflets may show excessive, restricted, or normal motion (Fig 9–4), each of which may be associated with regurgitation.[31, 32] Two-dimensional echo is used to detect leaflet thickness, mobility, and calcification; annular dilatation and calcification; subvalvular disease; and chordal elongation and rupture. TEE visualization of the chordae is sometimes impaired by shadowing and their far-field position.[33] IOE information about the mitral valve generally improves the accuracy of TTE data. The echocardiographic distinction between various mechanisms helps direct the surgeon's method of valve repair[31, 34] and reduces the learning curve for performing mitral valvuloplasty.[35]

Most mitral valve procedures are performed in patients with rheumatic and degenerative disease. Luckily, degenerative mitral valve disease is the most amenable to repair, which is successful in 75% of cases.[2, 36] Degenerative (myxomatous) disease is distinguished by variable degrees of chordal elongation or rupture, symmetric annular dilatation, or myxomatous billowing of the leaflets toward the left atrium during systole. The posterior leaflet, especially the middle scallop, is most commonly involved, which is fortunate because such abnormalities are the most easily repaired.[37] Resection of chordae or their transfer to unsupported portions of the leaflet is the mode of repair in these patients. In our series of patients with degenerative disease, repair was performed on 88% of patients with posterior chordal rupture, 81% with chordal elongation, 59% with anterior chordal rupture, 48% with annular dilatation, and 29% with severe ruptured chordae to both leaflets.[2]

Mitral insufficiency resulting from coronary atherosclerosis can be repaired in approximately 68% of patients.[2] Ischemic mitral insufficiency may result from one of two mechanisms: ventricular and annular dilatation secondary to wall motion abnormalities or aneurysm formation causing central regurgitation with normal mitral leaflets. This phenomenon is also found in patients with dilated cardiomyopathy. Repair may include annuloplasty. In contrast, mitral regurgitation from papillary muscle elongation or disruption causing valvular prolapse is repaired by reimplantation of the ruptured papillary muscles.[38] Ischemic mitral regurgitation with excessive leaflet motion has a more favorable prognosis after repair than does ischemic regurgitation due to ventricular dilation.[39]

Mitral insufficiency of a congenital, rheumatic, or infectious etiology can be repaired less frequently, or in about 50% of cases.[2] Rheumatic mitral disease is characterized by chordal and leaflet thickening, calcification, and retraction; commissural fusion; and sometimes asymmetric annular dilatation, especially of the posteromedial portion. Commissurotomy, debridement of calcium or fibrous tissue, and annuloplasty may be selectively applied to patients with rheumatic mitral regurgitation to relieve the regurgitation.

Doppler Studies Before Cardiopulmonary Bypass

Doppler echocardiographic evaluation of mitral regurgitation should also be performed in a complete and methodological fashion. Continuous-wave Doppler during TEE permits verification of the mitral diastolic gradient.[24] The left atrium should be carefully scanned to determine the extent of the flow disturbance, particularly in patients with jets deflected along the left atrial wall, because the size of the jet may seem smaller.[40, 41] Care should be taken that instrument settings are appropriately adjusted and that the pulse repetition frequency is high enough that the Nyquist aliasing limit is at least 0.45 m/sec. Severe regurgitation is suggested by a large jet on color Doppler that is more than 55% of the left atrial area[7] and extends near or to the posterior left atrial wall. Another helpful sign of significant regurgitation is the presence of color flow convergence on the ventricular side of the valve.[42–44] TEE criteria of the severity of mitral regurgitation must be adjusted to avoid overestimation relative to ventriculography.[45, 46] Assessment of pulmonic vein flow profiles provides an additional objective measure of left atrial flow dynamics as a correlate of the severity of mitral regurgitation.[47] (See Chapter 5 for a detailed discussion.)

The direction and origin of mitral regurgitation are useful in understanding the mechanism of dysfunction.[32, 34] By using long-axis views of the left ventricular inflow tract from either esophageal or epicardial imaging, one can determine which leaflet is most abnormal. In patients with excessive leaflet motion, the regurgitant jet is deflected opposite the leaflet with the most significant elongated or ruptured submitral support (Fig 9–5). Short-axis views are particularly important in defining medial vs. lateral relationships; here it is important to learn to use the transgastric short-axis image plane at the level of the mitral leaflets. In about 20% of all patients, this view is oblique during transverse TEE imaging,[48] a situation underscoring the importance of a good preoperative transthoracic examination or the availability of epicardial imaging, which often provides a better short-axis view of the mitral valve.

The mitral annulus is positioned at about 45 degrees with the sagittal plane, with antegrade flow pointing anteriorly and laterally toward the left ventricular apex. With this orientation of the mitral valve, changing the depth of TEE probe insertion allows one to pinpoint the site of regurgitation along the coaptation line. For example, if the continuity between flow convergence on the ventricular side and the regurgitant jet in the left atrium is well seen in a standard four-chamber view, a central origin of mitral regurgitation along the coaptation line is suggested. If probe withdrawal to a five-chamber TEE view provides better visualization of the origin of the jet, regurgitation originates closer to the anterolateral commissure. If a more inferior probe position

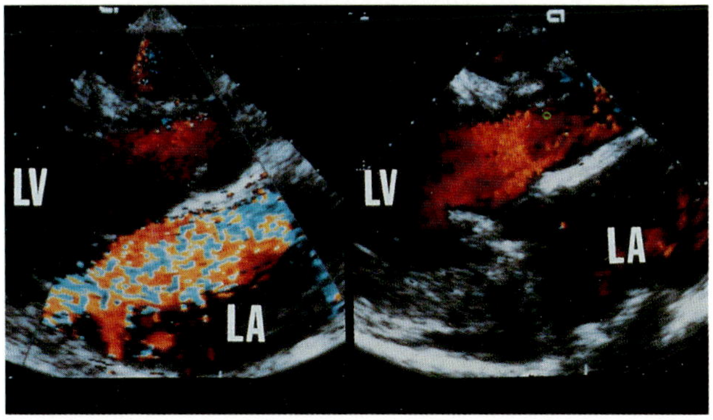

FIG 9–5.
Intraoperative parasternal long-axis–equivalent epicardial echocardiographic images before *(left)* cardiopulmonary bypass in a patient with severe prolapse of the posterior leaflet that is causing the regurgitant jet to be directed anteriorly. After successful repair for mitral regurgitation *(right)*, no regurgitation is seen on this systolic frame. *LA* = left atrium; *LV* = left ventricle. (From Stewart WJ, Kerber RD: Intraoperative echocardiography, in Marcus M, et al (eds): *Cardiac Imaging*. Philadelphia, WB Saunders, 1991, pp 619–633. Used by permission.)

near the level of the diaphragm shows the jet origin best, the regurgitation arises near the posteromedial commissure. Prosthetic regurgitation is further localized as valvular or perivalvular, and the location of the perivalvular jet is determined from a short axis of the valve ring. The prepump IOE may change the operative plan. Our experience can be summarized by a group of 426 patients having mitral repair over a 23-month period. Of these, 40 (9.4%) had a change in the operative technique as a result of the prebypass IOE study.

Intraoperative Echocardiography After Cardiopulmonary Bypass

During cardiopulmonary bypass for mitral valve repair, the surgeon tests the competence of the valve by insufflating the ventricle with fluid under pressure. Unfortunately, this method is fraught with inaccuracy.[6, 49] Methodical assessment of the surgical result begins with restoration of cardiac rhythm, discontinuation of cardiopulmonary bypass, and production of stable hemodynamics. If loading conditions are obtained that simulate ambulatory conditions, the amount of regurgitation assessed by echo is not systematically different from that seen on studies done in the echocardiography laboratory.[50]

The structure and motion of all portions of the mitral apparatus are examined during the postpump IOE. The entire left atrium is scanned in multiple planes with color flow mapping to compare with the prepump assessment of mitral regurgitation. Pulmonary vein flow is again recorded to document resolution of the systolic blunting or flow reversal caused by mitral regurgitation (Fig 9–6). The mechanism of residual mitral regurgitation is also assessed to determine what further repair is needed during the second pump run. The motion of the mitral valve within the ventricle during systole should also be observed closely.

Residual mitral regurgitation or other problems[1, 7, 51, 52] have been found in 8% of the 611 patients studied with IOE after mitral valve repair (Fig 9–7). Most of these patients (about 4% of the entire series) have persistent regurgitation that can be corrected with further repair (Fig 9–8) or, less commonly, valve replacement on the second pump run. In 2% to 3% of patients who undergo valvuloplasty for mitral valve prolapse, especially those with small ventricles and a large anterior leaflet who have repair with a stiff annular ring, systolic anterior motion of the mitral leaflets develops. This causes obstruction of the outflow tract during systole[53, 54] and significant residual regurgitation that is sometimes mild and sometimes so severe as to prevent weaning from the pump. The obstruction and the associated mitral regurgitation increase with hypovolemia (Fig 9–9) and catecholamine administration. Epicardial continuous-wave Doppler of the left ventricular outflow tract is useful to determine the severity of obstruction.[55–57]

Ventricular function is often mildly depressed immediately after cardioplegia, but it usually improves progressively.[58, 59] Ventricular function and wall motion abnormalities should be assessed from multiple transducer positions. In patients undergoing commissurotomy for mitral stenosis, the mitral

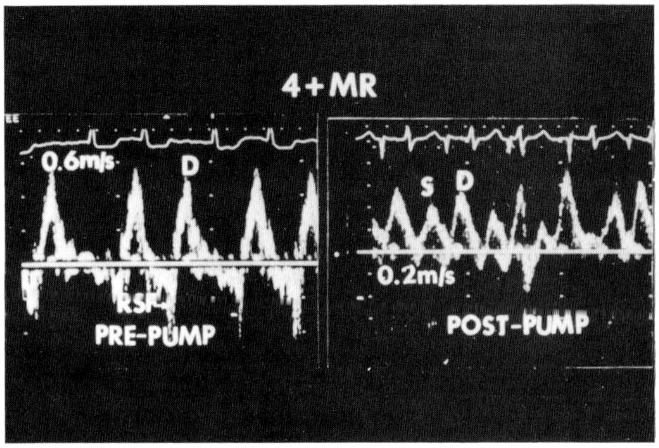

FIG 9–6.
Transesophageal pulsed-wave Doppler study of pulmonary venous flow. Reversal of systolic antegrade flow *(RSF)* in the prepump study *(left)* suggests the presence of significant mitral regurgitation *(MR)*. Diastolic *(D)* antegrade flow is prominent. After the repair *(right)*, systolic *(S)* antegrade flow is restored.

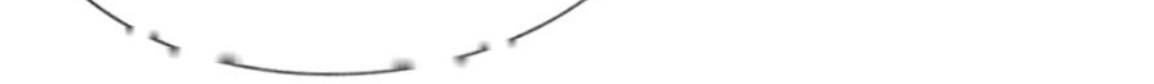
Persistent MR n = 33 (5.4%)
Persistent Flail n = 2 (0.4%)
Other n = 4 (0.6%)
Persistent MS n = 1 (0.2%)
LVOT Obstruction n = 14 (2.2%)
Successful Repairs n = 557 (91.2%)

FIG 9–7.
Frequency of second pump runs in 611 patients having IOE after mitral valve repair. *MR* = mitral regurgitation; *MS* = mitral stenosis; *LVOT* = left ventricular outflow tract. (From Stewart WJ, Salcedo EE, Cosgrove DM: *Cleve Clin J Med* 1991; 57:177–183. Used by permission.)

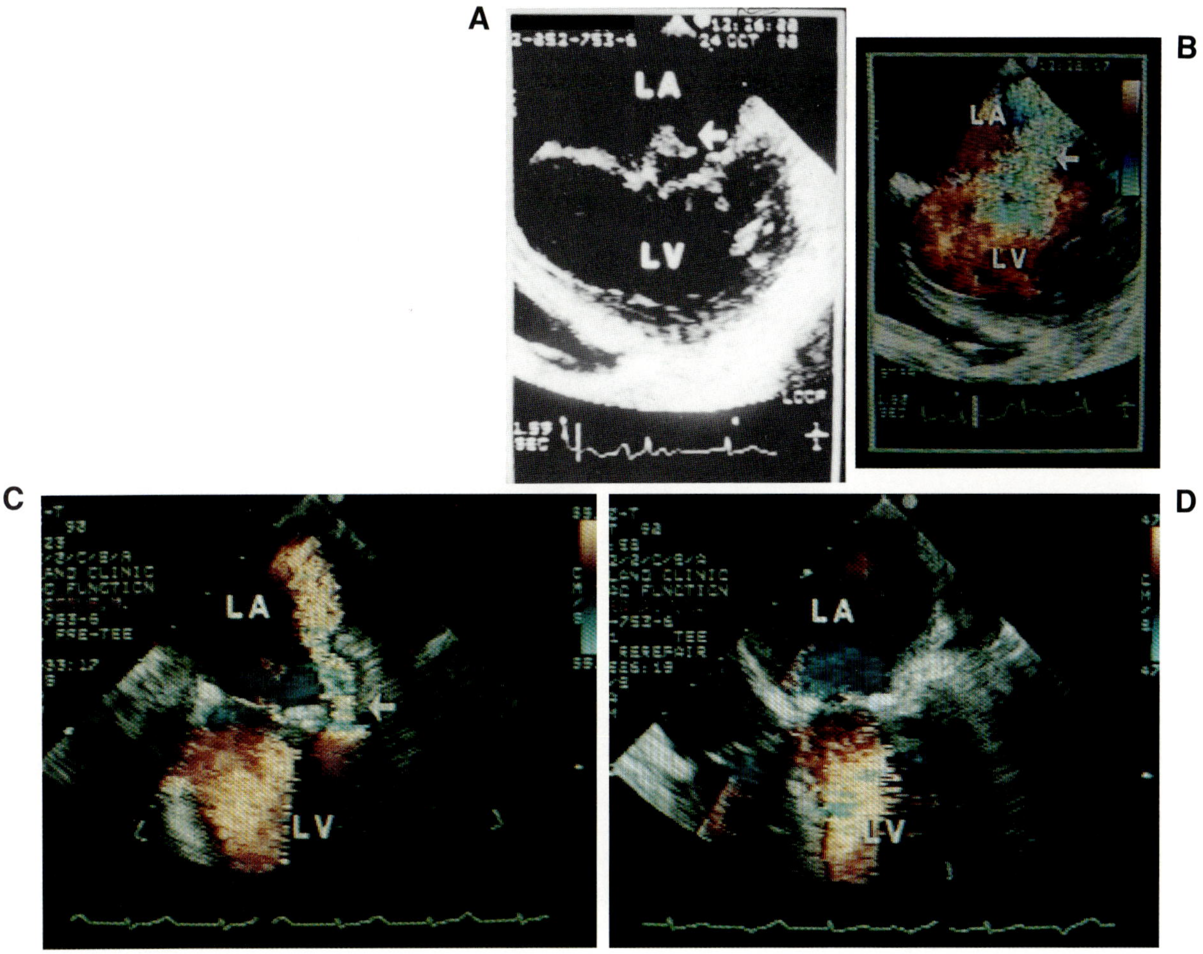

FIG 9–8.
A, TEE image of an anterior leaflet *(arrow)* flail in the left atrium *(LA)* due to myxomatous degeneration. **B,** severe mitral regurgitation is evident on color Doppler *(arrow)*. **C,** after quadrilateral resection of the anterior mitral leaflet and insertion of a Carpentier-Edwards ring, moderate mitral regurgitation was present due to a perforation between the ring and the lateral mitral annulus. **D,** after the patient was returned to cardiopulmonary bypass and the perforation was successfully repaired, no regurgitation remained. *LV* = left ventricle.

gradient before and immediately following bypass can be calculated by using TEE continuous-wave Doppler (Fig 9–10).

INTRAOPERATIVE ECHOCARDIOGRAPHY IN AORTIC VALVE DISEASE

New surgical techniques have been developed for repair of the aortic valve. These include triangular resection of prolapsing cusps, debridement of calcium and fibrotic tissue, resuspension of dislocated commissures, patch closure of perforations, commissural plication for annular dilatation, and reconstruction of congenital deformities.[60] However, aortic valve repair is technically more difficult and less commonly performed than aortic valve replacement or mitral valve repair. The art of repairing aortic valves is comparatively less advanced as compared with the depth of our understanding of mitral valve repair. IOE is therefore an integral part of the learning curve and an important feature of clinical success in aortic valve reconstruction.

For IOE examination of the aortic valve, multiple long- and short-axis projections should be utilized. Echocardiography aids the surgeon in understanding the severity and mechanism of aortic stenosis and regurgitation. Measurement of the aortic annulus on the outflow tract side of the valve in a long-axis view may guide the surgeon in choosing the

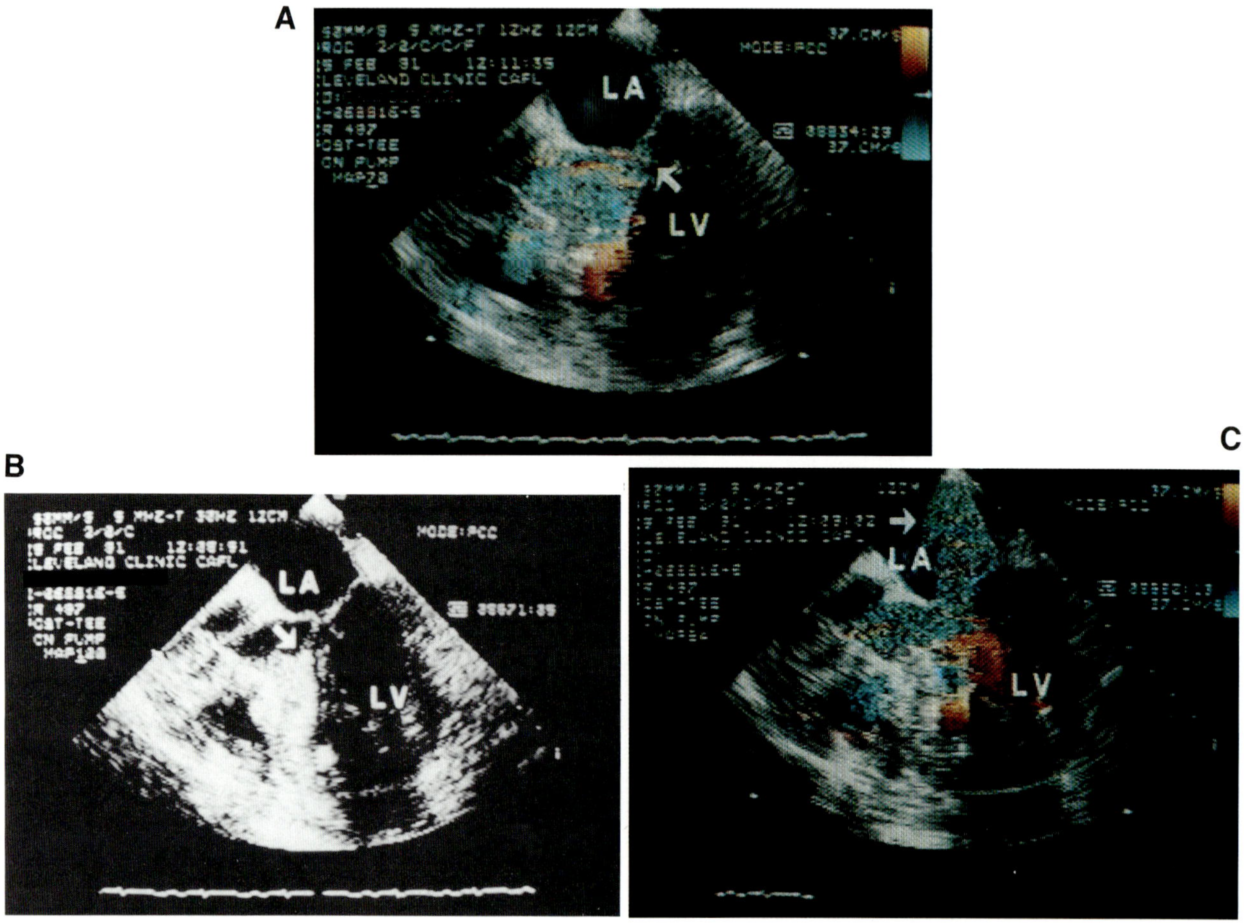

FIG 9–9.
A, transesophageal five-chamber image demonstrating dynamic changes in outflow obstruction after mitral valve repair with a Perigard ring annuloplasty and a quadrilateral resection of a posterior leaflet prolapse. Initially, no mitral regurgitation was present, and there was good coaptation of the leaflets *(arrow)*. **B,** with underfilling of the left ventricle, systolic anterior motion of the mitral leaflets developed, obstructed the left ventricular outflow tract, and resulted in **(C)** significant mitral regurgitation *(arrow)*.

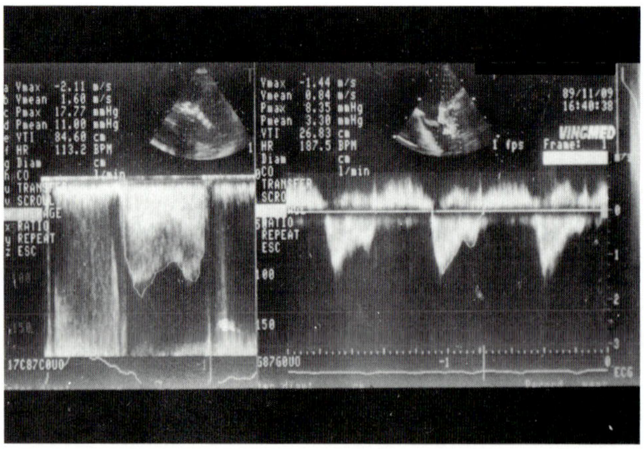

FIG 9–10.
Transesophageal continuous-wave Doppler recordings of mitral diastolic flow before *(left)* and after *(right)* commissurotomy for mitral stenosis show improvement in the mean mitral gradient from 11 to 3.3 mm Hg.

size of the prosthesis or homograft. An epicardial short-axis view of the valve is best to identify the number of cusps and their morphology as well as the location of calcification and its effect on leaflet mobility. In 90% of patients, a short-axis view of the aortic valve can be recorded either during transverse TEE imaging,[48] particularly by leftward flexion of the probe, or by rightward flexion during longitudinal imaging.

Intraoperative Echocardiography in Aortic Stenosis

Aortic stenosis is less amenable to valve repair than aortic regurgitation. In the 1980s, debridement techniques with the ultrasonic aspirator were developed, but early cusp retraction and surgery for aortic regurgitation proved to be a major limitation.[61] Preoperative TTE and catheterization measurements regarding the severity of stenosis should be utilized to decide whether to perform aortic valve surgery because such data are less affected by unusual loading conditions than are measurements made in the operating room.

Intraoperative two-dimensional echocardiography can visualize cusp thickening and restriction of motion, although we do not routinely use the two-dimensional image to planimeter aortic valve area as others have proposed.[62] Continuous-wave Doppler estimates of the aortic gradient (Fig 9–11) can be obtained during epicardial echocardiography by recording maximum valvular velocities with a continuous-wave probe applied against the right side of the ascending aorta (the aorta–superior vena cava sulcus transducer position) and the ultrasound beam pointing inferiorly.[14, 55–57, 63] From the same transducer location, pulse-wave Doppler can record outflow tract velocity. With the outflow tract diameter from the parasternal equivalent long axis view, the valve area can be calculated intraoperatively using the continuity equation.[64, 65] It is more difficult to align the continuous-wave Doppler cursor with the aortic valve (or left ventricular outflow) during TEE. In occasional patients, a transgastric view provides parallel orientation with the aortic valve flow.[25]

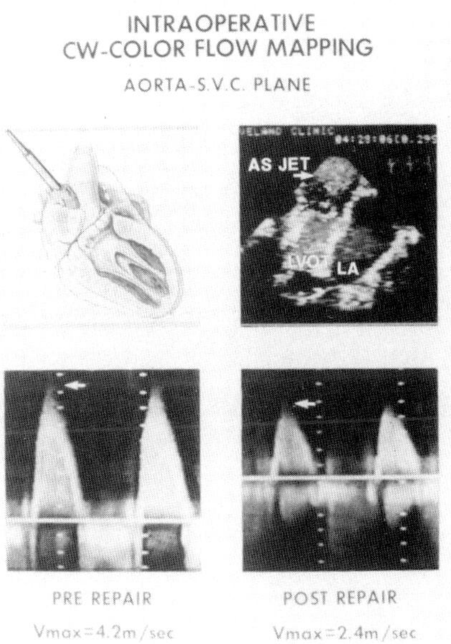

FIG 9–11.
Methods for measuring aortic valve velocity intraoperatively. **A,** position of the epicardial continuous-wave Doppler transducer in the aorta–superior vena cava transducer position. **B,** color flow image showing the aortic stenosis *(AS)* jet. **C,** the prepump maximum instantaneous gradient is 72 mm Hg. **D,** the gradient is reduced to 24 mm Hg after debridement of the aortic valve. *LVOT* = left ventricular outflow tract; *LA* = left atrium. (From Stewart WJ, Currie PJ, Schiavone WA, et al: Intraoperative echocardiography in patients with left ventricular outflow tract obstruction, in Maurer G, Mohl W (eds): *Proceedings of the First International Symposium on Echocardiography and Doppler in Cardiac Surgery.* New York, Igaku-Shoin Medical Publishers Inc, 1989, pp 337–345. Used by permission.)

Intraoperative Echocardiography of Aortic Regurgitation Before Cardiopulmonary Bypass

Techniques for repairing aortic regurgitation have been developed recently by ourselves and others.[60] Preoperative and prebypass IOE in patients with aortic regurgitation[55, 63] is useful to determine mobility, thickening, and the number of cusps present. Similar to the system used for understanding the mechanism of dysfunction of mitral valves, we categorize patients with aortic regurgitation by the presence of excessive, restricted, or normal leaflet motion. Color flow imaging to show the direction of the aortic regurgitation jet provides additional information regarding the type of regurgitation. Override, prolapse, flail, or asymmetric retraction of a cusp may divert the regurgitation anteriorly toward the septum or posteriorly toward the anterior mitral leaflet. A central jet commonly occurs with dilatation of the annulus, dilatation of the aortic root, or symmetric cusp retraction.

The valves most amenable to repair are those with prolapse of an aortic cusp[60,66] (Fig 9–12). This occurs commonly in patients with congenital bicuspid aortic valves[67] and in trileaflet valves with prolapse of the right coronary cusp. Other types of aortic regurgitation can be repaired in some cases (Fig 9–13). Central aortic regurgitation due to dilation of the aortic root can also be repaired with some certainty in the absence of significant valvular calcification. In patients with aortic aneurysms we often resuspend the aortic valve rather than replacing it if the valve tissue itself is unaffected by the disease process. The valve should be assessed by IOE prior to closing the chest to exclude residual aortic regurgitation.

The severity of aortic regurgitation is evaluated primarily according to jet width and length.[68] Severe aortic regurgitation is suggested by a jet width exceeding 60% of the outflow diameter or a jet area more than 60% of the outflow tract area. Color M-mode echocardiography of the left ventricular outflow tract just below the valve is often helpful to distinguish systolic from diastolic flow events. Flow convergence on the aortic side of the valve may also give a subjective hint of the presence of significant

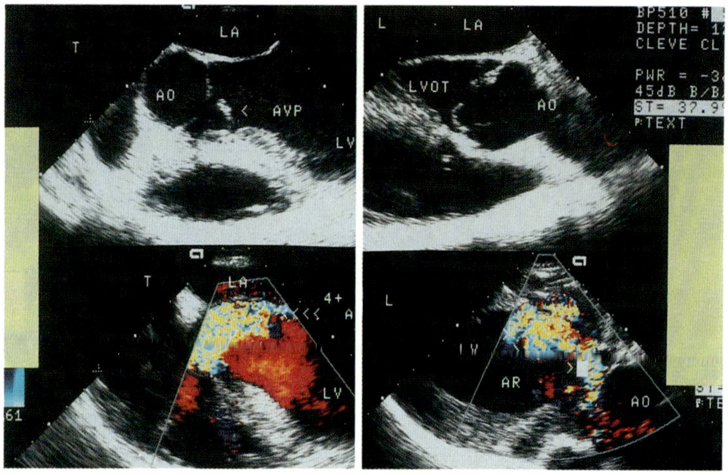

FIG 9–12.
Prepump intraoperative biplane transesophageal echo images in a patient with aortic regurgitation *(AR)* due to a prolapsing *(AVP)* bicuspid aortic valve demonstrate the ideal anatomy for successful repair. **A,** transverse *(T)* five-chamber two-dimensional echo image. **B,** longitudinal *(L)* two-dimensional echo image. **C,** transverse five-chamber color flow image. **D,** longitudinal color flow image.

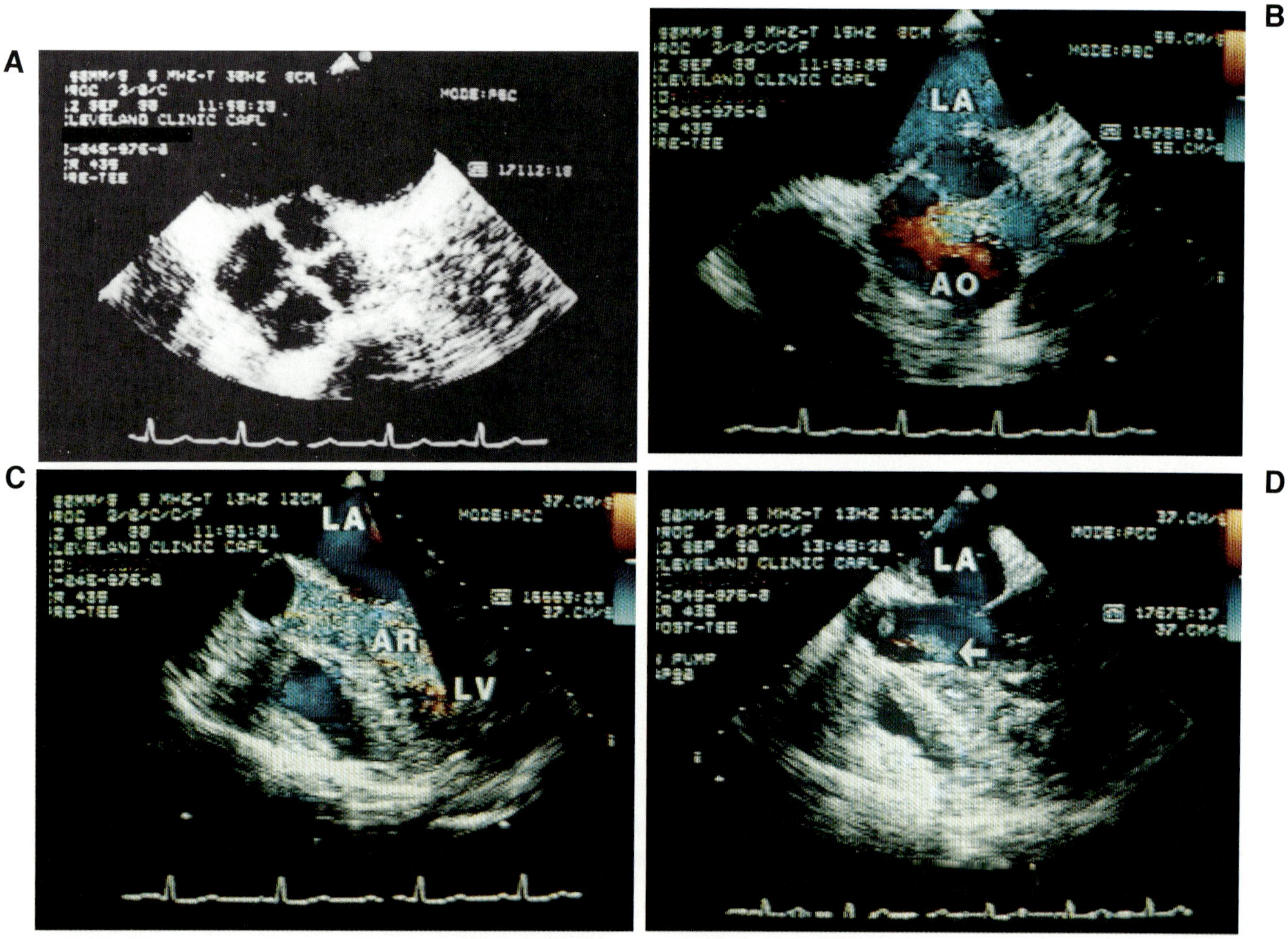

FIG 9–13.
A, TEE short-axis view of a quadricuspid aortic valve. In the closed position, the cusp's edges resemble the letter X. **B,** with color Doppler, failure of cusp coaptation centrally is indicated by the mosaic pattern of aortic regurgitation. **C,** in a TEE five-chamber view, severe aortic regurgitation *(AR)* fills the left ventricular outflow tract prior to repair. **D,** after repair of the quadricuspid valve, there is mild residual aortic regurgitation *(arrow)*. *AO* = aortic valve; *LA* = left atrium; *LV* = left ventricle.

regurgitation. Pressure half-time can be measured from continuous-wave recordings of the aortic regurgitation jet, either from an epicardial aorta–superior vena cava transducer position or from a transgastric TEE transducer position. Diastolic flow reversal as a function of severe aortic regurgitation (Fig 9–14) can be recorded from a TEE probe position near the aortic arch with the cursor aligned with flow in the ascending aorta.[69] Careful measurements of the hemodynamics of aortic regurgitation prior to attempted repair provide an important baseline with which to compare similar images following repair.

Intraoperative Echocardiography After Cardiopulmonary Bypass in Aortic Valve Repair

After aortic stenosis and regurgitation have been surgically corrected, IOE is employed to evaluate the results of surgery (Fig 9–15). In our series of 102 patients having aortic valve repair, 12% required a second pump run for further surgery[62] after IOE revealed persistent aortic regurgitation that was moderate or more in severity. During the same thoracotomy, further repair or aortic valve replacement can be successfully accomplished. In most patients studied intraoperatively after repair for aortic regurgitation, we also record pertinent data regarding the presence and severity of aortic stenosis. Even if the valve was not initially stenotic, the propensity of bicuspid or other abnormal aortic valves to undergo progressive fibrosis and calcification makes it important to obtain baseline postpump IOE and postoperative TTE data on the presence and severity of aortic stenosis.

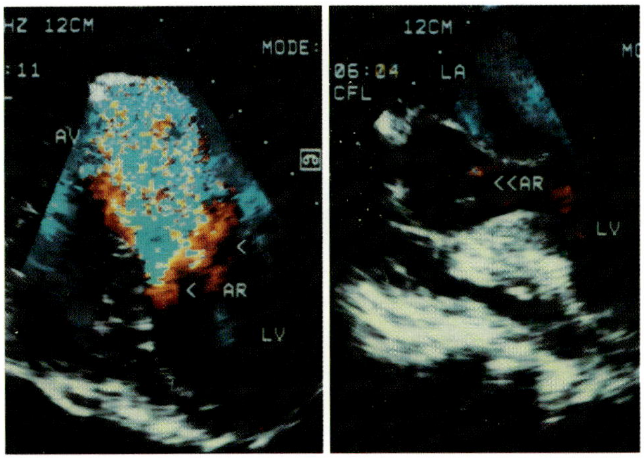

FIG 9–15.
TEE in a patient having successful valve repair shows severe aortic regurgitation *(AR)* before the repair **(A)** and trivial regurgitation afterward **(B).** *AV* = aortic valve; *LA* = left atrium; *LV* = left ventricle.

A

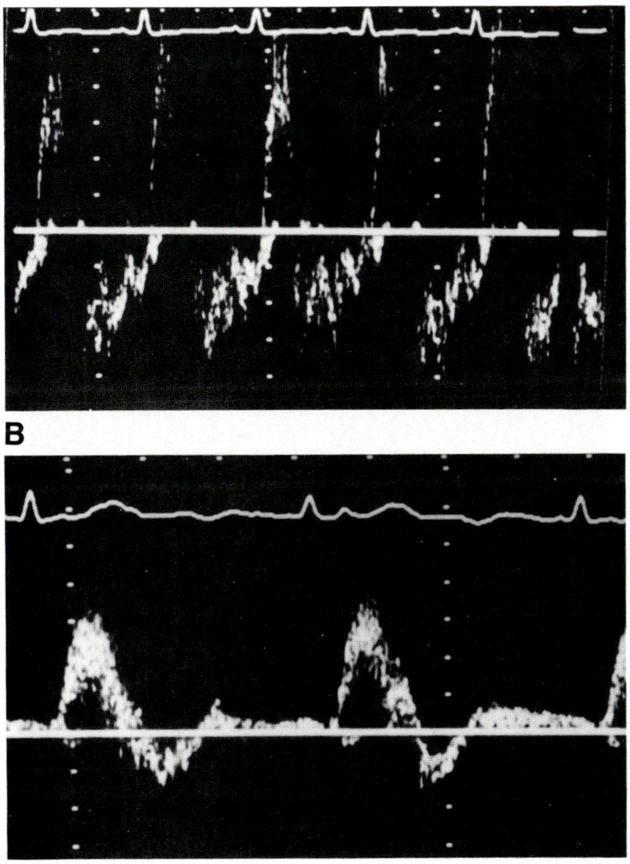

FIG 9–14.
Pulsed Doppler recordings of ascending aortic flow from the transesophageal approach with the transducer at the level of the aortic arch. Note the difference between the marked diastolic flow reversal in a patient with severe aortic regurgitation **(A)** and reversal only early in diastole in a patient with no aortic regurgitation **(B).**

INTRAOPERATIVE ECHOCARDIOGRAPHY AFTER CARDIOPULMONARY BYPASS IN PROSTHETIC VALVE SURGERY

We do not routinely perform IOE on patients undergoing prosthetic valve replacement because the frequency of changes in operative plans has been small. Out of a group of 171 aortic and 186 mitral prosthetic valves evaluated with IOE from 1987 to 1989, we found problems that led to a second pump run in only 4 aortic and 1 mitral valve patients (overall, 1.4%). This series was heavily weighted by situations in which we encountered difficulty in weaning patients from cardiopulmonary bypass,[70] and by patients in whom another valve was repaired.

Prosthetic valves of any type can be assessed for seating, leaflet motion, and regurgitation. A small jet of regurgitation is physiologic for most normally functioning prosthetic valves. TEE imaging of mitral prosthetic valves improves substantially on TTE because of less shielding of the left atrium.[12] This may also impede imaging of mitral regurgitation from some epicardial views. Likewise, shadowing of the left ventricular outflow tract by an aortic prosthesis during TEE sometimes makes assessment of aortic regurgitation difficult. When significant aortic regurgitation is suspected but not seen by TEE, epicardial imaging is necessary.

Localization of periprosthetic regurgitation by echocardiography is an important guide to operative management (Fig 9–16). In some patients, we have performed suture closure of the leak and used TEE or epicardial echocardiography to verify success of the procedure. Occasionally in patients,[71] the hole is sometimes so small as to be difficult to see on direct surgical inspection, yet TEE can verify that closure has led to resolution of the regurgitation, and ventricular volume overload. In patients with extensive calcification of the native annulus, successful suture closure may not be possible.

After implantation of an aortic valved conduit (the Bental procedure), the potential space between the native aorta and the conduit inside should be small. If it is larger and contains a hematoma, there should be no evidence of flow by color Doppler within the space. In rare cases, a connection from the left ventricular outflow tract into this potential space may compress the conduit and obstruct the left ventricular outflow.

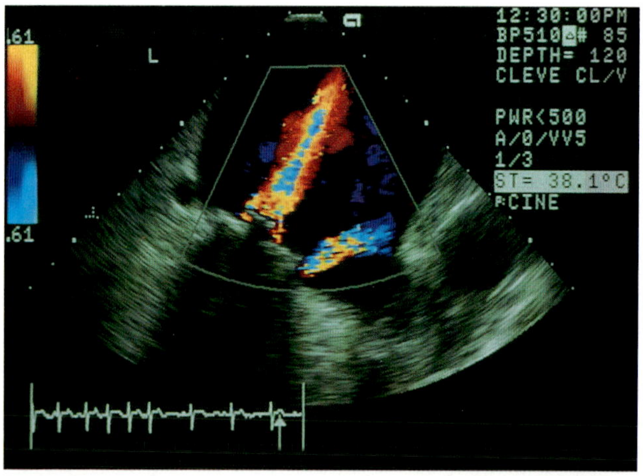

FIG 9–16.
A transesophageal longitudinal *(L)* image in a patient with a mechanical mitral prosthesis shows two jets of mitral regurgitation. The intraprosthetic jet is larger than the periprosthetic jet, which was located along the anterior portion of the mitral annulus. The perivalvular leak could not be imaged well with the standard transverse TEE image plane.

Implantation of a human valve (homograft) is an increasingly attractive alternative to valve replacement, particularly in young patients and those with infections. We image all aortic homografts after insertion to verify appropriate function. Regurgitation may occur due to inadequate commissural suspension. Hematoma between the layers of the homograft may cause outflow obstruction. In our experience with patients having postpump IOE after implantation of a homograft, 10% required a second pump run for further surgery due to suboptimal function defined by echocardiography.

INTRAOPERATIVE ECHOCARDIOGRAPHY IN HYPERTROPHIC CARDIOMYOPATHY AND DYNAMIC LEFT VENTRICULAR OUTFLOW OBSTRUCTION

In patients undergoing myectomy for hypertrophic cardiomyopathy, prepump IOE is useful to define the distribution of hypertrophy, the physiology of systolic anterior motion of the mitral valve and outflow tract obstruction, and the severity of mitral regurgitation. With the aortic annulus used as a reference point, the prepump IOE images identify the length and site of septal hypertrophy, the diameter of maximal septal thickness (Fig 9–17), and the location of systolic contact of the mitral valve with the septum. While TEE may be partially satisfactory, epicardial echocardiography is the preferred tool for assessment by continuous-wave Doppler of the outflow gradient and should be performed in all patients by using the epicardial aorta–superior vena cava transducer position.[56] The location of color Doppler aliasing at the point of contact between systolic anterior motion and the septum confirms that area as the site of maximal obstruction.

A five-chamber view during transverse TEE imaging or a longitudinal TEE view of the aortic valve and outflow tract may demonstrate the obstructive systolic anterior motion. In some patients, this view may be used to measure the obstructive gradient with TEE-derived continuous-wave Doppler.

Postpump epicardial echocardiography is the established method to assess the myectomy result.[56, 72] We measure outflow tract gradients in all

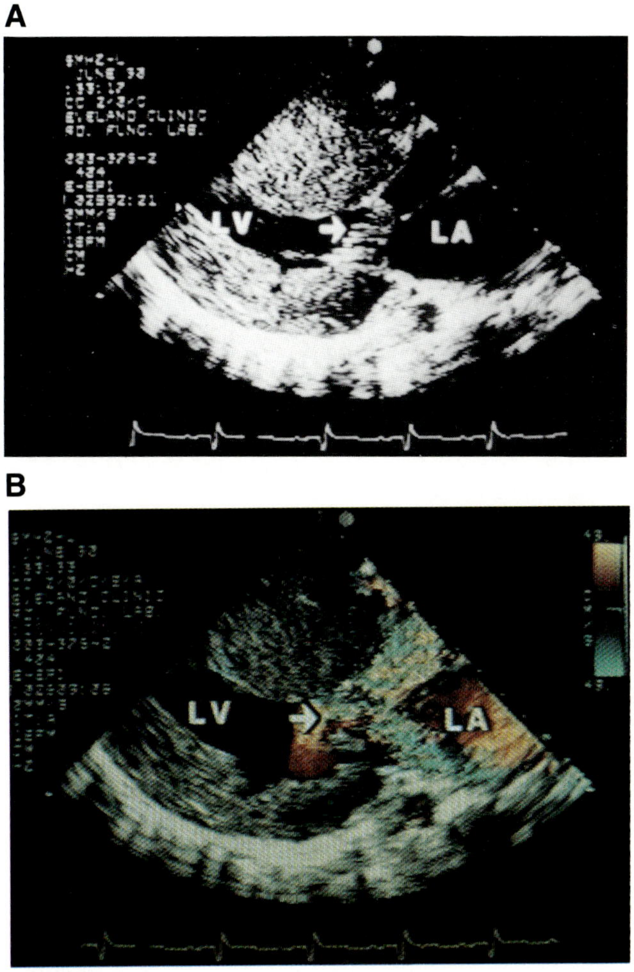

FIG 9–17.
Epicardial parasternal equivalent long-axis view **(A)** of hypertrophic cardiomyopathy. There is marked systolic anterior motion of the mitral leaflets *(arrow)* that is obstructing the left ventricular outflow tract and causing significant mitral regurgitation, which is evident on color Doppler **(B).** The parasternal epicardial view and a five-chamber transesophageal view are useful to define the area of septal hypertrophy that requires resection. *LV* = left ventricle; *LA* = left atrium.

patients by using epicardial continuous-wave Doppler at rest and with a challenge of intravenous isoproterenol. The presence and severity of systolic anterior motion of the mitral valve and mitral regurgitation are investigated with either epicardial or TEE imaging. The myectomy site can be evaluated from the long- and short-axis images (Fig 9–18). Color Doppler is used to exclude postoperative ventricular septal defects, intrinsic mitral regurgitation, or aortic regurgitation. In 20% of patients having myectomy, IOE has found suboptimal results due to persistent obstruction or persistent intrinsic mitral regurgitation.[72]

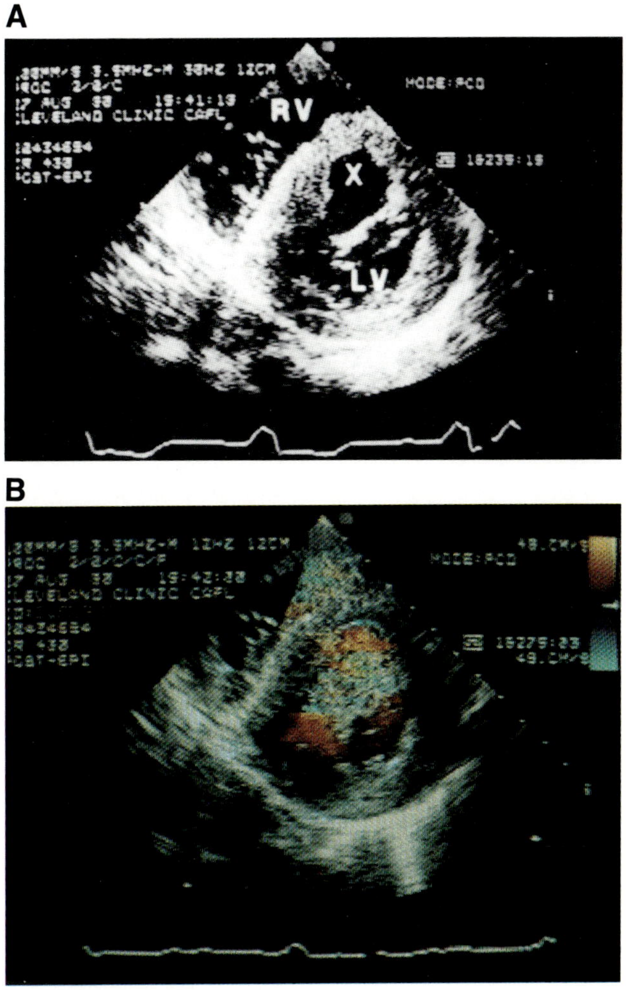

FIG 9–18.
An epicardial parasternal equivalent short-axis view **(A)** of the left ventricle shows the myectomy site *(X)* in a patient with hypertrophic cardiomyopathy. While outflow obstruction was successfully alleviated, color Doppler **(B)** revealed the presence of a small ventricular septal defect at the myectomy site. *LV* = left ventricle; *RV* = right ventricle.

INTRAOPERATIVE ECHOCARDIOGRAPHY IN TRICUSPID VALVE SURGERY

TEE permits adequate recognition of tricuspid regurgitation that is sometimes better than with transthoracic imaging. Biplane TEE often allows better alignment of the ultrasound beam with the tricuspid regurgitation jet during longitudinal imaging. It is useful to measure the diameter of the tricuspid and mitral annulus, which are normally about equal at 2.8 ± 0.5 cm (range, 2 to 4 cm) in a four-chamber view during diastole.[73] The presence of tricuspid annular dilation assessed by IOE, the patient's response to alterations in loading conditions, and other anatomic features are important components of the prepump evaluation of patients with tricuspid regurgitation. However, IOE assessment of the severity of tricuspid regurgitation is even more problematic than other valve lesions because multiple factors profoundly affect tricuspid valve closure. Annular dilatation or right ventricular dysfunction cause tricuspid regurgitation, and are markedly affected by pulmonary artery pressure volume status and myocardial ischemia.[6, 74] Intraoperative right ventricular injury or fluid overload may significantly increase tricuspid regurgitation which may quickly change in severity from moment to moment. Alternatively, hypovolemia and anesthesia itself may reduce the severity of tricuspid regurgitation relative to the ambulatory studies.[75] For this reason, we believe that prepump IOE should not overrule decisions for or against tricuspid valve surgery based on preoperative clinical and imaging evaluation during ambulatory conditions.

Epicardial imaging may also provide a more complete assessment when TEE images of the tricuspid valve are suboptimal. Marked atrial enlargement may also reduce the quality of TEE imaging of the tricuspid valve because of its position in the farfield. In this setting, epicardial detection of tricuspid regurgitation may be superior. Epicardial echocardiography is essential when shadowing of the tricuspid valve occurs by aortic and mitral prostheses. The subcostal-equivalent epicardial view brings the right heart into the near field of the echo image and improves resolution.

INTRAOPERATIVE ECHOCARDIOGRAPHIC ASSESSMENT OF VENTRICULAR FUNCTION

A major application of IOE is the monitoring of ventricular function. IOE is useful for routine monitoring during noncardiac surgery in patients at high risk for myocardial ischemia. Transverse and longitudinal transgastric views in various combinations are useful to determine chamber size, regional wall thickness and systolic thickening, and endocardial motion.

Intraoperative embolism of air or thrombi may also cause ventricular wall motion abnormalities.[76] The transverse TEE four-chamber view is also useful for assessment of right ventricular function. Diastolic function may be examined by carefully assessing mitral and tricuspid valvular and pulmonary and hepatic venous flow,[77–79] all of which can be accomplished during TEE. These maneuvers also demonstrate atrial function, cardiac rhythm, and venous flow reversal suggestive of tricuspid and mitral regurgitation.[47]

IOE is useful for serial monitoring of ventricular function, pre– and post–cardiopulmonary bypass status, and function after the administration of coronary vasodilators and inotropes. Digital storage and display of images facilitate comparative analysis. For a more detailed discussion, see Chapter 10, "Intraoperative Monitoring."

INTRAOPERATIVE ECHOCARDIOGRAPHIC EVALUATION OF THE THORACIC AORTA

IOE is a useful adjunct to operations for thoracic aortic aneurysms. Transesophageal and epicardial (or epiaortic) imaging demonstrates the dimensions of the aorta and the location of thrombus, intimal tears, and dissection. In patients with aortic dissection, TEE is highly sensitive and specific to determine its extent, quantitate aortic valve dysfunction, identify hemopericardium, and characterize ventricular function.[80] While aortic aneurysms are usually assessed before the patient reaches the operating room, the first echocardiographic assessment is sometimes intraoperative. In a hemodynamically unstable patient with clinical evidence of aortic dissection, TEE is the most rapid and reliable way to verify this diagnosis. While coronary arteriography may be essential to define coronary anatomy, TEE can document involvement of the proximal coronary arteries in the dissection and localize ventricular wall motion abnormalities.

During TEE evaluation of thoracic aortic aneurysms, it is important to measure the diameter of the aorta at the level of the aortic valve annulus, sinuses of Valsalva, ascending aorta, arch, and descending thoracic aorta. A short segment of the upper abdominal aorta is also visible. With longitudinal TEE imaging, a larger segment of the distal ascending aorta can be imaged that is otherwise shielded by the trachea during transverse TEE. Involvement of branch vessels of the arch is better visualized in the longitudinal than in the transverse plane.[17, 18, 20, 21] The echocardiographic findings are used to help anticipate the extent and nature of the aortic aneurysm and the decision to perform either aortic valve replacement or resuspension.

After repair of an aortic dissection with placement of a conduit, ventricular and aortic valve function are also reassessed with a IOE. If an ascending aortic tube graft has been implanted, the potential space between the conduit and native aortic wall is assessed for size and abnormal flow suggestive of leakage from the conduit. Of 19 patients imaged with postpump IOE, a change in surgical management resulting from IOE occurred in 2 patients (11%).[81] After replacement of the ascending aorta with a conduit, flow in the false lumen of the descending aorta may or may not be seen, but is ideally absent. The presence of flow rather than a thrombus may imply greater shear forces postoperatively, although prognostic implications are not known.

In patients undergoing standard coronary bypass surgery, preoperative visualization of atherosclerosis in the ascending aorta forewarns of the danger of disruption and embolization of plaque.[82] Identification of the location of plaques with echocardiography may change the methods or location chosen for cannulation of the aorta.[83] In all postpump IOE studies done for any reason, we routinely check the ascending and descending aorta for dissection that can occur iatrogenically at the site of the aortic cannulation.

HISTORICAL PERSPECTIVE AND CONCLUSIONS

While IOE has recently been expanding in popularity, M-mode echocardiography was used in the operating room as early as 1972.[84] IOE progressed further in the early 1980s by applying transthoracic two-dimensional echo transducers covered by sterile sheaths directly to the epicardial surface. With the addition of color flow imaging, IOE has become much more valuable. Since the initiation of IOE at the Cleveland Clinic in 1984,[85] epicardial imaging has gradually fallen to a plateau of 40% of all studies, in part because of the advent of TEE (Fig 9–19). TEE alone is performed in 60% of cases, 26% have epicardial imaging only, while both modalities are employed in 14% of patients.[50] However, epicardial echocardiography remains our "gold standard." When abnormalities requiring a return to cardiopulmonary bypass are suspected but not confirmed by TEE, we rely on epicardial imaging because of its greater numbers of transducer positions and imaging planes and the greater flexibility of epicardial Doppler.

Future advances in technology will likely increase the utility of intraoperative TEE. New dual-

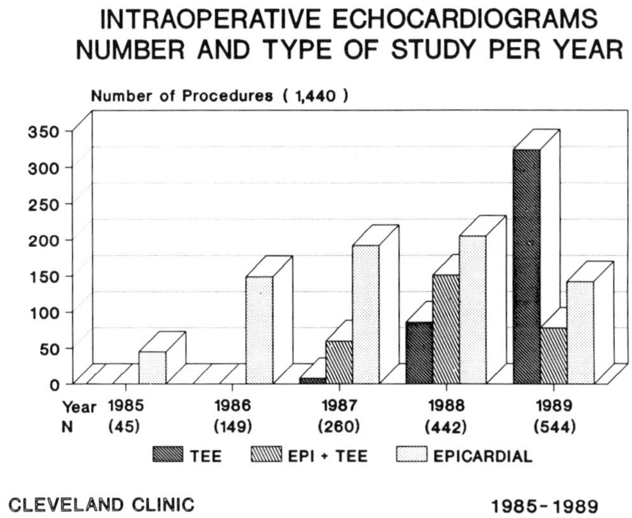

FIG 9–19.
Trends in the utilization of TEE vs. epicardial echo in the IOE service at the Cleveland Clinic from 1985 to 1989. TEE has gradually increased in usage, but epicardial imaging is still necessary for some indications (see the text).

frequency TEE transducers enhance far field resolution. Biplane and omniplane TEE increase the number of views available.[17–23] Continuous-wave Doppler during TEE permits a more complete hemodynamic assessment.[24, 25] Yet optimal application of IOE still depends on the availability of both TEE and epicardial echo.[86]

REFERENCES

1. Stewart WJ, Salcedo EE, Cosgrove DM: The value of echocardiography in mitral valve repair. *Cleve Clin J Med* 1991; 57:177–183.
2. Cosgrove DM, Stewart WJ: Mitral valvuloplasty. *Curr Probl Cardiol* 1989; 14:353–416.
3. Goldman ME, Mora F, Guarino R, et al: Mitral valvuloplasty is superior to valve replacement for preservation of left ventricular function: An intraoperative two-dimensional echocardiographic study. *J Am Coll Cardiol* 1987; 10:568–575.
4. Cohn LH, Couper GS, Kinchla NM, et al: Decreased operative risk of surgical treatment of mitral regurgitation with or without coronary artery disease. *J Am Coll Cardiol* 1990; 16:1575–1578.
5. David TE, Komeda M, Pollick C: Mitral valve annuloplasty: The effect of the type on left ventricular function. *Ann Thorac Surg* 1989; 47:524–528.
6. Maurer G, Czer L: Intraoperative color Doppler assessment of mitral and tricuspid valve repair, in *Echocardiography and Doppler in Cardiac Surgery*. New York, Igaku-Shoin Medical Publishers Inc, 1989, pp 243–257.

7. Stewart WJ, Currie PJ, Salcedo EE, et al: Intraoperative Doppler color flow mapping for decision-making in valve repair for mitral regurgitation. *Circulation* 1990; 81:556–566.
8. Hanrath P, Schluter M, Langenstein BA, et al: Transesophageal horizontal and sagittal imaging of the heart with a phased array system. Initial clinical results, in Hanrath P, Bleifeld W, Souquet J (eds): *Cardiovascular Diagnosis by Ultrasound.* The Hague, Martinus Nijhoff, 1982, pp 280–288.
9. Schluter M, Hinrichs A, Thier W, et al: Transesophageal two-dimensional echocardiography: Comparison of ultrasonic and anatomic sections. *Am J Cardiol* 1984; 53:1173–1178.
10. Seward JB, Khandheria BK, OH JK, et al: Transesophageal echocardiography: Technique, anatomic correlations, implementation, and clinical applications. *Mayo Clin Proc* 1988; 63:649–680.
11. Mitchell MM, Sutherland GR, Gussenhoven EJ, et al: Transesophageal echocardiography. *J Am Soc Echocardiogr* 1988; 1:362–377.
12. Nellessen U, Schnittger I, Appleton CP, et al: Transesophageal two-dimensional echocardiography and color Doppler flow velocity mapping in the evaluation of cardiac valve prostheses. *Circulation* 1988; 78:848–855.
13. Klein AL, Stewart WJ, Cosgrove DM, et al: Intraoperative epicardial echocardiography: Technique and imaging planes. *Echocardiography* 1990; 7:241–251.
14. Stewart WJ, Currie PJ, Agler DA, et al: Intraoperative epicardial echocardiography: Technique, imaging planes, and use in valve repair for mitral regurgitation. *Dynamic Cardiovasc Imaging* 1987; 1:179–186.
15. Currie PJ, Stewart WJ, Lytle BW, et al: Comparison of intraoperative transesophageal and epicardial color flow Doppler in mitral valve repair (abstract). *J Am Coll Cardiol* 1988; 11:2.
16. Salcedo EE, Stewart WJ, Klein AL, et al: Evolution of transesophageal and epicardial echocardiography for intraoperative decision-making (abstract). *J Am Soc Echocardiogr* 1990; 3:219.
17. Bansal RC, Shakudo M, Shah PM, et al: Biplane transesophageal echocardiography: Technique, image orientation, and preliminary experience in 131 patients. *J Am Soc Echocardiogr* 1990; 3:350–366.
18. Seward JB, Khandheria BK, Edwards WD, et al: Biplanar transesophageal echocardiography: Anatomic correlations, image orientation, and clinical applications. *Mayo Clin Proc* 1990; 65:1193–1213.
19. Flachskampf FA, Hoffmann R, Hanrath P: Experience with a transesophageal echotransducer allowing full rotation of the viewing plane: The omniplane probe (abstract). *J Am Coll Cardiol* 1991; 17:34.
20. Cohen GI, Chan KL: Anatomic correlations of the long-axis views in biplane transesophageal echocardiography. *Am J Cardiol* 1990; 66:1007–1010.
21. Cohen GI, Chan KL: Biplane transesophageal echocardiography: Clinical applications of the long-axis plane. *J Am Soc Echocardiogr* 1991; 4:155–163.
22. Khandheria BK, Seward JB, Edwards WD, et al: Biplane transesophageal echocardiography: Anatomic correlation, new imaging planes, and clinical utility (abstract). *Circulation* 1990; 82(suppl 3):551.
23. Bansal RC, Shakudo M, Shah PM, et al: Biplane transesophageal echocardiography: Technique, image orientation, and preliminary experience in 131 patients. *J Am Soc Echocardiogr* 1990; 3:348–366.
24. Weintraub A, Pandian N, Simoneti J, et al: CW Doppler in transesophageal echocardiography allows analysis of high velocity flows and enhances the utility of transesophageal echo (abstract). *Circulation* 1991; 82(suppl 3):669.
25. Samdarshi T, Fan PH, Chouinrd M, et al: Intraoperative transesophageal color Doppler guided continuous wave Doppler assessment of aortic valve stenosis (abstract). *Circulation* 1990; 82(suppl 3):551.
26. Geibel A, Kasper W, Behroz A, et al: Risk of transesophageal echocardiography in awake patients with cardiac diseases. *Am J Cardiol* 1988; 62:337–339.
27. Daniel WG, Erbel R, Kasper W, et al: Safety of transesophageal echocardiography. *Circulation* 1991; 83:817–821.
28. Foster E, Kusumoto FM, Sobol SM, et al: Streptococcal endocarditis temporally related to transesophageal echocardiography. *J Am Coll Cardiol* 1990; 3:424–427.
29. Lam HC, Ranganathan N, Wigle ED, et al: Morphology of the human mitral valve. *Circulation* 1970; 41:449–458.
30. Ranganathan N, Lam JHC, Wigle ED, et al: Morphology of the human mitral valve. *Circulation* 1970; 41:459–467.
31. Stewart WJ, Chavez AM, Currie PJ, et al: Echo determination of mitral pathology and feasibility of repair for mitral regurgitation (abstract). *Circulation* 1986; 76(suppl 4): 448.
32. Stewart WJ, Agler DA, Homa DA, et al: Predicting the mechanism of mitral regurgitation prior to repair: A system using leaflet motion and color Doppler jet direction (abstract). *Circulation* 1990; 82(suppl 3):551.
33. Marwick T, Obarski T, Salcedo E, et al: Transesophageal echo evaluation of mitral stenosis may underestimate "splitability score" (abstract). *J Am Coll Cardiol* 1990; 3:211.
34. Stewart WJ, Currie PJ, Salcedo EE, et al: Jet direction by color flow mapping accurately depicts the mechanism of mitral regurgitation. (abstract). *Circulation* 1988, 78(suppl 2):131.
35. Antunes MJ, Colsen PR, Kinsley RH: Mitral valvuloplasty: A learning curve. *Circulation* 1983; 68(suppl 2):70–75.
36. Cosgrove DM, Chavez AM, Lytle BW, et al: Results of mitral valve reconstruction. *Circulation* 1986; 74(suppl 1):82–86.
37. Spencer FC, Colvin SB, Culliford AT, et al: Experi-

ences with Carpentier techniques of mitral valve reconstruction in 103 patients. *J Thorac Cardiovasc Surg* 1985; 90:341–350.

38. Carpentier A, Chauvaud S, Fabiani JN: Reconstructive surgery of mitral valve incompetence. *J Thorac Cardiovasc Surg* 1980; 79:338–348.
39. Hendren WG, Nemec JJ, Lytle BW, et al: Mitral valve repair for ischemic mitral insufficiency. *Ann Thorac Surg*, in press.
40. Cape EG, Yoganathan AP, Weyman AE, et al: Adjacent solid boundaries alter the size of regurgitant jets on Doppler color-flow maps. *J Am Coll Cardiol* 1991; 17:1094–1102.
41. Newman BG: The deflection of plane jets by adjacent boundaries: Coanda effect, in Lachmann GV (ed): *Boundary Layer Control Principles and Application.* New York, Pergamon Press Inc, 1961, pp 232–264.
42. Cohen GI, Davison MB, Klein AL, et al: Transthoracic Doppler of prosthetic mitral regurgitation: The utility of color Doppler flow convergence. (abstract). *J Am Coll Cardiol* 1991; 17:359.
43. Bargiggia GS, Tronconi L, Raisaro A, et al: Color Doppler diagnosis of mechanical prosthetic mitral regurgitation: Usefulness of the flow convergence region proximal to the regurgitant orifice. *Am Heart J* 1990; 120:1137–1141.
44. Po-Hoey F, Kapur KK, Krishan AK, et al: Utility of color flow acceleration in differentiating valvar from paravalvar prosthetic mitral regurgitation. (abstract). *Circulation* 1987; 76(suppl 4):448.
45. Cohen GI, Chan KL: Comparison of transesophageal echocardiography and angiography in the assessment of mitral regurgitation (abstract). *Circulation* 1990; 82(suppl 3):550.
46. Yoshida K, Yoshikawa J, Yamaura Y, et al: Assessment of mitral regurgitation by biplane transesophageal color Doppler flow mapping. *Circulation* 1990; 82:1121–1126.
47. Klein AL, Obarski TP, Stewart WJ, et al: Transesophageal Doppler echocardiography of pulmonary venous flow. A new marker of mitral regurgitation severity. *J Am Coll Cardiol* 1991; 18:518–526.
48. Davison M, Cohen G, Marwick T, et al: The frequency of acquisition and quality of images obtained by transesophageal echocardiography. A prospective study of 100 consecutive cases (abstract). *J Am Soc Echocardiogr* 1991; 4:288.
49. King H, Csicsko J, Leshnower A: Intraoperative assessment of the mitral valve following reconstructive procedures. *Ann Thorac Surg* 1980; 29:81–83.
50. Salcedo EE, Davison MB, Agler D, et al: Comparison of intraoperative and outpatient transesophageal echo for the assessment of mitral regurgitation severity (abstract). *J Am Soc Echocardiogr* 1991; 4:298.
51. Marwick T, Currie PJ, Stewart WJ, et al: Echocardiographic evaluation of immediate and late failed mitral valve repair (abstract). *J Am Coll Cardiol* 1989; 3:114.
52. Goldman ME, Mindich BP, Teichholz LE, et al: Intraoperative contrast echocardiography to evaluate mitral valve operations. *J Am Coll Cardiol* 1984; 4:1035–1040.
53. Mihaileanu S, Marino JP, Chauvaud S, et al: Left ventricular outflow obstruction after mitral valve repair (Carpentier's technique). *Circulation* 1988; 78(suppl 1):78–84.
54. Kreindel MS, Schiavone WA, Lever HM, et al: Systolic anterior motion of the mitral valve after Carpentier ring valvuloplasty for mitral valve prolapse. *Am J Cardiol* 1986; 57:408–412.
55. Stewart WJ, Currie PJ, Schiavone WA, et al: Intraoperative echocardiography in patients with left ventricular outflow tract obstruction, in Maurer G, Mohl W (eds). *Proceedings of the First International Symposium on Echocardiography and Doppler in Cardiac Surgery.* New York, Igaku-Shoin Medical Publishers Inc, 1989, pp 331–345.
56. Stewart WJ, Schiavone WA, Salcedo EE, et al: Intraoperative Doppler echocardiography in hypertrophic cardiomyopathy: Correlations with the obstructive gradient. *J Am Coll Cardiol* 1987; 19:327–335.
57. Currie PJ, Stewart WJ: Intraoperative echocardiography for surgical repair of the aortic valve and left ventricular outflow tract. *Echocardiography* 1990; 7:273–288.
58. Pitarys CJ, Forman MB, Panayiotol H, et al: Long-term effects of excision of the mitral apparatus on global and regional ventricular function in humans. *J Am Coll Cardiol* 1990; 15:557–561.
59. Carabello BA, et al: Preservation of left ventricular function in patients with mitral regurgitation: A realistic goal for the nineties. *J Am Coll Cardiol* 1990; 15:564–565.
60. Cosgrove DM, Rosenkranz ER, Hendren WG, et al: Valvuloplasty for aortic insufficiency. *J Thoracic Cardiovasc Surg* 1991; 102:571–576.
61. Freeman WK, Schaff HV, Orszulak TA, et al: Ultrasonic aortic valve decalcification: Serial Doppler echocardiography follow-up. *J Am Coll Cardiol* 1990; 16:623–630.
62. Chandrasekaran K, Foley R, Weintraub A, et al: Evidence that transesophageal echocardiography can reliably and directly measure the aortic valve area in patients with aortic stenosis—A new application that is independent of LV function and does not require Doppler data (abstract). *J Am Coll Cardiol* 1991; 17:20.
63. Stewart WJ, Currie PJ, Salcedo EE, et al: Intraoperative echo in aortic valve repair (abstract). *Circulation* 1988; 78(suppl 2):435.
64. Warth DC, Stewart WJ, Block P, et al: A new method to calculate aortic valve area without left heart catheterization. *Circulation* 1984; 70:978–983.
65. Skjaerpe T, Hagrenaes L, Hatle L: Noninvasive estimation of valve area in patients with aortic stenosis

by Doppler ultrasound and two-dimensional echocardiography. *Circulation* 1985; 72:810.
66. Edwards JE: The congenital bicuspid aortic valve. *Circulation* 1961; 23:485–488.
67. Stewart WJ, King ME, Gillam LD, et al: Prevalence of aortic valve prolapse with bicuspid aortic valve and its relation to aortic regurgitation: A cross-sectional echocardiographic study. *Am J Cardiol* 1984; 54:1277.
68. Perry GJ, Helmcke F, Nanda NC, et al: Evaluation of aortic insufficiency by Doppler color flow mapping. *J Am Coll Cardiol* 1957; 9:952.
69. Boughner DR: Assessment of aortic insufficiency by transcutaneous Doppler ultrasound. *Circulation* 1975; 52:874–879.
70. Jacobs LE, Kotler MN, Ioli A: Left ventricular outflow tract obstruction following mitral valve replacement with Carpentier-Edwards prosthesis. *Echocardiography* 1990; 7:147–153.
71. Davison M, Burstow DJ: Transesophageal echocardiography in the assessment of hemolytic anemia following mitral valve surgery (abstract). *J Am Soc Echocardiogr* 1990; 3:221.
72. Marwick T, Stewart WJ: Intraoperative echocardiography guides extent of myectomy in hypertrophic cardiomyopathy (abstract). *Circulation* 1989; 80(suppl 2):268.
73. Cohen GI, White M, Sochowski RA, et al: Normal reference measurements obtained from transesophageal echocardiographic studies (abstract). *Circulation* 1990; 82(suppl 3):30.
74. Czer LS, Maurer G, Bolger A, et al: Tricuspid valve repair. *J Thorac Cardiovasc Surg* 1989; 98:101–111.
75. Stevenson JG, Sorensen GK: Significant reduction in intraoperative color Doppler tricuspid regurgitation jet area from effects of anesthesia prior to actual surgical repair (abstract). *J Am Coll Cardiol* 1991; 17:19.
76. Obarski TP, Cosgrove DM, Loop FD, et al: Increased incidence of perioperative myocardial infarction in valve repair for mitral regurgitation (abstract). *J Am Coll Cardiol* 1990; 15:236.
77. Hatle LK, Appleton CP, Popp RL: Differentiation of constrictive pericarditis and restrictive cardiomyopathy by Doppler echocardiography. *Circulation* 1989; 79:357–370.
78. Nishimura RA, Housmans PR, Hatle LK, et al: Assessment of diastolic function of the heart: Background and current applications of Doppler echocardiography. Part I. Physiologic and pathophysiologic features. *Mayo Clin Proc* 1989; 64:71–81.
79. Nishimura RA, Housmans PR, Hatle LK, et al: Assessment of diastolic function of the heart: Background and current applications of Doppler echocardiography. Part II. Clinical studies. *Mayo Clin Proc* 1989; 64:71–81.
80. Erbel R, Daniel W, Visser C, et al: Echocardiography in diagnosis of aortic dissection. *Lancet* 1989; 1:457–461.
81. Stewart WJ, Salcedo EE: Intraoperative echocardiography in thoracic aortic aneurysm. Presented at the fourth meeting of the International Society of Ultrasound in Cardiac Surgery. Innsbruck, Austria, May 1991.
82. Karalis DG, Chandrasekaran K, Victor MF, et al: Recognition and embolic potential of intraaortic atherosclerotic debris. *J Am Coll Cardiol* 1991; 17:73–78.
83. Barzilai B, Marshall WG, Saffitz JE, et al: Avoidance of embolic complications by ultrasonic characterization of the ascending aorta. *Circulation* 1989; 80(suppl 1):277–279.
84. Johnson ML, Holmes JH, Spangler RD, et al: Usefulness of echocardiography in patients undergoing mitral valve surgery. *J Thorac Cardiovasc Surg* 1972; 64:922.
85. Stewart WJ, Gill CC, Currie PJ, et al: Intraoperative Doppler color flow mapping in valve conservation surgery (abstract). *Circulation* 1986; 74(suppl 2):145.
86. Stewart WJ, Kerber RD. Intraoperative echocardiography, in Marcus M, et al (eds): *Cardiac Imaging*. Philadelphia, WB Saunders Co, 1991, pp 619–633.

Chapter 10

Intraoperative Monitoring

Michael K. Cahalan, M.D.

Two-dimensional transesophageal echocardiography (TEE) provides remarkably revealing images of cardiovascular anatomy and physiology. Patients and physicians should benefit from these images because they offer more information and less risk than do alternative monitoring techniques. Indeed, information derived from TEE can dramatically alter anesthetic and surgical management. This chapter will focus on the basic technique needed by the anesthesiologist for intraoperative monitoring with TEE and the supporting studies that delineate the clinical advantages of TEE over customary alternatives.

BASIC TECHNIQUE OF TEE

With the introduction in West Germany of a phased-array transducer that could be positioned in the esophagus, intraoperative two-dimensional echocardiography became a practical tool for anesthesiologists.[1] A typical esophageal transducer has 64 piezoelectric elements; is 42 mm long, 13 mm wide, and 11 mm thick; operates at 5 MHz; and is mounted on the tip of a 9-mm-diameter gastroscope (see Fig 2–3). Once the transducer has been inserted through the mouth and advanced 30 to 35 cm and the controls of the gastroscope retroflexed to angle the ultrasound beam downward (10 to 30 degrees caudad), a view of the left atrium, left ventricle, and left ventricular outflow tract including the aortic valve and right ventricle is easily obtained (see Fig 2–6,D). This cross section is ideal for rapid detection of gross morphologic abnormalities of the mitral valve, masses in the left atrium, and with color Doppler, mitral stenosis and mitral and aortic regurgitation. When the transducer is advanced 1 to 2 cm deeper into the esophagus and the beam again angled downward 10 to 30 degrees, the four cardiac chambers can be seen (see Fig 2–10,A). This position is ideal for evaluation of relative left and right ventricular size and function as well as color Doppler evaluation of tricuspid regurgitation. The transducer is advanced another 2 to 7 cm and then angled upward 10 to 30 degrees to obtain the short-axis cross section of the left ventricle at the level of the papillary muscles (see Fig 2–8,A). For the following three reasons, this cross section is ideal for monitoring left ventricular filling and ejection. First, all major coronary arteries supply the myocardium viewed in this cross section (Fig 10–1). The right coronary artery supplies the inferior wall and part of the septum. The left anterior descending artery supplies part of the septum and anterior wall, while the circumflex artery usually supplies the remainder of the anterior and posterior (free wall) of the left ventricle at this midpapillary muscle level. Thus, if a single monitoring position is to be used during surgery (the usual situation given the many other tasks of the anesthesiologist), the short-axis cross section at the midpapillary muscle level is ideally suited for detection of ischemia (see the studies below). Second, changes in preload cause larger changes in the short-axis dimension than in the long-axis dimension of the left ventricle. Thus, changes in filling are more easily appreciated by viewing the short-axis cross section. Third, movement of the probe from its monitoring position at the short-axis, midpapillary muscle level is immediately apparent because the morphology of the papillary muscles changes as they extend from their origins in the wall of the ventricle to their insertions into the chordae. Relative changes in filling and ejection are assessed during surgery, and to make such evaluations valid, the same cross section must be viewed.

In our experience, inserting and positioning the TEE probe usually requires less than 5 minutes. After insertion of the probe, we record cross sections of the aortic and mitral valves on videotape with and without color Doppler imaging. These images reveal valvular pathology that when present might alter

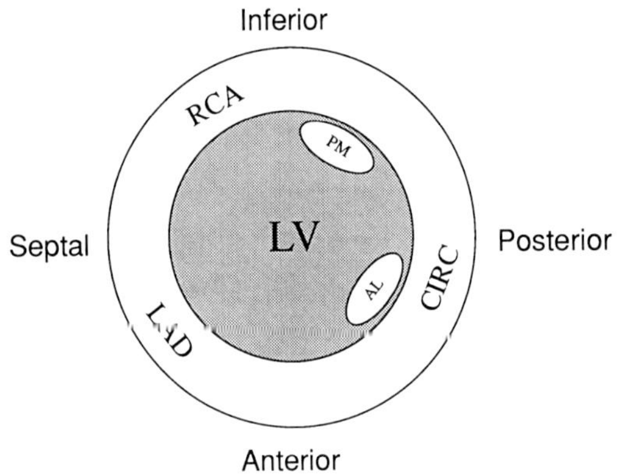

FIG 10–1.
Diagrammatic short-axis TEE at the midpapillary muscle level. *LV* = ventricular cavity *(shaded area); AL* and *PM* = anterior lateral and posterior medial papillary muscles. The LV is divided into four segments or walls by two perpendicular lines bisecting the papillary muscles. The walls are by convention named anterior, posterior, septal, and inferior. Coronary blood flow is supplied to these walls as indicated by the left anterior descending coronary artery *(LAD)*, the circumflex coronary artery *(CIRC)*, and the right coronary artery *(RCA)*.

surgical and anesthetic management. If possible, it is important to record a complete TEE study. Information regarding such details as valvular morphology may become invaluable postoperatively as a baseline, particularly in patients who, after surgery, are suspected of having endocarditis. Thereafter, we monitor the short-axis view of the left ventricle at the level of the papillary muscles and have done so for up to 12 hours. These images are recorded prior to surgical incision, at the conclusion of surgery, and at strategic intervals during surgery, for instance, during unclamping of the abdominal aorta or whenever hemodynamic or cardiac problems develop. The real-time interpretations ("preliminary TEE note") are placed in the patient's chart by the anesthesiologist after completion of surgery. The videotape is subsequently evaluated by an echocardiographer who issues a formal report with a copy to the anesthesiologist. In approximately 8% to 10% of patients, the short-axis view cannot be obtained because of horizontal displacement of the heart by the contents of the abdomen. Other views, such as a four-chamber view, must then be monitored, but changes in left ventricular filling and segmental contraction are not as easily assessed.

We have obtained high-resolution echocardiograms in 97% of the more than 2,700 anesthetized patients we have studied with TEE. In 3 patients, suspected complications have been noted. In 1 patient, the esophageal stethoscope was buried in the esophagus and not removed until the third postoperative day. In the second patient, upper gastrointestinal bleeding (about 1 L) was noted after coronary artery surgery. This bleeding resolved spontaneously, and its exact site was not determined. In the third patient, a splenic injury was noted during abdominal aortic aneurysmectomy and not thought to be due to surgical retraction. An incidental splenectomy was performed because heparinization was planned. In all three cases, insertion and manipulation of the echocardiographic probe were accomplished without apparent difficulty. As a precaution, we do not perform TEE monitoring in patients with a history of swallowing complaints or esophageal disease. One published report describes two patients who suffered temporary unilateral vocal cord paralysis after TEE monitoring during "sitting" craniotomies.[2] Both of these patients were positioned with nearly full neck flexion. The authors of this report believe (personal communication) that the recurrent laryngeal nerve was injured when the larynx, endotracheal tube, and shaft of the gastroscope were compressed between the chin and vertebral column.

MONITORING LEFT VENTRICULAR FILLING AND GLOBAL EJECTION

TEE provides more reliable information on left ventricular filling in patients undergoing cardiovascular surgery than does the pulmonary artery catheter. For instance, Harpole et al. studied 12 patients during resection of abdominal aortic aneurysms.[3] At multiple times during surgery, hemodynamics, echocardiograms, and first-pass radionuclide studies were recorded simultaneously. The correlation coefficients between echocardiographic and radionuclide estimates were $r = 0.84$ for end-diastolic volume and $r = 0.84$ for ejection fraction. In contrast, no significant correlation was found between pulmonary artery diastolic pressure and either the echocardiographic or radionuclide estimates of left ventricular filling. Thus, TEE provides the anesthesiologist with a direct method to assess left ventricular preload and ejection.

In practical terms, however, the quantitative analysis of the echocardiograms, as it has traditionally been performed, was too time-consuming to be of value in the operating room. For that reason, we have used qualitative estimates of left ventricular filling and ejection in real time to guide our administration of fluids and inotropes (Table 10–1). Marked changes in filling and ejection can occur before, si-

TABLE 10–1.
Diagnosis of Hypotension With TEE

EDA*	EF_a*	MR*	Diagnosis
⇓	⇑	0	Hypovolemia
⇑	⇓	0	Myocardial depression
⇔	⇑	0	Low systemic resistance
⇔	⇑	+2–4	Mitral regurgitation
⇑	0	0	Cardiac arrest

*EDA = end-diastolic cross-sectional area, or the size of the left ventricle at end diastole; EF_a = area ejection fraction, or the fractional change in the cross-sectional area of the left ventricle during systole; MR = mitral regurgitation and is graded on a 0 (none) to +4 (severe) scale.

multaneously with, or in the absence of changes in blood pressure or filling pressures. A video processing computer converts the echocardiographic images from one cardiac cycle into digital code and then plays the cycle repeatedly for comparison with other cardiac cycles captured at other times during surgery. This juxtapositioning of images greatly facilitates the qualitative evaluation of changes in left ventricular filling, ejection, and left ventricular segmental wall motion. In patients who might require

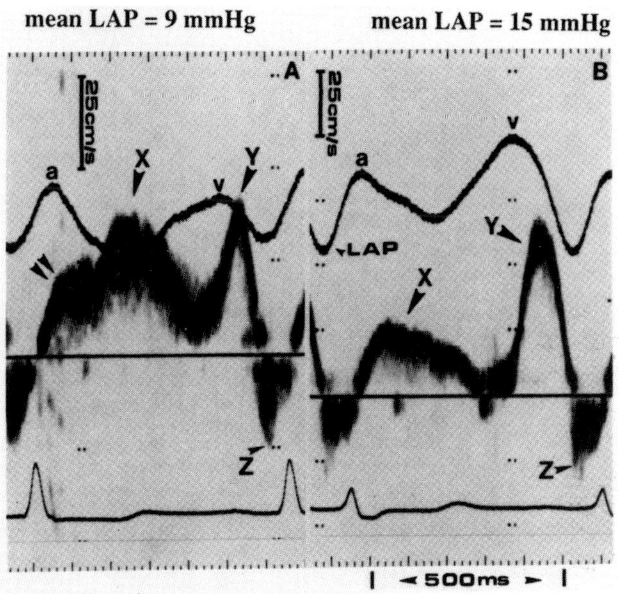

FIG 10–2.
Effect of increased mean left atrial pressure *(LAP)* on pulmonary venous flow velocities. The tracings from top to bottom are LAP, pulmonary venous flow velocity (with a zero velocity reference superimposed as a straight horizontal line), and electrocardiogram (ECG). *Left,* tracings from a patient with a LAP of 9 mm Hg show predominance of the systolic flow velocities (labeled with a *double arrow* and *X*). *Right,* tracings from a patient with a LAP of 15 show diastolic predominance (labeled with *Y*). (From Kuecherer HF, Muhiudeen IA, Kusumoto FM, et al: *Circulation* 1990; 82:1127–1139. Used by permission.)

pulmonary artery catheterization primarily for intraoperative monitoring, we now use TEE instead. When estimates of left atrial pressure are necessary, TEE can provide them indirectly by Doppler interrogation of pulmonary venous inflow patterns, a technique recently developed at the University of California, San Francisco (Fig 10–2).[4] Even when both TEE and a pulmonary artery catheter are in place, we preferentially consult the TEE images in critical situations such as acute hypotension because the information we need most (preload and ejection status) are instantly apparent from TEE but not from the pulmonary artery tracing.

Technological improvements are likely to further improve the intraoperative assessment of ventricular filling and function. Recently, Hewlett-Packard, Inc., one of the ultrasound manufacturers, has introduced a new application, "AQ, acoustic quantification," that uses the radio frequency signal from ultrasound to detect endocardium in an automated fashion. Short-axis images of the left ventricle by TEE are obtained, and area-time plots are generated on a real-time basis. This estimate of ventricular size and function (percent change in area), although limited by viewing the left ventricle from only one imaging plane, has an important potential for quantitatively following serial changes in left ventricular filling and function in real time.

DETECTION OF LEFT VENTRICULAR ISCHEMIA

Detection of myocardial ischemia is also more reliable with TEE than with traditional monitors. Since Tennant and Wiggers first described the association of segmental wall motion abnormality (SWMA) and ischemia,[5] many others have proved that ischemic segments of human and animal hearts do not exhibit normal inward wall motion or thickening during systole. SWMAs have been shown to occur within seconds of the onset of regional ischemia, before or in the absence of changes in the ECG.[6] The presence of an akinetic (noncontracting) or dyskinetic (paradoxically moving) segment of the left ventricle usually indicates an old infarction. However, the development of a new SWMA during examination, e.g., during intraoperative monitoring, is likely to be caused by myocardial ischemia.

Smith et al. utilized TEE in 50 patients undergoing coronary artery or major vascular surgery.[7] At predetermined intervals, echocardiograms and multilead ECGs (limb leads, augmented leads, and V5) were recorded, both of which were evaluated by "blinded" observers. Intraoperatively, 6 patients had ST segment changes diagnostic of myocardial ischemia (0.1-mV or greater deviation), while 24 had new SWMAs diagnostic of myocardial ischemia (Table 10–2). No patient experienced an ST segment change before or in the absence of a new SWMA. In 3 of the 6 patients who experienced ST segment change, the SWMA occurred minutes before the ECG change. Three of the 50 patients suffered intraoperative myocardial infarctions, and all had SWMAs develop and persist until the end of surgery in the corresponding area of myocardium. Only 1 of these patients had an intraoperative ST segment change diagnostic of ischemia. During the course of surgery, 24 patients had a total of 32 new SWMAs. Two patients had baseline hypokinetic segments that subsequently became dyskinetic. The remaining 22 had normal baseline wall motion in a segment that subsequently developed an abnormality. Of these 22, 4 had segmental dyskinesis, 9 had segmental akinesis, and 9 had severe segmental hypokinesis. Four of the 5 patients with double-vessel disease had new SWMAs, and these changes were in regions of myocardium supplied by the diseased coronary arteries and never in the "risk-free" myocardium.

In a similar study in which continuous TEE and two-lead Holter recordings were utilized, Leung et al. found comparable results.[8] Six of their 50 patients had major adverse outcomes (2 deaths from cardiac causes, 3 myocardial infarctions, and 1 ventricular failure). All 6 of these patients had new SWMAs detected after cardiopulmonary bypass that persisted to the conclusion of surgery. Two of the 6 had new ST segment change after bypass, and 3 others had uninterpretable ST segments due to bundle branch block or ventricular pacing. No patient without a new SWMA occurring after cardiopulmonary bypass had a major adverse outcome. In neither study were hemodynamics predictive of myocardial ischemia, that is, the majority of ischemia was noted during apparently normal hemodynamics. Thus, myocardial ischemia was detected more frequently with TEE than with ECG, usually in the presence of apparently normal hemodynamics, and new SWMAs that persisted were important prognostic signs for cardiovascular complications.

TABLE 10–2.
Segmental Wall Motion Analysis System*†

Motion	Radial Shortening‡	Myocardial Thickening§
Normal motion	>30%	+++
Mild hypokinesis	10–30%	++
Severe hypokinesis	>0, <10%	+
Akinesis	0	0
Dyskinesis	Systolic lengthening	Systolic thinning

*Adapted from Smith JS, Cahalan MK, Benefiel DJ, et al: *Circulation* 1985; 72:1015–1021.
†The diagnosis of myocardial ischemia requires worsening of segmental function (in the absence of comparable global changes) by two classes from normal or mild hypokinesis to at least severe hypokinesis or akinesis.
‡Radial shortening is defined as the decrease in length during systole of an imaginary radius from the endocardium to the center of the left ventricular cavity in the midpapillary muscle short-axis cross section. A floating reference system is used (see the text).
§Myocardial thickening is defined as the increase in distance between the endocardial and epicardial borders during systole.

Recently, van Daele et al. confirmed the insensitivity of hemodynamic monitoring, specifically, pulmonary capillary wedge pressure (PCWP) monitoring, for the detection of myocardial ischemia.[9] In 98 patients anesthetized with high-dose narcotics, 12-lead ECG and TEE identified 14 patients experiencing ischemia before the start of coronary artery surgery (all 14 had TEE-detected SWMAs, and 10 also had ST segment change). Concomitant with the onset of ischemia, PCWP increased 3.5 ± 4.8 mm Hg. However, many patients without ischemia experienced similar increases in PCWP. In fact, an increase of 3 mm Hg in the PCWP had a sensitivity of 33% and a positive predictive value of only 16% for the detection of myocardial ischemia in this patient population. Thus, the risk and expense of pulmonary artery catheterization can hardly be justified solely or primarily for the detection of intraoperative myocardial ischemia.

These "intraoperative" studies in fact used postoperative interpretations of the echocardiograms. In addition, they did not explore many inherent difficulties in the utilization of TEE as a monitor for intraoperative myocardial ischemia. In their patients, Smith et al.,[7] Leung et al.,[8] and van Daele et al.[9] used TEE to monitor the midpapillary muscle short-axis cross section of the left ventricle. Ischemia confined to the right ventricle or base or apex of the left ventricle would have been missed. This fact may in part explain why Leung et al found six episodes of significant ST change unaccompanied by new SWMAs.[8] One solution is to frequently reposition the probe to view other cross sections, but this is impractical when one anesthesiologist is responsible for both patient care and TEE monitoring. Another potential solution is provided by the biplane transesophageal probe, which has two transducers with their ultrasound beams oriented at right angles to each other. With this probe ideally positioned, the operator can immediately switch from the midpapillary muscle short-axis cross section to a long-axis cross section and view portions of the left ventricular base and apex. However, both cross sections cannot be viewed simultaneously in real time, and no studies are yet available that document an improved rate of ischemia detection with this new probe.

Even when an area of myocardium is clearly in view, its segmental contraction can be difficult to evaluate if the entire heart rotates or translates markedly during systole or if dysynergic contraction occurs due to bundle branch block or ventricular pacing. Consequently, a valid system for assessing an SWMA must first compensate for global motion of the heart (usually done by a "floating" frame of reference) and then evaluate both regional endocardial motion and myocardial thickening.[10] Unfortunately, no currently available automated wall motion analysis system has proved adequate for TEE images. Interpretation of septal motion is most often confounded by dysynergic contraction. When the septum is viable and nonischemic, it will appreciably thicken during systole, although its inward motion may begin slightly before or after inward motion of the other walls of the ventricle. Thus, new SWMAs can be detected during bundle branch block, ventricular pacing, and marked global movements of the heart, but not by assessment of endocardial motion alone.

Even when performed by experts, analysis of segmental wall motion is subjective; therefore, in our research studies we require at least two expert readers to *independently* review the echocardiograms. Other investigators have relied upon the simultaneous interpretation of two readers (consensus interpretations) or the interpretation of a single reader. Although more time-consuming than the other approaches, independent interpretations should be performed to minimize the risk that the bias or misinterpretation of a single observer could profoundly alter the results of the study. Interestingly, I have noted that the correlation between ECG and TEE evidence of ischemia seems better when two independent readers are used to diagnosis new SWMAs[7, 9, 11] and worse when only one reader is used.[12]

However, are all SWMAs indicative of myocardial ischemia or infarction? Clearly, they are not. Owing to biologic differences in normal patients, not all hearts contract normally, and not all parts of the same heart contract to the same degree.[13] However, an acute decrease or cessation of segmental contraction, for example, a new SWMA during surgery, is almost certainly due to myocardial ischemia. One exception to this rule is myocardial stunning, or prolonged, postischemic ventricular dysfunction.[14] When ischemia has been prolonged, full restoration of blood flow may occur minutes to hours before the return of normal segmental contraction. Does a new SWMA detected immediately after bypass represent inadequate revascularization and ongoing ischemia or stunned myocardium from inadequate preservation during bypass? Inadequate revascularization may require placement of additional grafts, while stunned myocardium requires only supportive measures until its function returns. When we are faced with this clinical dilemma, graft status is re-evaluated and the new SWMA watched for signs of improvement. If worsening occurs, if graft status is questionable, or if hemodynamics are tenuous, then additional revascularization is provided if possible.

Alternatively, ultrasound contrast agents may prove helpful in this area. A recent report by Aronson et al. demonstrated the potential of ultrasound contrast agents during myocardial revascularization.[15] In this study, patients undergoing coronary artery bypass grafting were imaged with TEE while sonicated Renografin was injected into the aortic root before grafting or directly into the proximal portion of vein grafts while on cardiopulmonary bypass. Contrast images provided information about the distribution of vein graft runoff (Fig 10–3). More importantly, by obtaining contrast-enhanced images with the patient on cardiopulmonary bypass, the investigators were able to identify poorly perfused myocardial regions that were associated with SWMAs detected after separation from cardiopulmonary bypass. The ability to detect inadequate revascularization of patients still on cardiopulmonary bypass has important clinical implications for individuals undergoing revascularization.

New ultrasound contrast agents with uniformity and a long shelf life, combined with new technology such as ultrasound backscatter analysis, may ultimately lead to an easy and accurate means of assessing not only myocardial perfusion but also viability. Much work is currently underway in these areas. It is anticipated that initial clinical application of this new technology will take place in the intraoperative setting during revascularization procedures.

Another conceivable cause of acute SWMA is unmasking areas of scarring by changes in afterload. For instance, a marked increase in blood pressure might retard contraction in an already damaged segment of myocardium more than in a normal segment. Three observations make this an unlikely explanation for the acute SWMAs reported in the stud-

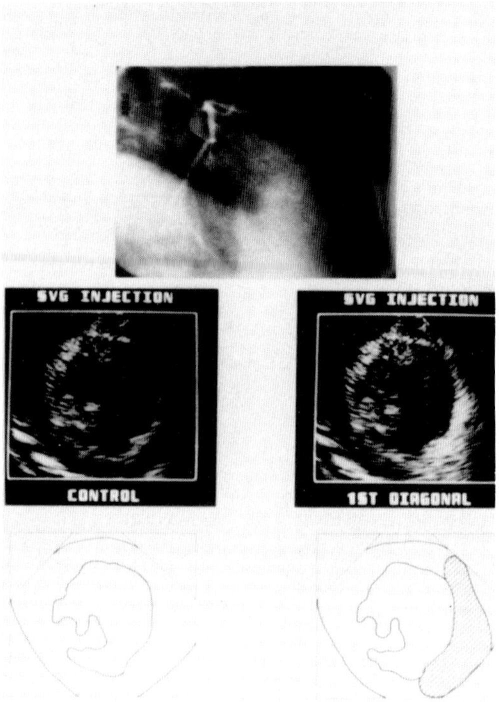

FIG 10–3.
Shown is an arteriogram *(top center)* of the left coronary artery obtained before surgery that demonstrates poor blood supply to the septal region by either septal branches or collateral vessels. The control TEE image *(center left)* was obtained before contrast. In these images, unlike standard images, the septum is to the viewer's right, and the lateral wall is to the left. The contrast-enhanced image *(center right)* was obtained while sonicated Renografin was injected directly into the proximal end of a saphenous vein graft *(SVG)* to the first diagonal branch. Note the opacification in the septal region as compared with the unopacified control image. Note also the attenuation *(black area)* lateral to the opacified region. (Courtesy of Dr. Solomon Aronson, University of Chicago.)

ies above. First, only marked changes in segmental contraction were taken as indicative of ischemia. It is hard to imagine that a sudden increase in afterload would cause one segment to cease or nearly cease contracting in the absence of changes in the other segments. Second, none of the above-mentioned intraoperative studies demonstrated any consistent correlation between hemodynamic aberrations and new SWMAs. In general, anesthesiologists prevent marked changes in loading conditions. Third, the vast majority of new SWMAs occurred in segments of myocardium with normal contraction at baseline (after induction of anesthesia). Thus, acute changes in left ventricular loading probably require an intervention by the anesthesiologist, can cause myocardial ischemia, but alone are not an explanation for new SWMAs.

Tethering, or systolic dysfunction of nonischemic myocardium adjacent to ischemic or infarcted myocardium, is also commonly mentioned as another cause of "artifactual" SWMAs. Tethering probably accounts for the consistent overestimation of infarct size by echocardiography when compared with postmortem studies. However, Force et al. used an improved analysis system and found that segmental contraction is normal to within 1 cm of the ischemic area.[16] Thus, tethering may actually help the intraoperative detection of myocardial ischemia by making a new SWMA involve an area of myocardium slightly larger than the true area of ischemia. However, tethering does not create new SWMAs in the absence of acute myocardial ischemia.

Even if TEE can be refined to image all new SWMAs, anesthesiologists must recognize them in real time in order to institute appropriate, timely therapy. Clements and de Bruijn found that after 20 minutes of instruction, 53 clinicians correctly identified 95% of SWMAs replayed for them from videotape.[17] However, Saada et al. reported a much lower recognition rate when anesthesiologists were asked to evaluate segmental wall motion in real time while they were administering anesthesia.[18] In this latter study in 29 patients, 6 severe SWMAs occurred intraoperatively, and neither anesthesiologists (resident or faculty) recognized 3 of them. In the 3 other ischemic episodes, a quad screen system was used that allowed the juxtapositioning of the baseline echocardiogram (the images from one cardiac cycle played continuously) and subsequent echocardiograms on the same video screen. With this technique, both anesthesiologists recognized 2 of the ischemic episodes, and 1 recognized the third. Clearly, new SWMAs can be missed by the anesthesiologist if recall of baseline wall motion is inadequate. Quad screen systems are commercially available and in my experience definitely help in the recognition of SWMAs as well as changes in global ejection and filling.

OTHER APPLICATIONS

TEE also can detect small quantities of intravascular air that may enter the circulation during surgery. Moreover, two-dimensional TEE provides a nearly ideal examination of the intra-atrial septum and, during contrast studies, can reliably diagnose atrial septal defects.[19] Two-dimensional TEE is thus the first intraoperative monitor that can identify patients at risk of experiencing paradoxical emboli. Cucchiara monitored 12 patients during suboccipital craniotomy in a sitting position by using two-dimensional TEE and precordial nonimaging Doppler.[2] All 8 cases of Doppler-detected air were visualized by TEE. In 2 of the cases, air was noted first on the echocardiogram. In 2 more cases, a questionable Doppler change was noted, and the presence of air was verified by the echocardiogram. For 1 severe episode of embolization, air could be seen to cross from the right to the left atrium and pass to the left ventricle and aorta. The precordial Doppler monitor did not detect this event because it does not image the heart and, thus, cannot localize an air embolism within the atria. A subsequent study in animals confirmed that TEE is more sensitive for the detection of venous air embolism than is monitoring the precordial Doppler, pulmonary artery pressure, end-tidal carbon dioxide concentration, or arterial oxygen tension.[20]

Intraoperative TEE functions primarily as a monitoring tool for the anesthesiologist, but primarily as a diagnostic tool for surgeons and cardiologists. Together with color Doppler, it is an ideal technique for evaluating mitral and aortic diseases because of the proximity of the transesophageal transducer to the left atrium, mitral valve, aortic valve, and aorta. For instance, Sheikh et al. found that TEE provided a clinically relevant evaluation of the adequacy of mitral valve repair: patients with minimal or no residual regurgitation had a sixfold lower incidence of major postoperative complications or death.[21] In selected patients, TEE and color Doppler evidence of persistent regurgitation after valvuloplasty (even in the absence of hemodynamic abnormalities) will necessitate immediate reinstitution of cardiopulmonary bypass and revision or replacement of the repair. In so doing, subsequent reoperation, morbidity, and an increased risk of mortality may be avoided (see Chapter 9).

SUMMARY

TEE provides a window to the heart through which anesthesiologists, surgeons, and cardiologists can see anatomy, physiology, and the effects of anesthesia and surgery on the heart with a clarity not previously possible. Multiple studies have proved that TEE is a more sensitive and reliable method to detect changes in left ventricular filling and ejection than are traditional intraoperative monitors. Few authorities would contest these results. However, the most important work remains: to translate this superior monitoring technology into direct patient benefit.

REFERENCES

1. Schluter M, Langenstein BA, Polster J, et al: Transoesophageal cross-sectional echocardiography with a phased array transducer system. Technique and initial clinical results. *Br Heart J* 1982; 48:67–72.
2. Cucchiara RF, Nugent M, Seward JB, et al: Air embolism in upright neurosurgical patients: Detection and localization by two-dimensional transesophageal echocardiography. *Anesthesiology* 1984; 60:353–355.
3. Harpole DH, Clements FM, Quill T, et al: Right and left ventricular performance during and after abdominal aortic aneurysm repair. *Ann Surg* 1989; 209:356–362.
4. Kuecherer HF, Muhiudeen IA, Kusumoto FM, et al: Estimation of mean left atrial pressure from transesophageal pulsed Doppler echocardiography of pulmonary venous flow. *Circulation* 1990; 82:1127–1139.
5. Tennant R, Wiggers C: The effect of coronary occlusion on myocardial contraction. *Am J Physiol* 1935; 112:351–361.
6. Battler A, Froelicher VF, Gallagher KP, et al: Dissociation between regional myocardial dysfunction and ECG changes during ischemia in the conscious dog. *Circulation* 1980; 62:735–744.
7. Smith JS, Cahalan MK, Benefiel DJ, et al: Intraoperative detection of myocardial ischemia in high-risk patients: Electrocardiography versus two-dimensional transesophageal echocardiography. *Circulation* 1985; 72:1015–1021.
8. Leung JM, O'Kelly B, Browner WS, et al: Prognostic importance of postbypass regional wall-motion abnormalities in patients undergoing coronary artery bypass graft surgery. *Anesthesiology* 1989; 71:16–25.
9. van Daele ME, Sutherland GR, Mitchell MM, et al: Do changes in pulmonary capillary wedge pressure adequately reflect myocardial ischemia during anesthesia? A correlative preoperative hemodynamic, electrocardiographic, and transesophageal echocardiographic study. *Circulation* 1990; 81:865–871.
10. Lehmann KG, Lee FA, McKenzie WB, et al: Onset of altered interventricular septal motion during cardiac surgery. Assessment by continuous intraoperative transesophageal echocardiography. *Circulation* 1990; 82:1325–1334.
11. Smith JS, Roizen MF, Cahalan MK, et al: Does anesthetic technique make a difference? Augmentation of systolic blood pressure during carotid endarterectomy: Effects of phenylephrine versus light anesthesia and of isoflurane versus halothane on the incidence of myocardial ischemia (see comments). *Anesthesiology* 1988; 69:846–853.

12. London MJ, Tubau JF, Wong MG, et al: The "natural history" of segmental wall motion abnormalities in patients undergoing noncardiac surgery. *Anesthesiology* 1990; 73:644–655.
13. Pandian NG, Skorton DJ, Collins SM, et al: Heterogeneity of left ventricular segmental wall thickening and excursion in 2-dimensional echocardiograms of normal human subjects. *Am J Cardiol* 1983; 51:1667–1673.
14. Braunwald E, Kloner RA: The stunned myocardium: Prolonged, postischemic ventricular dysfunction. *Circulation* 1982; 66:1146–1149.
15. Aronson S, Lee B, Wiencek J, et al: Assessment of myocardial perfusion during CABG surgery with two-dimensional transesophageal contrast echocardiography. *Anesthesiology* 1991; 75:433–440.
16. Force T, Kemper A, Perkins L, et al: Overestimation of infarct size by quantitative two-dimensional echocardiography: The role of tethering and of analytic procedures. *Circulation* 1986; 73:1360–1368.
17. Clements FM, de Bruijn NP: Perioperative evaluation of regional wall motion by transesophageal two-dimensional echocardiography. *Anesth Analg* 1987; 66:249–261.
18. Saada M, Cahalan MK, Lee E, et al: Real-time evaluation of echocardiograms (abstract). *Anesthesiology* 1989; 71:344.
19. Hanrath P, Schluter M, Langenstein BA, et al: Detection of ostium secundum atrial septal defects by transesophageal cross-sectional echocardiography. *Br Heart J* 1983; 49:350–358.
20. Glenski JA, Cucchiara RF, Michenfelder JD: Transesophageal echocardiography and transcutaneous O_2 and CO_2 monitoring for detection of venous air embolism. *Anesthesiology* 1986; 64:541–545.
21. Sheikh KH, de Bruijn NP, Rankin JS, et al: The utility of transesophageal echocardiography and Doppler color flow imaging in patients undergoing cardiac valve surgery. *J Am Coll Cardiol* 1990; 15:363–372.

Chapter 11

The Role of Transesophageal Echocardiography in Critical Care

Elyse Foster, M.D.

Nelson B. Schiller, M.D.

The applications of transesophageal echocardiography (TEE) have expanded since its initial development in the early 1980s.[1, 2] In the critically ill patient there are several distinct advantages to TEE. It can be performed at the patient's bedside, and the imaging capability is far superior to transthoracic echocardiography (TTE), especially in an intubated patient, who is often difficult to position for adequate surface imaging. Usually only mild to moderate sedation and local anesthesia are required. TEE provides anatomic, functional, and hemodynamic information in an average of 10 to 20 minutes without the need for additional computer processing.

Common indications for TEE in the critically ill patient include (1) evaluation of ventricular function; (2) exclusion of significant valvular disease, including mitral regurgitation, prosthetic valve dysfunction, and endocarditis; (3) investigation of a cardiac embolic source; (4) suspicion of pericardial tamponade or constriction; (5) evaluation of hypoxemia to exclude right-to-left shunting across a patent foramen ovale; (6) evaluation of chest pain and post–myocardial infarction complications; (7) exclusion of mediastinal bleeding; and (8) use as an adjunct to radiologic techniques in chest trauma.

We have evaluated the previous 63 TEE studies performed in the critical care setting within the past 24 months at the University of California, San Francisco. A review of the indications and clinical characteristics of these patients follows. The studies were performed in the following locations: (1) medical-surgical intensive care unit, 51%; (2) cardiac care unit, 44%; (3) neurologic intensive care unit, 1.5%; (4) emergency room, 1.5%; and (5) cardiac catheterization laboratory, 1.5%. There were 28 men and 23 women; their ages ranged from 18 to 85 with a mean age of 56 years. Eight patients had multiple studies. The indications are summarized in Figure 11–1. Our findings are similar to those reported by other institutions,[3–5] although the percentage of patients in our series who were studied for suspected endocarditis or pyogenic complications was higher.

Findings were unexpected in 19 of 63 studies and led to a change in clinical management in 16%. Based on the results of TEE, 13 of 61 (21%) patients had further evaluation by a more invasive technique (i.e., cardiac catheterization or angiography), and 10 of 61 patients had surgical intervention without further study. Other clinical interventions included (1) further fluid resuscitation, (2) a change in cardiac medications, (3) the addition or discontinuation of antibiotic therapy, (4) thrombolytic or anticoagulant therapy, and (5) other.

In the series by Oh et al., two patients were felt to have had complications of TEE.[4] One patient with severe left ventricular dysfunction developed respiratory difficulty, and another patient had worsening hypoxemia despite mechanical ventilation. Pearson et al. reported complications in three patients that were easily remedied.[3] No major complications attributable to TEE were noted in our critical care patients, and the overall rate of complications during TEE is acceptably low.[6] In our ambulatory population we did encounter one case of streptococcal endocarditis that was temporally related in onset to recent TEE, and we therefore administer antibiotic

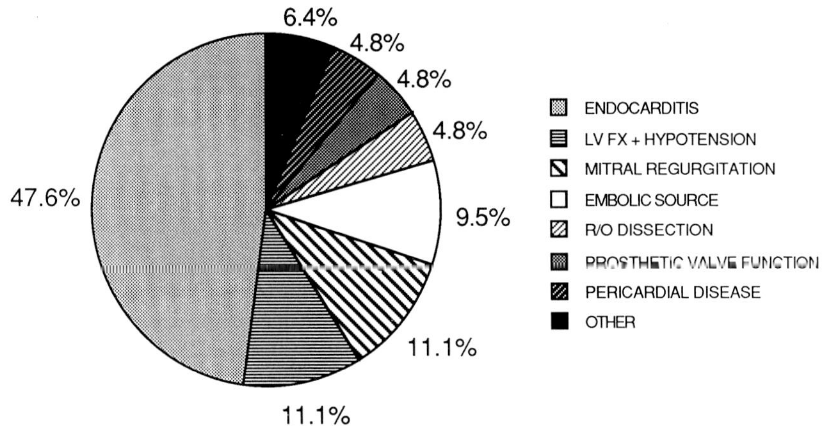

FIG 11–1.
UCSF experience: indications for TEE in 63 critical care patients. *LV FX* = left ventricular function; *R/O* = rule out.

prophylaxis according to current guidelines for endoscopy in moderate- and high-risk patients.[7, 8] Bacteremia has been reported to occur during TEE, although the incidence is variable,[9–11] and the issue remains unsettled (see Chapter 3).

The remainder of this chapter addresses the hemodynamic data available from TEE and specific indications for the procedure in critically ill patients.

HEMODYNAMICS

The combination of two-dimensional evaluation of left ventricular function with Doppler recordings from the pulmonary artery, pulmonary vein, and mitral inflow can provide valuable information regarding systolic and diastolic function. These data are both qualitative and quantitative and permit estimation of the left ventricular ejection fraction, left atrial pressure, and cardiac output. Although most of this information can be acquired with the first generation of monoplane TEE instruments with pulsed-wave and color Doppler capabilities, the availability of continuous-wave Doppler in the emerging generation of biplane TEE probes should substantially increase our capability for making hemodynamic measurements.

Left Ventricular Systolic Function

In the critical care setting, knowledge of the left ventricular systolic function is often a keystone of management. As mentioned previously, catheterization and left ventricular angiography are often precluded by the need to transport the patient and the presence of renal impairment. Portable nuclear scans provide accurate ejection fractions and are certainly useful, but they require time-consuming computer processing and provide little information regarding the presence of associated valvular disease or hemodynamics. TTE studies may be technically inadequate due to the presence of respiratory disease and the inability to position the patient adequately.

As discussed in Chapter 10 on intraoperative monitoring, the optimal view for evaluating left ventricular function is the transgastric transverse short-axis view at the papillary muscle level (see Fig 2–6, A).[12, 13] Segmental analysis of endocardial wall motion and systolic thickening is an important guide to the presence, extent, and distribution of coronary artery disease. In this view, the myocardial distribution of all three major coronary arteries is represented. The American Society of Echocardiography recommends dividing the heart into six myocardial segments at this level, with the anterior septum and the anterolateral walls in the left anterior descending distribution, the lateral and posterolateral walls in the circumflex distribution, and the inferior and inferior septum in the right coronary distribution (see Fig 10–1).[14] By using frame grabbers and computerized analysis systems, continuous cine loops obtained at this level can assist in measurement of an analog of the ejection fraction, the fractional area change (normal, greater than 36%).[12, 15] This view is also useful in estimating the left ventricular volume to detect hypovolemia, although in the paper by Urbanowicz et al., the correlation between end-diastolic area on TEE and end-diastolic volume index by scintigraphy was only fair.[15]

The biplane longitudinal view at the gastric level (see Fig 2–10,B and C) will provide confirmatory evidence of ischemic involvement and is useful for qualitative evaluation of basal descent, an additional measure of left ventricular systolic function.[16, 17] If the second plane is unavailable, the esophageal four-chamber transverse view (see Fig 2–10,A) can be examined for this parameter. Unfortunately, even severe apical wall motion abnormalities can be overlooked on TEE because foreshortening of the left ventricle is inherent in esophageal views, especially in dilated hearts. The inability to obtain a true long-axis measurement of the left ventricle has hampered our ability to perform two-dimensional quantitation of left ventricular volumes and mass when using TEE.[14, 18] However, the cross-sectional area can be measured from the transverse short-axis gastric views and provides an estimation of mass.[14]

Cardiac Output

Estimation of cardiac output is possible when using TEE. The basal transverse view of the main pulmonary artery and pulmonary artery bifurcation provides a window for pulsed Doppler interrogation that is nearly parallel to pulmonary flow. In a study by Muhiudeen et al., the pulsed-wave Doppler sample volume was placed just above the level of the pulmonic valve, and the signal was recorded.[19] The pulmonary artery diameter (PAd) was measured at the same level to calculate the cross-sectional area (CSA) of the vessel by using the equation: CSA = $(PAd/2)^2$. The pulmonary artery velocity/time integral (VTI) was measured by using an off-line analysis system, and Doppler cardiac output was calculated with the following equations:

$$SV\ (mL) = VTI\ (cm) \times CSA\ (cm^2)$$

$$CO\ (L/min) = [SV\ (mL) \times HR\ (beats/minute)]/1{,}000$$

where SV is the stroke volume, CO is the cardiac output, and HR is the heart rate. This was modestly correlated with thermodilution cardiac outputs (r = .65) over a wide range of cardiac outputs. Furthermore, increases in cardiac output correlated with thermodilution (r = .71), but decreases did not.[19]

Thus there may be limitations to measurement of cardiac output by TEE Doppler, but the proportion of these due to the known limitations of the thermodilution method is unclear.[20] Nevertheless, this method provides a useful guide to stroke volume measurements. Recent attempts to measure cardiac output by using the mitral flow velocity integral and biplane measurements of the mitral annulus show promise but require somewhat cumbersome mathematics.[21]

A simpler method of estimating cardiac output is to measure the velocity/time integral of the pulmonary artery flow, which is a measure of stroke distance (cm).[22] The normal stroke distance for the pulmonary artery is 13 to 15 cm. This technique, which uses pulmonary artery flow as a guide to total forward cardiac output, is invalid in the presence of a significant left-to-right shunt and in pulmonary stenosis. In these cases, cardiac output can be estimated by using the velocity/time integral of aortic flow, which is normally 18 to 20 cm.[23] In using pulmonary artery or aortic Doppler flow signals, interrogation angles should be within 20 degrees of being axial to the flow. The steerable continuous-wave Doppler technology available in the latest TEE probes may offer a more reproducible method of estimating cardiac output.[23]

An infrequent but extremely useful sign of reduced forward stroke volume is the presence of spontaneous contrast in the ascending and descending aortas. We have occasionally noted this sign in patients with severe mitral regurgitation or severely reduced left ventricular ejection fractions.

Estimation of Left Atrial Pressure

Normal pulmonary venous flow patterns from pulsed-wave Doppler recordings of the left upper pulmonary vein demonstrate biphasic inflow with a predominant systolic phase (S wave) and a secondary (i.e., lower peak velocity and flow velocity integral) diastolic phase (D wave) (see Fig 2–23,C). This pattern can be readily recognized on color flow Doppler imaging by its uniform orange color (see Fig 2–23,A), with greatest intensity during systole and little if any reverse flow. Recent work has shown that the systolic flow predominates when left atrial or pulmonary capillary wedge pressure is 15 mm Hg or less. At pressures greater than 15 mm Hg the peak flow velocity and the flow velocity integral during diastole is predominant.[24] High levels of positive end-expiratory pressure have also been shown to decrease pulmonary vein systolic flow, which may in part explain the decreased cardiac output associated with this intervention.[25, 26]

Several technical considerations are important. The pulsed Doppler sample volume should be placed 1 to 2 cm within the pulmonary vein and measurements made from end-expiratory tracings. Color flow Doppler with biphasic forward flow (in red) can be useful in guiding placement of the pulsed sample volume. There is normally a brief phase of late diastolic flow reversal corresponding to atrial systole (ar wave, see Figure 2–23,C). Systolic flow reversal is indicative of severe mitral regurgitation[27] (see Fig 9–6). Because severe mitral regurgitant jets are often eccentric, there can be differential flow into the right and left pulmonary veins.[28, 29] Although flow in the right pulmonary vein is more difficult to sample because it is usually perpendicular to the Doppler beam, it should be interrogated in the presence of a mitral regurgitation jet directed toward the interatrial septum, which is usually associated with a flail posterior leaflet.[29] In a recent study, Klein et al. demonstrated that approximately one third of patients with severe (4+) mitral regurgitation show reverse flow in the right pulmonary vein only.[28] In summary, routine sampling of pulmonary vein flow provides important hemodynamic information.

During the expiratory phase in the mechanically ventilated patient, there is increased venous return to the right-heart chambers, and the atrial septum will transiently reverse its normal left-to-right curvature in systole. Kusumoto et al. have shown that in the presence of pulmonary capillary wedge pressures greater than 15 mm Hg, the atrial septum fails to reverse curvature during positive-pressure ventilation.[30] This sign can be used in conjunction with the pulmonary venous flow pattern to estimate filling pressures.

The pulsed Doppler mitral inflow signal is obtained in the four-chamber view at the tips of the mitral leaflet by following similar guidelines as for TTE. It has become clear that the components of the mitral inflow signal result from a complex interplay of left ventricular relaxation, chamber compliance, and left atrial pressures.[31–33] Changes in preload and afterload have also been shown to alter Doppler characteristics of the mitral inflow.[34] In patients older than 50 years of age, reduced preload and low atrial pressures are often associated with a predominant atrial filling phase (A wave dominant) of the mitral inflow signal. Alternately, high left atrial pressures are associated with a high E wave velocity, rapid deceleration time, and diminished A wave velocity (i.e., restrictive physiology). Since this picture can resemble the normal pattern of youth, the change has been called "pseudonormalization." A predominant early filling phase and increased E wave velocity are also characteristic of significant mitral regurgitation.

An additional echocardiographic sign of elevated left atrial pressures is the presence of spontaneous contrast in the left atrium. This is most commonly present when there is also an associated stagnant flow state, specifically mitral stenosis and atrial fibrillation. The presence of spontaneous contrast usually excludes significant mitral regurgitation and is commonly found in patients with embolic events.

Even when technical considerations limit optimal imaging, TTE and Doppler imaging can complement the TEE. For example, subcostal imaging of the inferior vena cava is usually possible in the critical care patient and can predict right atrial pressure with fair accuracy, except in the mechanically ventilated patient.[35] A plethoric inferior vena cava (greater than 2 cm in diameter) with reduced inspiratory collapse (less than 50%) is found when the right atrial pressure exceeds 15 mm Hg. Alternatively, a small inferior vena cava with spontaneous collapse is consistent with right atrial pressures of close to 0 mm Hg. The pending availability of continuous-wave Doppler will permit us to evaluate pulmonary artery systolic pressure from the tricuspid regurgitant jet, and this will contribute powerful additional data. Until then, continuous-wave Doppler of these jets should be attempted from the surface study to estimate pulmonary artery pressures.[36]

In summary, a plethora of hemodynamic information is available from a carefully executed TEE study, which can complement invasive hemodynamic measurements and in certain situations eliminate their need. The remainder of this chapter addresses the specific indications for TEE in the critical care patient.

SPECIFIC INDICATIONS

Evaluation of the Hypotensive Patient

In the evaluation of the hypotensive mechanically ventilated patient in the critical care setting it may be extremely difficult to adequately evaluate volume status. The jugular venous pressure may appear elevated on physical examination, and cardiac auscultation is limited. A pulsus paradoxus is often noted in the absence of cardiac tamponade. Wide fluctuations in pressure recordings from pulmonary artery catheters are often present due to the effects of positive-pressure ventilation. Since TTE data are frequently fragmentary in this population, TEE can be diagnostic.

The finding of a small hypercontractile left ventricle with a normal pulmonary venous flow pattern and an A wave–dominant mitral inflow pattern is consistent with hypovolemia. Cardiogenic shock is associated with global hypokinesis or segmental wall motion abnormalities and a reduced overall left ventricular ejection fraction. The pulmonary venous flow pattern would be expected to reflect high left atrial pressures with diastolic predominance of the flow.[24] Pericardial effusion usually improves the precordial window, so pericardial tamponade can generally be diagnosed by TTE, but occasionally this can be an unsuspected finding on TEE (Fig 11–2). Here, right ventricular and right atrial collapse may be overt and suggest the diagnosis.[37, 38]

A massive pulmonary embolus with acute right ventricular failure is frequently unrecognized as an etiology of hypotension. Findings on TEE can include emboli in transit, right atrial and ventricular dilatation, and severely reduced right ventricular function. There are occasional reports of a thromboembolus identified within the pulmonary artery.[39] In a prospective study by Wittlich et al., TEE detected pulmonary artery thrombi in 8 out of 24 patients with pulmonary emboli. In the other 16 patients, thrombi in the pulmonary artery could not be identified by either TEE or angiography.[40] Right ventricular dysfunction is nonspecific[41] and may need to be differentiated from a right ventricular infarction, which is almost always seen in conjunction with an inferoposterior myocardial infarction (see below).[42–44]

The immediate availability of the hemodynamic and anatomic information gained from this technique allows critical care personnel to rapidly institute or alter therapy for correction of hypotension.

Evaluation of Dyspnea and Pulmonary Edema

The etiology of acute dyspnea may not be readily apparent on physical examination and routine laboratory testing. The differentiation of cardiogenic from noncardiogenic pulmonary edema is difficult by portable chest x-rays, which may exaggerate cardiac dimensions. The electrocardiogram is nonspecific unless there is an acute myocardial infarction; even the information from a right-heart catheterization may be difficult to interpret. In the acutely dyspneic patient, it may be difficult to auscultate a new murmur of mitral regurgitation or aortic insufficiency, and an acoustic window for TTE is often unavailable.

The patient must be stabilized with medical therapy and intubated if necessary before TEE can be performed. Sedation with morphine sulfate may be sufficient; however, if necessary, midazolam and vecuronium can be administered. Potential findings on TEE include acute severe mitral regurgitation due to flail leaflet and chordal rupture; acute severe aortic regurgitation due to endocarditis, trauma, or dissection; myocardial infarction or ischemia with an unrevealing electrocardiogram; and pulmonary embolus. The finding of acute aortic or mitral valvular regurgitation can lead to rapid lifesaving surgical in-

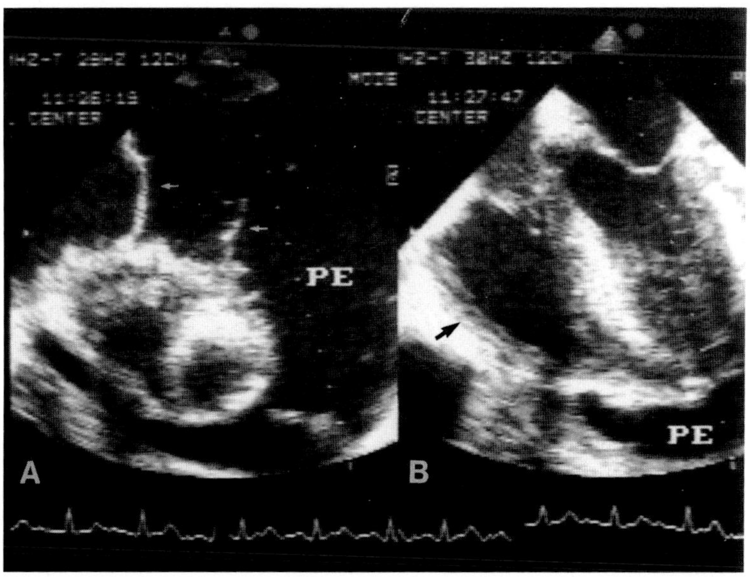

FIG 11–2.
TEE in a patient who had aortic valve replacement for endocarditis. A large pericardial effusion *(PE)* with adhesion to the right ventricular free wall *(black arrow)* and fibrinous strands *(small arrows)* are seen on transverse gastric **(A)** and esophageal four-chamber **(B)** views.

tervention, and catheterization may be avoided in certain instances. The finding of a right atrial thrombus (or embolus in transit) in the presence of right ventricular dysfunction provides strong circumstantial evidence for a pulmonary embolus in the patient with acute respiratory failure as discussed above.[39, 40]

In Figure 11–3,A, a large highly mobile right atrial thrombus was visualized in a patient with acute dyspnea and chest pain. His pulmonary artery peak systolic pressure, estimated from the surface Doppler of his tricuspid regurgitation jet, was 60 mm Hg. There was right ventricular dilation and a reduced ejection fraction. A lung scan showed a high probability for a pulmonary embolus. In Figure 11–3,B, a saline contrast study shows evidence of right-to-left shunting across a patent foramen ovale that was associated with the increased right atrial pressures. He received intravenous streptokinase, which resulted in a reduction in the size of his thrombus, and he was eventually discharged on a regimen of warfarin. He returned 2 weeks later with a right cerebrovascular infarct, presumably on the basis of an embolus, and died of complications of his stroke.

Evaluation of Chest Pain and Complications of Myocardial Infarction

The differential diagnosis of chest pain in the absence of diagnostic electrocardiographic changes is a challenge to both emergency room physicians and cardiologists. The consequences of a misdiagnosis of acute myocardial infarction or aortic dissection can be catastrophic. Following TTE to exclude obvious segmental wall motion abnormalities and pericardial effusion, TEE can be performed safely at the bedside to investigate possible thoracic aortic dissection.[45, 46] In the European cooperative study of TEE in aortic dissection that was discussed in more detail in Chapter 7, two false-positive results were found to be due to aortic ectasia.[46] Aortic insufficiency was found in 29 of 44 patients with types I and II dissection.[46] An example of a type I dissection with severe aortic insufficiency from our laboratory is shown in Figure 11–4. The intimal tear was found in 40 of 82 (49%) patients by two-dimensional imaging alone.[46] Color flow Doppler imaging may improve localization of the site of an intimal tear (see Figs 7–10 and 7–11). False-negatives can result early on when a thrombus fills the false lumen and there is no evidence of flow on color Doppler imaging.[47] The diagnosis of dissection is discussed in greater detail in Chapter 7.

We have found TEE to be useful in evaluating suspected complications of acute myocardial infarction. In our experience the procedure is generally well tolerated, although a large series of patients with acute myocardial infarction has not been published. Potentially correctable causes of cardiogenic shock are often apparent on TTE, but when technical limitations produce inadequate images, these can

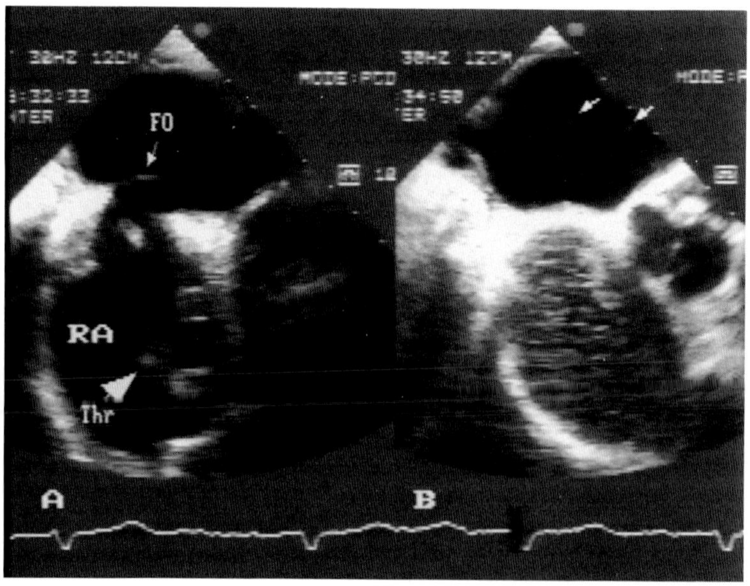

FIG 11–3.
Four-chamber view **(A)** showing a lobulated right atrial thrombus (*Thr*) and a stretched foramen ovale (*FO*) bowing toward the left atrium. A saline contrast study **(B)** shows microbubbles in the left atrium that crossed the atrial septum via a patent foramen ovale (see the text). *RA* = right atrium.

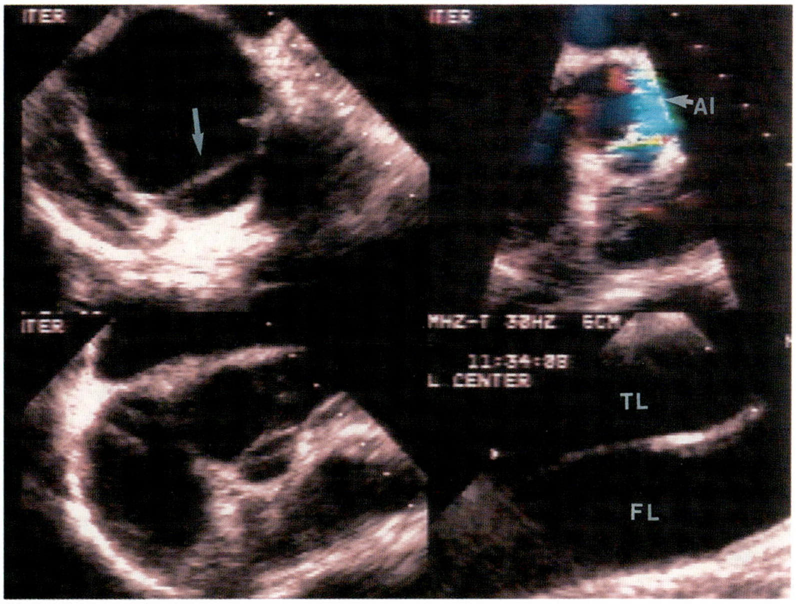

FIG 11–4.
Type I aortic dissection showing the intimal flap *(large arrow)* and severe aortic insufficiency *(AI)*. The true *(TL)* and false *(FL)* lumina were identified on real-time imaging by the characteristic systolic expansion of the true lumen.

easily be diagnosed by TEE. The mechanism of mitral regurgitation, whether due to papillary muscle rupture or segmental contraction abnormalities, may be apparent.[48] In the series of Pearson et al. from St. Louis University, six patients with acute myocardial infarctions were examined. Two of the six patients had severe mitral regurgitation due to a ruptured papillary muscle head and associated flail leaflet.[3]

The site of a ventricular septal defect can be accurately localized to guide surgical correction[49] (Fig 11–5). Left ventricular free wall rupture is usually catastrophic, but occasionally it is contained by the pericardium, and a pseudoaneurysm results.[50] Biplane technology should be extremely helpful in identifying this rare but life-threatening complication. There are characteristic pulsed and color flow

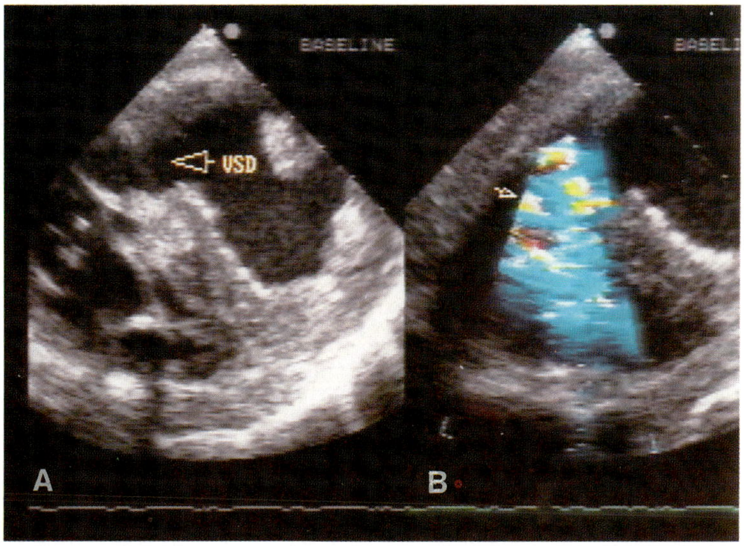

FIG 11–5.
A large ventricular septal defect *(VSD)* is seen on the transverse gastric view **(A)** in a patient with a recent inferoposterior myocardial infarction. The tear is seen in the posterior septum. Color flow Doppler imaging **(B)** demonstrates high-velocity systolic flow from left to right.

Doppler findings consisting of antegrade flow into the pseudoaneurysm during early systole and retrograde flow in early diastole.[51, 52] This pattern is helpful in differentiating between a pseudoaneurysm and a loculated pericardial effusion.

The right ventricle is well visualized in the transverse views on TEE, and although usually apparent on electrocardiography and physical examination, the diagnosis of right ventricular infarct can be made by TEE when surface echocardiography is technically inadequate.[42–44] In the presence of severe segmental wall motion abnormalities with an ejection fraction of less than 30% and involvement of more than 40% of the left ventricle, the prognosis is usually poor.[53, 54] Recent investigations in the use of dobutamine and pacing to identify not only ischemic but also "viable" myocardium may lead to techniques that can guide revascularization in the future.[55, 56] Coronary imaging and Doppler flow velocity measurements of the left anterior descending artery have been studied recently and hold promise for rapid identification of proximal coronary stenoses.[57–59]

It should again be emphasized that even with biplane probes the apex is poorly visualized by TEE and apical infarction with aneurysm formation and thrombi can be overlooked. This blind spot can also lead to an overestimation of the left ventricular ejection fraction when the most severe ischemic involvement is in the apex and basal function is preserved. Therefore, in conjunction with TEE, it is important to attempt apical transthoracic imaging in the patient with myocardial infarction by using transducers with optimal near-field resolution to identify apical wall motion abnormalities and mural thrombi.[60, 61]

Evaluating Complications of Cardiac Surgery

The cause of hemodynamic instability in the cardiac surgical patient during the initial days in the intensive care unit may be uncertain. The presence of a pericardial or mediastinal hematoma is easily established by TEE.[62, 63] Chan reported seven consecutive patients in whom hypotension developed within the first 48 hours following cardiac surgery.[62] TTE was inadequate in each case, and TEE revealed evidence of clots compressing the right atrium or right ventricle in three patients. In three other patients, there was evidence of severe myocardial dysfunction, and one patient had the unexpected finding of a ventricular septal rupture following aortic valve replacement.

Perioperative myocardial infarction has been reported in approximately 5% of patients following coronary artery bypass grafting.[64] This is not always associated with acute graft closure, and diagnosis is often difficult.[65] The patient may be unable to differentiate ischemic chest pain from incisional pain, and the electrocardiogram is often nondiagnostic. Cardiac enzyme determinations are delayed. TEE can accurately identify new wall motion abnormalities, particularly when a baseline study has been obtained following coronary bypass surgery in the operating room, and appropriate treatment can be initiated.

In the patient who has had valve replacement, TEE can identify periprosthetic regurgitation, especially in the mitral position.[66, 67] Because of acoustic shadowing, periprosthetic leaks involving the aortic valve may be better visualized on transthoracic imaging.[66, 68] Periprosthetic regurgitation must be differentiated from the normal seating regurgitation present in mechanical prostheses. Mohr-Kahaly et al. found early systolic regurgitant flow in 95% of mitral prostheses by TEE as compared with 44% of aortic prostheses.[68]

With the advent of early surgery for endocarditis, evaluation of prosthetic function and residual infection by TEE may be indicated.[69, 70] One patient in our series with a history of intravenous drug abuse and *Staphylococcus aureus* endocarditis had an initial TEE showing aortic valve endocarditis, severe aortic insufficiency, an annular abscess, and pericardial effusion. He had successful surgical debridement and aortic valve replacement with a St. Jude's mechanical prosthesis. Eleven days postoperatively he developed hemodynamic instability; repeat TEE showed moderate periprosthetic regurgitation, enlargement of the abscess cavity, and shunting from the aorta to the right ventricle. At reoperation the abscess was successfully patched, and a second valve was inserted. He recovered from his endocarditis.

Vegetations on prosthetic valves are usually not apparent on TTE due to acoustic shadowing. The superior resolution on TEE greatly improves the sensitivity for detection of early (as well as late) prosthetic valve endocarditis[71, 72] (Fig 11–6). This is especially true for small vegetations less than 1 cm in diameter and for the detection of abscesses.[73] However, TEE can be frustrated in many cases of double-valve replacement because the mitral prosthesis shadows the aortic prosthesis.

Fortunately, disruption of valve repair is an infrequent complication, but we have seen one patient in whom dehiscence of a Duran ring led to severe mitral regurgitation and pulmonary edema. In con-

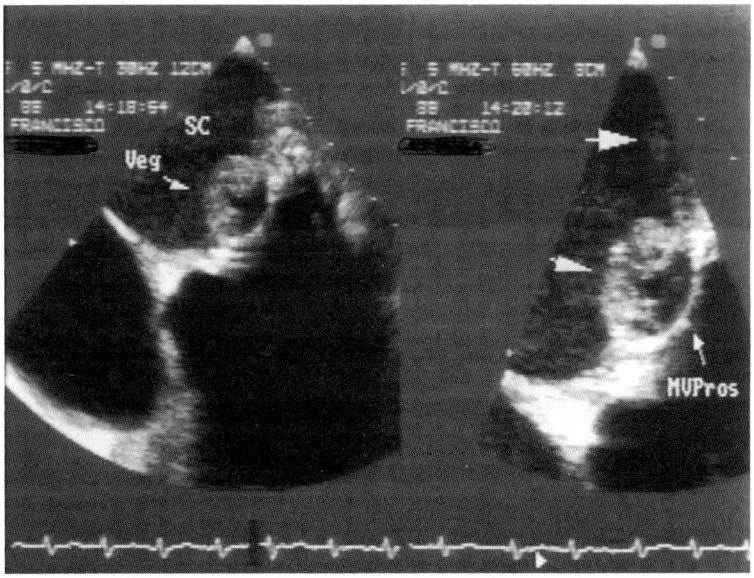

FIG 11–6.
Multilobulated vegetation *(Veg)* due to *Staphylococcus epidermidis* in a patient with a recent mitral valve replacement *(MVPros)*. This was associated with obstruction to left ventricular inflow and spontaneous contrast *(SC)*.

genital heart disease, residual shunts can be identified by using color flow Doppler imaging and saline contrast following repairs of ventricular and atrial septal defects. Occasionally unexplained hypoxemia may be due to right-to-left shunting across a patent foramen ovale. This diagnosis can be made by the venous injection of microbubbles during TEE with visualization of the fossa ovalis.

Pericardial tamponade due to persistent bleeding and early postoperative pericardial or mediastinal constriction due to hematoma and inflammation can be diagnosed on TEE when surface imaging is inadequate and invasive information is ambiguous.[62, 63] Kochar et al. recently reported four patients who became hypotensive following heart surgery.[63] Poor-quality transthoracic images and elevated right atrial and pulmonary capillary wedge pressures on right-heart catheterization led to TEE. In each case they found a localized hematoma causing right atrial compression that was subsequently confirmed and successfully drained at reoperation.

In summary, there is mounting evidence that TEE can add substantial diagnostic information to the evaluation of the postoperative cardiac surgical patient with hemodynamic instability or unexplained fever.

Evaluation of Endocarditis and Embolic Sources

The most frequent indication for TEE among our critical care population is to exclude endocarditis or evaluate pyogenic complications. The findings in the patients who were studied for endocarditis are shown in Figure 11–7. The sensitivity for detection of vegetations on TEE is greater than 90% as compared with approximately 60% on TTE.[71, 72] The incremental diagnostic gain is greatest for small vegetations and for growths located on prosthetic valves. In our series, of the 14 patients who were evaluated for unexplained fever or bacteremia without a source, 3 had definite vegetations, 5 had possible small vegetations, and in 6 patients there was no evidence of endocarditis. Unfortunately, it is difficult to distinguish on echocardiography between vegetations and other valvular masses such as localized thickening due to myxomatous changes, Lambdl's excrescences, and sutures in the region of a prosthetic valve. We have found the downstream location of the mass, the liverlike texture, and the independent motion to be helpful in making the diagnosis of vegetation.

The additional advantage of TEE in endocarditis is the improved detection of abscesses (see Chapter 6). These have been reported in up to 30% of cases coming to surgery or autopsy.[74] A recent prospective study by Daniel et al.[73] of 44 patients with 46 regions of abscess formation demonstrated that TEE had a high sensitivity (87%) for the detection of abscesses as compared with 28% for TTE. Specificity was similar (95% vs. 97%). False-positive diagnoses resulted most commonly from sclerotic changes associated with the mitral valve. Patients with aortic

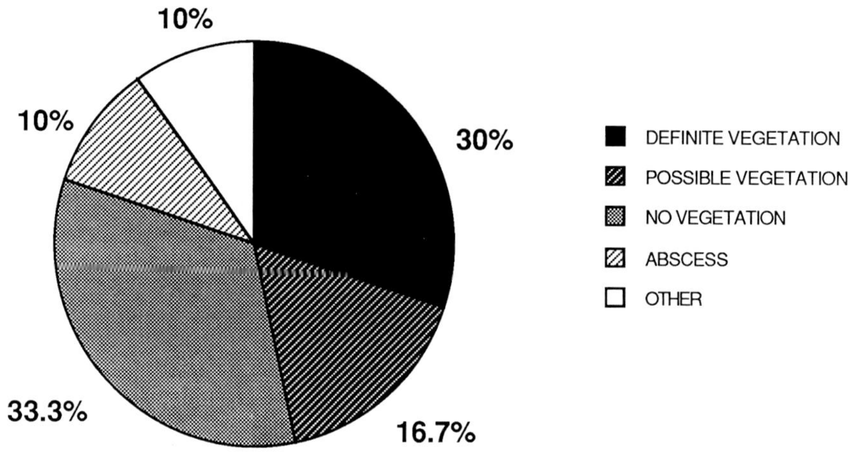

FIG 11–7.
TEE findings in 30 critically ill patients with endocarditis.

valve endocarditis, either native or prosthetic, and staphylococcal infection were more likely to have pyogenic complications. The location of these abscesses included the aortic root, prosthetic valve ring, interventricular septum, mitral apparatus, and papillary muscle. The latter was not detected by either TTE or TEE. The mortality for patients with pyogenic complications was nearly twice that for uncomplicated endocarditis (22.7% vs. 13.5%). In our series, 11 studies were performed to exclude abscess formation in 6 patients with known endocarditis. TEE was positive in 3 of the 11 studies. Five of the 6 patients died.

A number of investigators have examined the prognostic value of echocardiography, both transthoracic and transesophageal, in predicting the need for early surgical intervention and valve replacement in endocarditis.[71, 75] In a recent study using two-dimensional echocardiography, Jaffe et al. reported a slightly increased risk of embolism in patients with vegetations larger than 10 mm in size, and increased mortality was associated with prosthetic valve endocarditis, systemic embolism, and staphylococcal infection.[75] Mügge et al. showed an increased embolic rate with mitral vegetations greater than 10 mm in size but not for aortic vegetations.[71] Vegetation size did not appear to predict mortality or heart failure.

In summary, it is well established that TEE is more sensitive than TTE for the detection of vegetations and ring abscess. Whether all patients with endocarditis should be studied by TEE and when they should be studied are major questions remaining to be answered. It does not appear that echocardiographic predictors alone will dictate early surgery. However, once the clinical situation demands surgical intervention, most patients can undergo valve replacement for endocarditis without cardiac catheterization based on the results of combined TTE and TEE.

Investigating a noninfectious embolic source is a less common indication in the critical care patient than in the ambulatory patient. This was the indication in only 4% of our patients, 5% of the Mayo Clinic series, and 26% of the St. Louis patients.[3, 4] Similar to ambulatory patients, the potential etiologies include a left atrial thrombus and spontaneous contrast, a patent foramen ovale, and marantic vegetations and other cardiac masses.[76–78] As mentioned above, atherosclerotic debris and thrombi within the aortic arch and descending aorta are important potential sources of emboli that may be overlooked.[78, 79] The finding of atheromatous and thombotic debris in the descending aorta appears to be an important predictor of embolic complications of interarterial catheterization.[79] The role of interatrial septal aneurysm remains controversial, although it is commonly found in patients who are studied for embolic sources. In the critically ill patient with intracardiac catheters, a thrombus can appear fairly rapidly and may be a source for both pulmonary and systemic emboli in patients with an intracardiac communication.

Miscellaneous Indications

An important indication is the evaluation of potential cardiac transplant donors. Because of mechanical ventilation in the brain-dead patient and frequent coexistence of multiple trauma, TTE may be technically difficult. Two of the five patients investigated by using TEE for this indication by Oh et. al.[4] were excluded as possible transplant donors. One had a right ventricular contusion, and another had evidence of anteroseptal myocardial infarction; both diagnoses were confirmed at autopsy.

The role of TEE in the evaluation of cardiac trauma has not been fully investigated, although this is a potentially important area.

TECHNICAL CONSIDERATIONS

Several technical considerations deserve special mention. When called to perform TEE in a mechanically ventilated patient, assistance from an anesthesiologist or intensivist is often advisable. Esophageal intubation may be complicated by the presence of an endotracheal tube, and special care must be taken not to extubate the patient while manipulating the tube to gain access to the esophagus. Direct laryngoscopy was necessary in a small percentage of our patients who could not be adequately positioned for the usual method of esophageal intubation. An uncooperative mechanically ventilated patient may require a paralytic agent such as vecuronium in addition to adequate analgesia and sedation. We have occasionally found it necessary to deflate the cuff of the endotracheal tube momentarily to permit passage of the TEE probe. A nasogastric tube may prevent good esophageal contact and impede imaging and thus may need to be removed. If possible, it is advisable to administer an antipyretic and use other cooling methods in a febrile patient to prevent overheating of the probe and shutdown of the equipment. This problem can be significant but is being addressed by the manufacturers of ultrasound equipment who are supplying lower transmit energy levels for TEE that can limit overheating of the probe.

SUMMARY

TEE with its markedly improved resolution has substantially improved the diagnostic capabilities of the echocardiographer. This is highly apparent in the critical care setting where TTE is often extremely limited. Morphologic, physiologic, and hemodynamic information is available on-line and permits the intensivist to make rapid changes in clinical management. Although there is no proof that application of this technique has improved overall survival in this group of patients, anecdotal experience and recently published series suggest that otherwise inapparent diagnoses have been made that have led to overall clinical improvement.

REFERENCES

1. Seward JB, Khandheria B, Oh J, et al: Transesophageal echocardiography: Technique, anatomic correlations, implementation, and clinical applications. *Mayo Clin Proc* 1988; 63:649–680.
2. Matsuzaki M, Toma Y, Kusukawa R: Clinical applications of transesophageal echocardiography. *Circulation* 1990; 82:709–722.
3. Pearson AC, Castello R, Labovitz A: Safety and utility of transesophageal echocardiography in the critically ill patient, *Am Heart J* 1990; 119:1083–1089.
4. Oh JK, Seward J, Khandheria B, et al: Transesophageal echocardiography in critically ill patients, *Am J Cardiol* 1990; 66:1492–1495.
5. Sanfilippo AJ, Weyman AE: The role of echocardiography in managing critically ill patients, *J Crit Illness* 1988; 3:27–44.
6. Daniel WG, Erbel R, Kasper W, et al: Safety of transesophageal echocardiography: A multicenter survey of 10,419 examinations. *Circulation* 1991; 83:817–821.
7. Foster E, Kusumoto F, Sobol S, et al: Streptococcal endocarditis temporally related to transesophageal echocardiography. *J Am Soc Echocardiogr* 1990; 3:424–427.
8. Dajani AS, Bisno A, Chung K, et al: Prevention of bacterial endocarditis: Recommendations by the American Heart Association, *JAMA* 1990; 264:2912–2922.
9. Gorge G, Erbel R, Henrichs K, et al: Positive blood cultures during transesophageal echocardiography. *Am J Cardiol* 1990; 65:1404–1405.
10. Dennig K, et al: Bacteremia with transesophageal echocardiography. *Circulation* 1989; 80(suppl 2):473.
11. Chandrasekaran K, Bansal R, Mintz G, et al: Impact of transesophageal color flow Doppler echocardiography in current cardiology practice. *Echocardiography* 1990; 7:115–145.
12. Leung JM, Schiller NB, Mangano DT: Transesophageal echocardiographic assessment of left ventricular function. *Int J Card Imaging* 1989; 5:63–70.
13. Schiller NB, Cahalan MK, Lee E: Intraoperative assessment of left ventricular function and wall motion by transesophageal echocardiography. *Echocardiography* 1989; 6:79–86.
14. Schiller NB, Shah P, Crawford M, et al: Recommendations for quantitation of the left ventricle by two-dimensional echocardiography. *J Am Soc Echocardiogr* 1989; 2:358–367.
15. Urbanowicz JH, Shaaban M, Cohen N, et al: Compar-

ison of transesophageal echocardiographic and scintigraphic estimates of left ventricular end-diastolic volume index and ejection fraction in patients following coronary artery bypass grafting. *Anesthesiology* 1990; 72:607–612.
16. Seward JB, Khandheria B, Edwards W, et al: Biplane transesophageal echocardiography: Anatomic correlations, image orientation, and clinical application. *Mayo Clin Proc* 1990; 65:1193–1213.
17. Simonson JS, Schiller NB: Descent of the base of the left ventricle: An echocardiographic index of left ventricular function. *J Am Soc Echocardiogr* 1989; 2:25–35.
18. Lenhoff SJ, MacPhail B, Smith M, et al: Value and limitations of biplane transesophageal echocardiography in the estimation of left ventricular volumes and ejection fraction (abstract). *J Am Coll Cardiol* 1991; 17(suppl 2):35.
19. Muhiudeen IA, Kuecherer H, Lee E, et al: Intraoperative estimation of cardiac output by transesophageal pulsed Doppler echocardiography. *Anesthesiology* 1991; 74:9–14.
20. Levett JM, Replogle RL: Thermodilution cardiac output: A critical analysis and review of the literature. *J Surg Res* 1979; 27:393–404.
21. Griffin BP, Hore P, Davison K, et al: Determination of cardiac output with single and biplane transesophageal echocardiography (abstract). *J Am Coll Cardiol* 1991; 17(suppl 2):35.
22. Haites NE, McLennan F, Mowat D, et al: How far is the cardiac output? *Lancet* 1984; 2:1025–1027.
23. Bouchard A, Blumlein S, Schiller N, et al: Measurement of left ventricular stroke volume using continuous wave Doppler echocardiography of the ascending aorta and M-mode echocardiography of the aortic valve. *J Am Coll Cardiol* 1987; 9:75–83.
24. Kuecherer HK, Muhiudeen I, Kusumoto F, et al: Estimation of mean left atrial pressure from transesophageal pulsed Doppler echocardiography of pulmonary venous flow. *Circulation* 1990; 82:1127–1139.
25. Hoffman R, Lambertz H, Jutten H, et al: Mitral and pulmonary venous flow under influence of PEEP analyzed by transesophageal echocardiography. *Circulation* 1990; 82(suppl 3):722.
26. Akamatsu S, Terazawa E, Kagawa K, et al: Effect of PEEP on left atrial filling dynamics assessed by transesophageal pulsed Doppler echocardiography, *Circulation* 1990; 82(suppl 3):722.
27. Klein AL, Obarski T, Stewart W, et al: Transesophageal Doppler echocardiography of pulmonary venous flow: A new marker of mitral regurgitation severity. *J Am Coll Cardiol* 1991; 18:518–526.
28. Klein AL, Cohen G, Davison M, et al: Importance of sampling both pulmonary veins in the transesophageal assessment of severity of mitral regurgitation (abstract). *J Am Coll Cardiol* 1991; 17(suppl 2):199.
29. Himelman RB, Kusumoto F, Oken K, et al: The flail mitral valve: Echocardiographic findings by precordial and transesophageal imaging and Doppler color flow mapping. *J Am Coll Cardiol* 1991; 17:272–279.
30. Kusumoto FM, Muhiudee I, Cahalan M, et al: The interatrial septal response to transatrial pressure gradients and its potential for predicting pulmonary capillary wedge pressure. *Circulation* 1990; 82(suppl 3):722.
31. Nishimura RA, Housmans P, Hatle L, et al: Assessment of diastolic function of the heart: Background and current applications of Doppler echocardiography, Part I. Physiologic and pathophysiologic features. *Mayo Clin Proc* 1989; 64:71–81.
32. Nishimura RA, Abel M, Hatle L, et al: Assessment of diastolic function of the heart: Background and current applications of Doppler echocardiography, Part II. Clinical studies. *Mayo Clin Proc* 1989; 64:181–204.
33. Devereux R: Left ventricular diastolic function: Early diastolic relaxation and late diastolic compliance. *J Am Coll Cardiol* 1989; 13:337–339.
34. Nishimura RA, Abel M, Housmans P, et al: Mitral flow velocity curves as a function of different loading conditions: Evaluation by intraoperative transesophageal Doppler echocardiography. *J Am Soc Echocardiogr* 1989; 2:79–87.
35. Kircher BJ, Himelman RB, Schiller NB: Noninvasive estimation of right atrial pressure from the inspiratory collapse of the inferior vena cava. *Am J Cardiol* 1990; 66:493–496.
36. Yock PG, Popp RL: Noninvasive estimation of right ventricular systolic pressure by Doppler ultrasound in patients with tricuspid regurgitation. *Circulation* 1984; 70:657–662.
37. Gillam LD, Guyer D, Gibson T, et al: Hydrodynamic compression of the right atrium: A new echocardiographic sign of cardiac tamponade. *Circulation* 1983; 68:294.
38. Levine MJ, Lorell B, Divei D, et al: Implications of echocardiographically assisted diagnosis of pericardial tamponade in contemporary medical patients: Detection before hemodynamic embarrassment. *J Am Coll Cardiol* 1991; 17:59–65.
39. Nixdorf U, Erbel R, Drexler M, et al: Detection of thromboembolus of the right pulmonary artery by transesophageal two-dimensional echocardiography. *Am J Cardiol* 1988; 61:488–489.
40. Wittlich N, Erbel R, Todt M, et al: Detection of pulmonary artery thrombi by transesophageal echocardiography in patients with pulmonary embolism. *Eur Heart J* 1989; 10(suppl):21.
41. Hurford WE, Zapol WM: The right ventricle and critical illness: A review of anatomy, physiology and clinical evaluation of its function. *Intensive Care Med* 1989; 14:448–457.
42. Baigre RS, Haq A, Morgan C, et al: The spectrum of right ventricular involvement in inferior wall myocardial infarction: A clinical hemodynamic and noninvasive study. *J Am Coll Cardiol* 1983; 1:1396.
43. Lopez-Sendon J, Garcia-Fernandez M, Coma-Conella

I, et al: Segmental right ventricular function after acute myocardial infarction: Two-dimensional echocardiographic study in 63 patients. *Am J Cardiol* 1983; 51:390.
44. Jugdutt BI, Sussex B, Sivaram C, et al: Right ventricular infarction: Two-dimensional echocardiographic evaluation. *Am Heart J* 1984; 107:505.
45. Erbel R, Boerner N, Steller D, et al: Detection of aortic dissection by transesophageal echocardiography. *Br Heart J* 1987; 58:45–51.
46. Erbel R, Engberding R, Daniel W, et al: Echocardiography in diagnosis of aortic dissection. *Lancet* 1989; 1(B636):457–461.
47. Mohr-Kahaly S, Puth M, Erbel R, et al: Intramural hematoma visualized by transesophageal echocardiography—an early sign of aortic dissection (abstract). *J Am Coll Cardiol* 1991; 17(suppl 2):20.
48. Nishimura RA, Schaff H, Shub C, et al: Papillary muscle rupture complicating acute myocardial infarction: Analysis of 17 patients. *Am J Cardiol* 1983; 51(1):373–377.
49. Hill JD, Stiles QR: Acute ischemic ventricular septal defect. *Circulation* 1989; 79(suppl 1):112–115.
50. Vlodaver Z, Coe JI, Edwards JE: True and false left ventricular aneurysms. Propensity of the latter to rupture. *Circulation* 1975; 51:567–572.
51. Loperfido F, Pennestri F, Mazzari M, et al: Diagnosis of left ventricular pseudoaneurysm by pulsed Doppler echocardiography. *Am Heart J* 1985; 110:1291–1298.
52. Roelandt JRTC, Sutherland G, Yoshida K, et al: Improved diagnosis and characterization of left ventricular pseudoaneurysm by Doppler color flow imaging. *J Am Coll Cardiol* 1988; 12:807–811.
53. Page DL, Caulfield N, Kastor J, et al: Myocardial changes associated with cardiogenic shock. *N Engl J Med* 1971; 285:133.
54. Alonso DR, Scheidt S, Post M, et al: Pathophysiology of cardiogenic shock: Quantification of myocardial necrosis, clinical, pathologic, and electrocardiographic correlations. *Circulation* 1973; 48:588.
55. Lambertz H, Kreis A, Trümper H, et al: Simultaneous transesophageal atrial pacing and transesophageal two dimensional echocardiography: A new method of stress echocardiography. *J Am Coll Cardiol* 1990; 16:1143.
56. Pierard LA, DeLandsheere C, Berthe C, et al: Identification of viable myocardium by echocardiography during dobutamine infusion in patients with myocardial infarction after thrombolytic therapy: Comparison with positron emission tomography. *J Am Coll Cardiol* 1990; 15:1021–1031.
57. Yamagishi M, Yasu T, Ohara K, et al: Detection of coronary blood flow associated with left main coronary artery stenosis by transesophageal Doppler color flow echocardiography. *J Am Coll Cardiol* 1991; 17:87–93.
58. Iliceto S, Marangelli V, Memmola C, et al: Transesophageal Doppler echocardiography evaluation of coronary blood flow velocity in baseline conditions and during dipyridamole-induced coronary vasodilation. *Circulation* 1991; 83:61–68.
59. Pearce FB, Sheikh K, deBruijn N, et al: Imaging of the coronary arteries by transesophageal echocardiography. *J Am Soc Echocardiogr* 1989; 2:276–283.
60. Visser CA, Kan G, Lie K, et al: Incidence and one-year follow-up of left ventricular thrombus following acute myocardial infarction. An echocardiographic study of 96 patients (abstract). *J Am Coll Cardiol* 1983; 1(2):648.
61. Asinger RW, Mikell F, Elsperger J, et al: Incidence of left ventricular thrombosis after acute transmural myocardial infarction. Serial evaluation of two-dimensional echocardiography. *N Engl J Med* 1981; 305:297.
62. Chan KL: Transesophageal echocardiography for assessing cause of hypotension after cardiac surgery. *Am J Cardiol* 1988; 62:1142–1143.
63. Kochar GS, Jacobs LE, Kotler MN: Right atrial compression in postoperative cardiac patients: Detection by transesophageal echocardiography. *J Am Coll Cardiol* 1990; 16:511–516.
64. CASS Principal Investigators and their Associates: Coronary Artery Surgery Study (CASS): A randomized trial of coronary artery bypass surgery: Survival data. *Circulation* 1983; 68:939.
65. Brindis RG, Brundage B, Vllyot D, et al: Graft patency in patients with coronary artery bypass operation complicated by perioperative myocardial infarction. *J Am Coll Cardiol* 1984; 3:55.
66. Nellessen U, Schnittger I, Appleton C, et al: Transesophageal two-dimensional echocardiography and color Doppler flow velocity mapping in the evaluation of cardiac valve prostheses. *Circulation* 1988; 78:848–855.
67. Van den Brink RBA, Visser CA, Basart DC, et al: Comparison of transthoracic and transesophageal color Doppler flow imaging in patients with mechanical prostheses in the mitral valve position. *Am J Cardiol* 1989; 63(20):1471–1474.
68. Mohr-Kahaly S, Kupferwasser I, Erbel R, et al: Regurgitant flow in apparently normal valve prostheses: Improved detection and semiquantitative analysis by transesophageal two-dimensional color-coded Doppler echocardiography. *J Am Soc Echocardiogr* 1990; 3:187–195.
69. Kay PH, Christiansen F, Dawkins R, et al: The results of surgery for active endocarditis of the native aortic valve. *J Cardiovasc Surg* 1984; 25:231–240.
70. Richardson JV, Karp R, Kirklin J, et al: Treatment of infective endocarditis: A ten-year comparative analysis. *Circulation* 1978; 58:589.
71. Mügge A, Daniel W, Frank G, et al: Echocardiography in infective endocarditis: Reassessment of prognostic implications of vegetation size determined by

the transthoracic and the transesophageal approach. *J Am Coll Cardiol* 1989; 14:631–638.
72. Erbel R, Rohmann S, Drexler, et al: Improved diagnostic value of echocardiography in patients with infective endocarditis by transesophageal approach. A prospective study. *Eur Heart J* 1988; 9:43–53.
73. Daniel WG, Mügge A, Martin R, et al: Improvement in the diagnosis of abscesses associated with endocarditis by transesophageal echocardiography. *N Engl J Med* 1991; 324:795–800.
74. Arnett EN, Roberts WC: Valve ring abscess in infective endocarditis: Frequency, location and clues to clinical diagnosis from the study of 95 necropsy patients. *Circulation* 1976; 54:140–145.
75. Jaffe WM, Morgan D, Pearlman A, et al: Infective endocarditis, 1983–1988: Echocardiographic findings and factors influencing morbidity and mortality. *J Am Coll Cardiol* 1990; 15:1227–1233.
76. Pearson AC, Labovitz A, Tatinenis S, et al: Superiority of transesophageal echocardiography in detecting cardiac source of embolism in patients with cerebral ischemia of uncertain etiology. *J Am Coll Cardiol* 1991; 17:66–72.
77. Daniel WG, Engberding R, Erbel R, et al: Transesophageal echocardiography in arterial embolism and cerebral ischemic events—A European multicenter study in patients without pre-known cardiac disease. *Eur Heart J* 1989; 10(suppl):204.
78. Pop G, Sutherland G, Koudstaal P, et al: Transesophageal echocardiography in the detection of Intracardiac embolic sources in patients with transient ischemic attacks. *Stroke* 1990; 21:560–565.
79. Karalis DG, Chandrasekaran K, Victor M, et al: Recognition and embolic potential of intraaortic atherosclerotic debris. *J Am Coll Cardiol* 1991; 17:73–78.

PART IV

Future Directions

Chapter 12

Recent and Future Technological Advances

David J. Sahn, M.D.

BACKGROUND

After the initial development of first M-mode[1] and later mechanical[2] and subsequently phased-array[3] imaging of the heart from the esophagus, commercially available 32-element transverse-probe phased-array (Diasonics) and biplane prototypes were explored for use in cardiac diagnosis and in anesthesia monitoring both in Europe (mainly Germany) and in the United States (mainly at the University of California, San Francisco). There were few advancements in technologies for transesophageal imaging until Lancee and associates in Rotterdam produced and evaluated a 5.5-MHz, 64-element phased array capable of very high resolution imaging of cardiac anatomy.[4] A major impetus to transesophageal echocardiography (TEE) occurred with the capability of performing Doppler color flow mapping so as to substantially increase the amount of imaging information gained during a time-limited semi-invasive echocardiographic examination. This major stimulation to further development of the field was due in large measure to the pioneering work of Omoto and colleagues,[5] who first reported and incorporated single-plane TEE and color Doppler into perioperative management and then rapidly rekindled interest in biplane TEE. If we now would consider color biplane TEE state-of-the-art, the following new and future technological innovations will and should be addressed in this chapter:

1. Technology for and specific advantages of simultaneous matrix biplane TEE
2. Technology for and advantages of omniplane or varioplane TEE
3. Technologies for smaller endoscopes for infants, and for adults, new connector and cable technologies; single of two-plane steerability on endoscopes; higher frequencies for higher resolution, and other aspects of miniaturization
4. Opportunities for using TEE-type devices for monitoring, diagnostic, or interventional catheterization applications from an intravascular or intracardiac location
5. Opportunities for three-dimensional reconstruction of cardiac anatomy with TEE and its use for full rotational tomographic imaging of the mediastinum
6. Opportunities for the combination of TEE with other cardiac testing systems, intravascular imaging, and transesophageal atrial pacing

SIMULTANEOUS MATRIX BIPLANE VISUALIZATION

Omoto and his associates first reported the matrix biplane concept.[6] While two orthogonally arranged arrays could be rapidly switched to provide simultaneous biplane visualization, it has most often been found that fine changes in transducer and esophagoscope flexing are required to optimize visualization when the two arrays are offset and about 1 cm apart from each other on the tip of the esophagoscope. Also, since the locations of the arrays of a standard biplane system are offset, the orthogonal views differ in region and are not superimposable or reconstructible. The matrix concept represents a difficult feat in transducer fabrication that entails producing a fine crosscut in the array in the two orthogonal directions and then mounting separate connections to the longitudinal and transverse effective element sections (Fig 12–1). A "simultaneous" switched biplane visualization can be achieved in the planes by switching back and forth between scan planes, between completed scan lines, or between repeated scanned full frames many times each second. A major problem that arises, not so much in two-dimensional tissue visualization, but in color Doppler, is the resultant slow frame rates or low frame line densities because color Doppler interrogation requires a "packet" of up to 5 to 8 interrogations in each direction to solve for velocities (as opposed to single interrogations of each direction for tissue imaging). This problem is much less when interrogation distances or angles are limited for color Doppler or when new parallel processing methods are used that solve for two lines on the return of each burst of ultrasound. This process "doubles" the number of lines available for color or tissue imaging, thus facilitating the line sharing needed for simultaneous biplane visualization. Advantages of this method involve an immediate three-dimensional appreciation of spatial anatomy for decision making. We have found this most useful when the best visualization of a structure or location may be changing rapidly between the two planes either as a function of respiration, cardiac motion, or motion of an intracardiac target such as a double umbrella being placed in an atrial septal defect. Especially in these last catheter applications, biplane simultaneous matrix visualization is similar to biplane fluoroscopy during interventions. We have only recently begun work with a 6.8-mm TEE probe with matrix technology that is suitable for babies and we are quite encouraged by its initial applications.

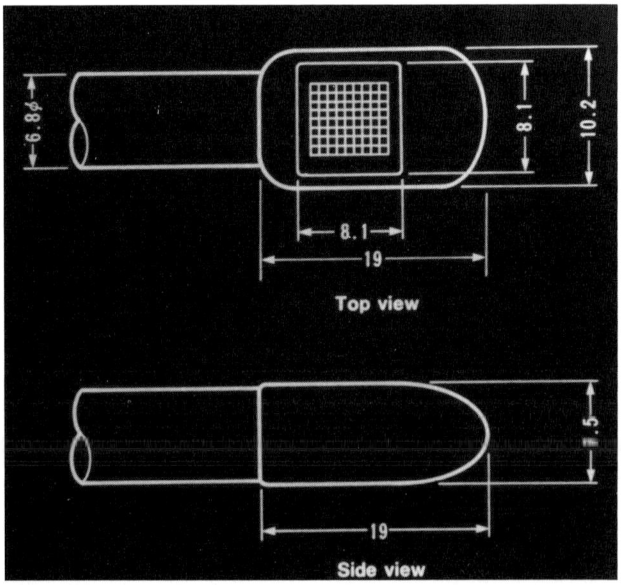

FIG 12–1.
Diagram of a matrix probe for simultaneous biplane TEE for pediatrics. (Courtesy of Professor Ryozo Omoto, Saitama, Japan.)

OMNIPLANE OR VARIOPLANE ESOPHAGEAL ECHOSCOPES

Sometimes neither the longitudinal nor the transverse plane of imaging provides the optimal visualization of relevant structures. Unlike transthoracic echocardiography, fine angulations or rotations of the probe cannot be undertaken. With an esophagoscope manipulation is limited to either forward-and-back angulation or side-to-side curvature of the probe tip. Another approach that may be less cumbersome and may also involve less cable tension on the probe or angulation pressure on the esophagus involves rotating the array at the tip of the esophagoscope to intermediate positions between the longitudinal and transverse planes. This rotation scheme requires unique connectors capable of moving with the array and a driving mechanism to turn the array that can be mechanically cable driven, either by hand or with a small motor. The array pallet is usually built and then cut to an oval shape, the end elements being foreshortened with some slight loss of resolution. Other constraints are that the connecting mechanism to the array and the turning mechanism takes up room in the scope shaft and in the tip, with a necessary increase in size. The first prototype was 16 mm at its tip.[7] Experience with this device suggests that new unique views and information can be obtained (Fig 12–2), but that almost 30% of awake patients studied in the U.S. evaluation center could or would not swallow a TEE probe this big. The concept has generated much excitement, however, and a smaller implementation, the so called "varioplane" probe, is under evaluation in Rotterdam with

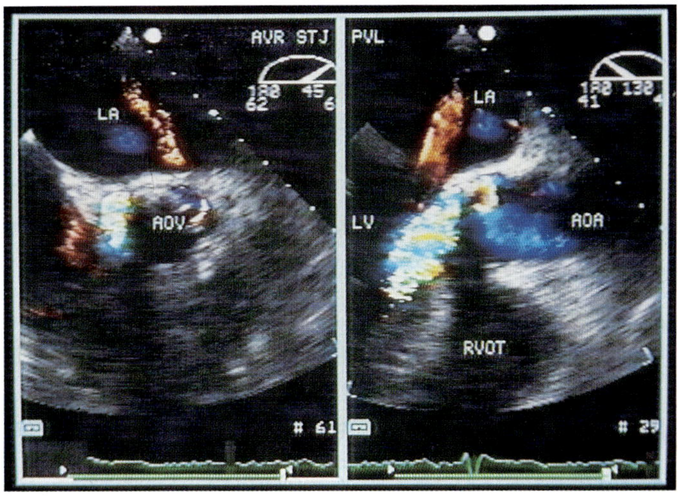

FIG 12–2.
OmniPlane images. This figure illustrates the advantages of multiple degrees of imaging planes. The *left panel* demonstrates at 45 degrees off-axis (see angle meter at top of image), the origin of aortic insufficiency at the aortic valve level (*AOV*). The *right panel* demonstrates the extent of aortic insufficiency in the left ventricular (*LV*) outflow tract at 130 degrees off-axis. *AOA* = ascending aorta; *LA* = left atrium; *RVOT* = right ventricular outflow tract. (Courtesy of Prof. Dr. P. Hanrath, University of Aachen.)

promising clinical results. Use of these probes will again further challenge efforts at image orientation and require an in-depth understanding of three-dimensional spatial anatomy of the heart by the user but promises new and optimized views for diagnostic purposes. Position sensing of the scan plane and acquisition and reconstruction of the ultrasonic tissue or even flow data from this approach hold significant promise as a method for deriving three-dimensional images of cardiac anatomy and flow.

SMALLER HIGHER-FREQUENCY ESOPHAGOSCOPES FOR INFANTS AND ADULTS

Little was available for performing TEE in infants undergoing corrective or palliative surgery for congenital heart disease until about 2 years ago. Before that time the 9- to 11-mm esophagoscopes available could not be inserted into babies under 7 to 8 kg in weight. Since the trend in pediatric cardiology and surgery was toward open heart correction of even severe defects in infancy, intraoperative monitoring of these children remained the realm of epicardial echo.[8] Again, because of the efforts of Kyo and Omoto from Saitama, Japan, first a 6.8-mm, 28-element, transverse-plane probe and later a 40-element, longitudinal-plane probe were developed that could be used in infants as small as 2 kg.[9] The initial approaches were to limit the number of elements to achieve probes 7 mm or less, which at 5 Mhz produced some limitation of resolution, most apparent beyond 4-cm depth. However, adequate results were obtained to allow monitoring of heart repairs in infants. Subsequently, 6.8-mm, 24-element (each plane) biplane and similar 24 × 24-element baby matrix probes have been produced as well as a 4-mm, 18-element array that can be introduced into unsedated newborns since they have little gag reflex. It has also been found in exploring these simple approaches to smaller probes that only angulation anteriorly and posteriorly has been required in baby biplane probes and it is rarely necessary to angulate from side to side. As a consequence, cable space in the endoscopic shaft can be limited. Recently, the ultrasound engineering group at Rotterdam and several other commercial groups have produced 7- to 8-mm, 48-element, transverse-plane or even biplane infant probes with moderately good resolution at 5 Mhz and suitable for use in most babies (Fig 12–3). There have been several spin-offs related to these pediatric efforts that may have relevance to general adult cardiology applications of TEE. Thus, if one had a smaller probe that had high resolution and adequate penetration, could TEE be performed in conscious adults with lower sedation requirements and less discomfort and risk? Even with compromised probes with small numbers of elements, Nanda and associates have reported that diagnostic TEE could be performed in adults by using a pediatric 6.8-mm probe.[10] Important information from this study included the fact that the probe used had only one plane of steerability, the anteroposterior plane. De-

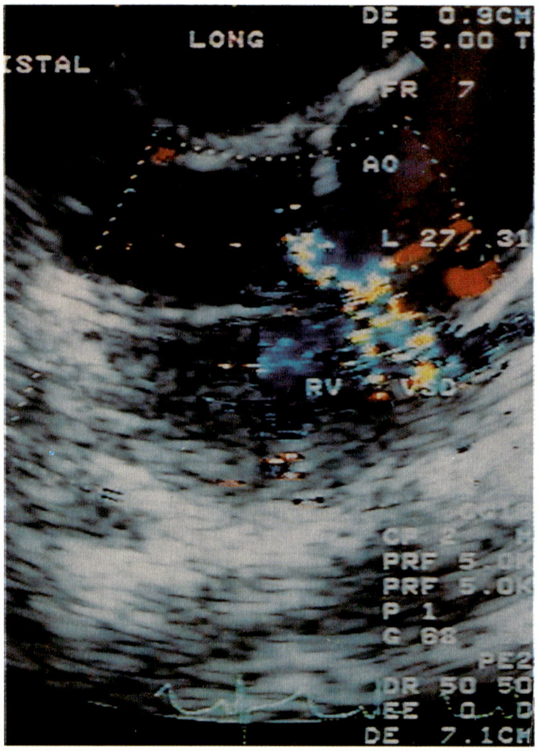

FIG 12–3.
Longitudinal-plane image of a directly subaortic supracristal ventricular septal defect *(VSD)* in a 4-month-old baby that was visualized with a new pediatric biplane probe. *RV* = right ventricle; *AO*= aorta.

spite this, adequate contact could be obtained in the adult esophagus, and adequate angulation could be obtained to derive the diagnostic views necessary. There was, of course, a difference in the resolution obtained when compared with the full-sized 48- or 64-element adult probes usually used.

In light of the above, it is germane to discuss the components necessary to produce a very high resolution miniaturized TEE probe. Smaller size of the shaft could be obtained from denser cabling to allow 64 to 68 individual shielded connector wires within the shaft of the scope. Obviously, once the optical fibers have been removed, and they have generally been found not to be necessary or even helpful in diagnostic TEE, then only the transducer connecting cables and the steering cables are within the shaft of the scope. We have seen very densely packed cables containing 64 fully shielded wires packed in a housing just under 3 mm in size. One could wire a fully enabled matrix probe with a 4.5-mm tube packed in this way. The other approach to reducing the volume of the array connecting wires would be to digitize and preamplify the information within the probe tip and use fewer wires. Efforts in this regard are also underway. There are also other efforts underway in Norway that are aimed at implementing very small motor-driven rotating probes for TEE at 6 to 7.5 MHz, even in an omniplane fashion. Finally, it is also appropriate to point out that there are ferromagnetic alloy materials that can produce tip flexion without cable connectors by electronically controlling heating and cooling of mixed alloy strips within the probe tip (Fig 12–4).

The next requirement for a miniaturized high-frequency probe involves raising the array frequency to 7.5 MHz or even to 10 MHz. Since most clinical indications for TEE scanning involve scanning to identify structures that are within 6 cm of the probe face, it is not necessary to require penetration to the apex for all probes used for adult TEE. Such a range of focus and sensitivity for imaging and for Doppler and color Doppler are within the range of penetration at 7.5 MHz. It would be expected that imaging

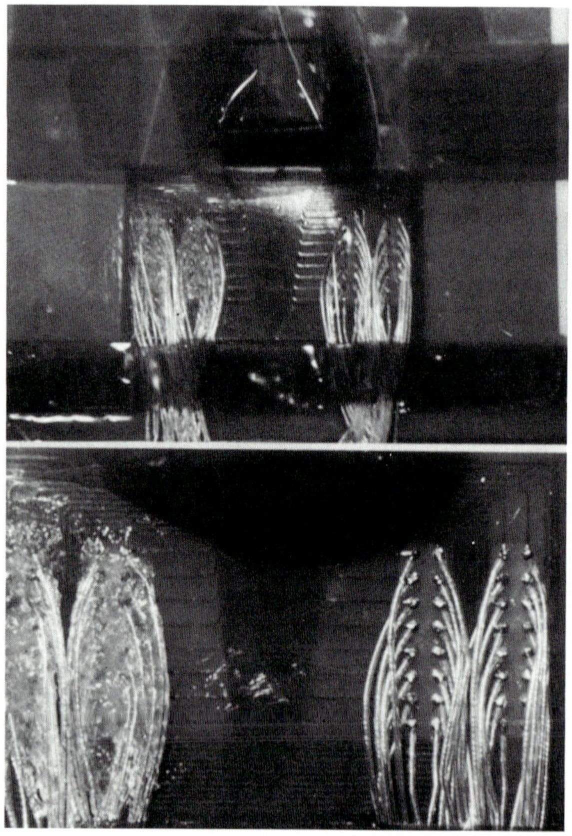

FIG 12–4.
Flexible connector strips are used to allow a foldable connection between the 64 wires in this probe and the 7.5-MHz array.

of the atrial septum, pulmonary veins, and the proximal coronary arteries could be greatly facilitated by using such an approach. Element size and spacing are smaller at higher frequency, and it becomes an art to cut high-frequency arrays with high yield. Nonetheless, efforts from our group have shown that with a 0.6 wavelength spacing at 7.5 MHz, 64-element arrays with pallet sizes around 7 × 7 mm can be produced, and these would be quite applicable to pediatric and potentially to some aspects of adult TEE. A high degree of electronic accuracy is required for steering and focusing of these high-frequency arrays, but this has now become almost state-of-the-art in industry.[11, 12]

The last area relevant to arrays, which has been accomplished by annular array, mechanically steered TEE probes and only recently with phased-array TEE probes, is the ability to derive continuous-wave Doppler information during TEE. While less important in the operating room where pressure measurements can be obtained directly, this is a very important feature for outpatient TEE if one wishes, on the same examination, to derive Doppler hemodynamics. This application may be especially useful for assessing right-heart hemodynamics in patients with lung disease who are difficult subjects to evaluate when using routine transthoracic echo Doppler methods.[13]

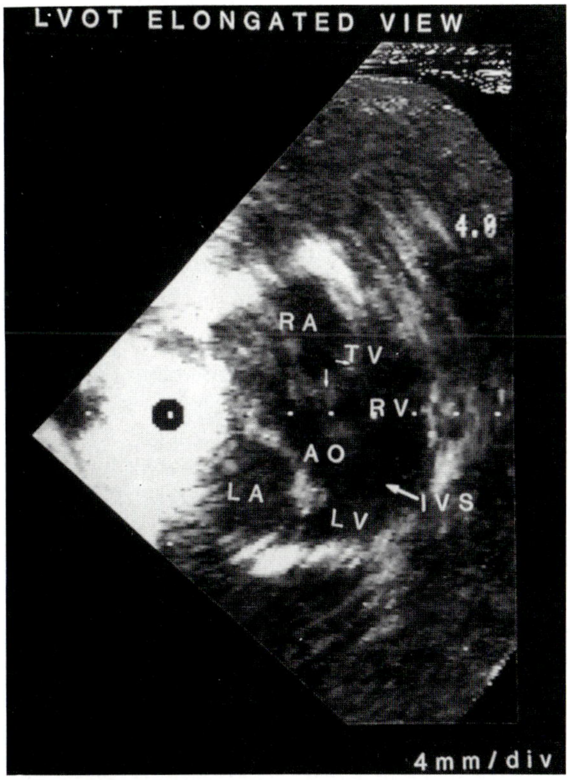

FIG 12–5.
Cardiac imaging performed from the esophagus of a 1.2-kg rabbit by using a 20-MHz catheter primarily designed for intravascular ultrasound. *RA/LA* = right/left atrium; *RV/LV* = right/left ventricle; *AO* = aorta; *IVS* = interventricular septum; *TV* = tricuspid valve.

POTENTIALS FOR INTRAVASCULAR USE OF SMALL TEE PROBES

A number of new applications of intravascular scanning in congenital and acquired heart disease seem to overlap areas where TEE has been helpful, such as the atrial septum and the aortic arch.[14] This is true because both are miniaturized high-frequency scanners designed for near-field high-resolution scanning. Just as an intravascular device can theoretically be used as an esophagoscope[15] (Fig 12–5), a miniaturized esophagoscope can be used from an intravascular route with the potential of allowing detailed cardiac imaging even if "parked" at the superior vena caval right atrial junction like a central venous pressure line[16] (Fig 12–6). While this could be possibly useful since it might be less uncomfortable than the esophagoscope, its more interesting potentials appear to lie with intraoperative and especially postoperative imaging where indwelling access might be quite interesting (Fig 12–7).

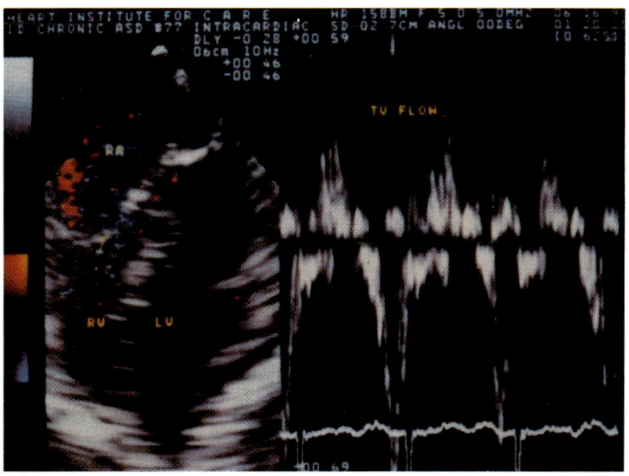

FIG 12–6.
Four-chamber view derived from a miniaturized 4-mm TEE probe inserted into the right atrium of a 12-kg pig from a superior vena caval location. The whole heart can be imaged. *LV* = left ventricle; *RA* = right atrium; *RV* = right ventricle.

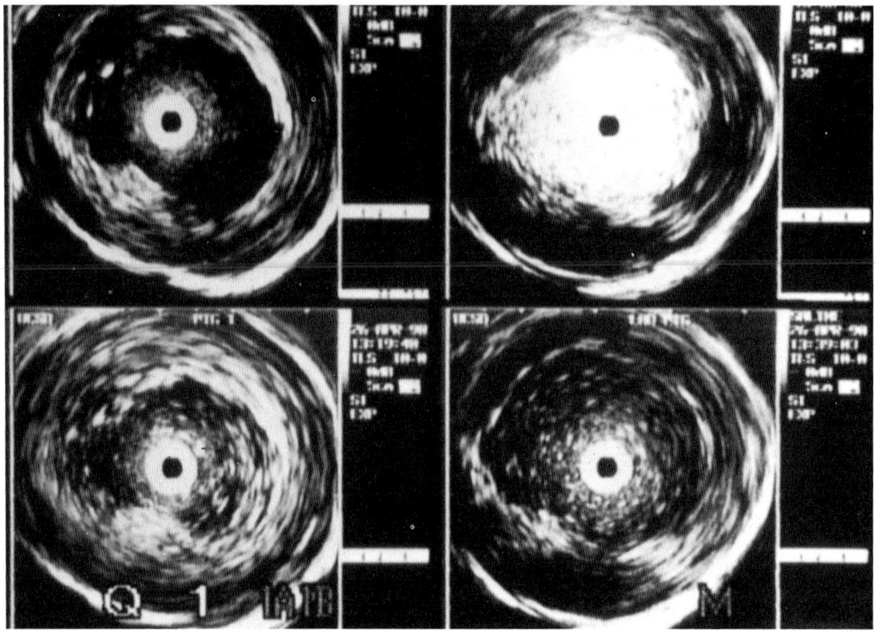

FIG 12–7.
Monitoring contrast study of the left ventricle by using a 12.5-MHz intravascular scanner placed in the left ventricle, which may prove less traumatic than TEE for the patient. *Upper left panel*: precontrast; *upper right panel*: peak contrast.

THREE-DIMENSIONAL RECONSTRUCTION OF CARDIAC ANATOMY FROM TEE IMAGES

Because of the quality of the window for rotated and angled views, a number of investigators have pursued reconstructing added and spatially oriented echotomographic views from transesophageal examinations in order to provide more extensive detail, complex cardiac relationships, or wall motion or chamber volumes. Complete 360-degree tomographic views of thoracic anatomy were shown by Seward and coworkers by rotating an esophagoscope without changing the plane of imaging.[17] Other investigators have either moved the transducer up and down or angulated it mechanically by using stepper motors in order to stack spaced segments, or they have angled oblique slices and achieved three-dimensional reconstruction by sensing the position of the plane of imaging.[18] It is apparent that these approaches will require faster computing or real-time calculation and display of data before they can be widely applied clinically. Nonetheless, some of the varioplane methodologies,[7] by pivoting the scan plane 180 degrees, can provide a unique and facilitated method for obtaining spatially correct, angulated planar data without the difficulty sometimes encountered when transducer contact is lost with the wall and a portion of the data is lost for reconstruction.

COMBINATIONS OF ESOPHAGEAL ECHOCARDIOGRAPHY WITH OTHER METHODS FOR VARIOUS STUDIES

Early esophagoscopes used for scanning also had their optical and suction systems in place. It was quickly found that ultrasound images gave enough orientation that optical imaging of internal landmarks was not necessary. Nonetheless, as catheter ultrasound systems are being combined with atherectomy and endoscopic, balloon, and localization systems, the same may occur for TEE. Balloon contact enhancing devices have been used from time to time in order to improve windows. For small endoscopes, inflation of a balloon **after** insertion might improve contact without being as uncomfortable at the time of insertion. Magnetic localization systems have been used for reconstruction of anatomy in vascular imaging and may aid three-dimensional reconstruction from TEE images.[19] In such systems, magnetic fields developed by coils mounted in the scope are sensed with substantial spatial accuracy by an external antenna system to provide spatial sensing of the position and orientation of the device inside the body. Other approaches to adding to the utility of TEE for detecting coronary disease have been to perform pharmacologic stress TEE for imaging of regional wall motion or changes in coronary flow dynamics[20] or the possibility of combining the TEE probe with pacing electrodes for TEE-monitored transesophageal atrial paced stress echocardiography.[21]

CONCLUSIONS

Advances in instrumentation will continue to provide new capabilities, new formats, new sizes, and new promise for TEE. Higher frequencies, higher resolution, and smaller, less "invasive" and multiplanar scopes are on the near horizon with the promise of three-dimensional acquisition and on-line three-dimensional display in the not too distant future.

REFERENCES

1. Frazin L, Talano JV, Stephanides L, et al: Esophageal echocardiography. *Circulation* 1976; 54:102.
2. Hisanaga K, Hisanaga A, Nagata K, et al: Transesophageal cross-sectional echocardiography. *Am Heart J* 1980; 100:605.
3. Souquet J: Phased array transducer technology for transesophageal imaging of the heart: Current status and future prospects, in Hanrath P, Bleifeld W, Souquet J (eds): *Cardiovascular Diagnosis by Ultrasound.* The Hague, Martinus Nijhoff, 1982, pp 251–259.
4. de Jong N, Lancee CT, Gussenhoven WJ, et al: Transesophageal echocardiography. *Med Biol Eng Comput* 1985; 23(suppl 1):64–72.
5. Kyo S, Takamoto S, Masumura M, et al: Immediate and early postoperative evaluation of results of cardiac surgery by transesophageal echocardiography *Circulation* 1987; 76(suppl 5):1121–1132.
6. Omoto R, Kyo S, Matsumura M, et al: On-line real time biplane transesophageal imaging technique (abstract). *Circulation* 1989; 80(suppl 2):475.
7. Flachkampf FA, Hoffmann R, Hanrath P: Experience with a transesophageal echo-transducer allowing a full rotation of the viewing plane: The omniplane probe (abstract). *J Am Coll Cardiol* 1991; 17:34.
8. Sahn DJ: Intraoperative applications of two-dimensional and contrast two-dimensional echocardiography for evaluation of congenital, acquired and coronary heart disease in open-chested humans during cardiac surgery, in Rijsterborgn H (ed): *Echocardiology.* The Hague Martinus Nijhof F, 1981.
9. Ritter SB: Pediatric transesophageal color flow imaging 1990: The long and the short of it. *Echocardiography* 1990; 7:713.
10. Mahan EF, Helmcke F, Nanda NC, et al: Use of the "pediatric" transesophageal probe in adults: A smaller probe for bigger hearts (abstract). *J Am Coll Cardiol* 1990; 42:670.
11. Sahn DJ: Advances in ultrasound imaging for congenital heart disease. Diagnosis and management, in Pongpanich B, Sueblinvong V, Vongprateep C (eds): *Pediatric Cardiology—Proceedings of the III World Congress of Pediatric Cardiology.* Amsterdam, Excerpta Medica, 1990, pp 3–8.
12. Sahn DJ, Tasker D, Hagen-Ansert S, et al: Miniaturized high frequency phased array devices for high resolution neonatal and intraoperative imaging (abstract). *J Am Coll Cardiol* 1990; 15:10.
13. Weintraub A, Pandian N, Simonetti J, et al: CW Doppler in transesophageal echocardiography allows analysis of high velocity flows and enhances the utility of transesophageal echo (abstract). *Circulation* 1990; 82:669.
14. Ricou F, Ludomirsky A, Weintraub RG, et al: Applications of intravascular scanning and transesophageal echocardiography in congenital heart disease: Trade-offs and the merging of technologies *Int J Card Imaging* 1991; 6:221.
15. Valdes-Cruz L, Sahn DJ, Yock P, et al: Experimental animal investigations of the potential for new approaches to diagnostic cardiac imaging of infants and small premature infants from intracardiac and transesophageal approaches using a 20 MHz real time ultrasound imaging catheter (abstract). *J Am Coll Cardiol* 1989; 13:137.
16. Valdes Cruz LM, Sideris E, Sahn DJ, et al: Transvascular intracardiac applications of a miniaturized phased array ultrasonic endoscope. *Circulation* 1991; 83:1023.
17. Seward JB, Kahnderia BK, Tajik AJ: Wide field transesophageal echocardiographic tomography, feasibility study. *Mayo Clin Proc* 1990; 65:31.
18. Wollschlager H, Zether AM, Klein HP, et al: Transesophageal echo computer tomography: A new method for dynamic 3-D imaging of the heart *(abstract). J Am Coll Cardiol* 1989; 13:68.
19. Aretz HT, Gregory KW, Martinelli OMA, et al: Ultrasonic guidance of laser atherectomy. *Int J Card Imaging* 1991; 6:231.
20. Iliceto S, Marangelli V, Memmola C, et al: Transesophageal Doppler echocardiography: Evaluation of coronary blood flow velocity in baseline conditions and during dipyridamole-induced coronary vasodilation. *Circulation* 1991; 83:61–68.
21. Lambaertz H, Kreis A, Trumper H, et al: Simultaneous transesophageal atrial pacing and transesophageal two dimensional echocardiography: A new method of stress echocardiography. *J Am Coll Cardiol* 1990; 16:1143.

Index

U

V

W